Contents

Foreword

In the past 20 years, micronutrients have assumed great public health importance. As a consequence, considerable research has been carried out to better understand their physiological role and the health consequences of micronutrient-deficient diets, to establish criteria for defining the degree of public health severity of micronutrient malnutrition, and to develop prevention and control strategies.

One of the main outcomes of this process is greatly improved knowledge of human micronutrient requirements, which is a crucial step in understanding the public health significance of micronutrient malnutrition and identifying the most appropriate measures to prevent them. This process also led to successive expert consultations and publications organized jointly by the Food and Agriculture Organization of the United Nations (FAO), the World Health Organization (WHO) and the International Atomic Energy Agency (IAEA) providing up-to-date knowledge and defining standards for micronutrient requirements in 1973[1], 1988[2] and in 1996[3]. In recognition of this rapidly developing field, and the substantial new advances that have been made since the most recent publication in 1996, FAO and WHO considered it appropriate to convene a new expert consultation to re-evaluate the role of micronutrients in human health and nutrition.

To this end, background papers on the major vitamins, minerals and trace elements were commissioned and reviewed at a Joint FAO/WHO Expert Consultation (Bangkok, 21–30 September 1998). That Expert Consultation was assigned three main tasks:

- Firstly, the Consultation was asked to review the full range of vitamin and mineral requirements—19 micronutrients in all—including their role in

---

[1] *Trace elements in human nutrition. Report of a WHO Expert Committee.* Geneva, World Health Organization, 1973 (WHO Technical Report Series, No. 532).

[2] *Requirements of vitamin A, iron, folate and vitamin B$_{12}$. Report of a Joint FAO/WHO Expert Consultation.* Rome, Food and Agriculture Organization of the United Nations, 1988 (FAO Food and Nutrition Series, No. 23).

[3] *Trace elements in human nutrition and health.* Geneva, World Health Organization, 1996.

normal human physiology and metabolism, and conditions of deficiency. This included focusing on and revising the requirements for essential vitamins and minerals, including vitamins A, C, D, E, and K; the B vitamins; calcium; iron; magnesium; zinc; selenium; and iodine, based on the available scientific evidence.

- Secondly, the Consultation was asked to prepare a report that would include recommended nutrient intakes for vitamins A, C, D, E, and K; the B vitamins; calcium; iron; magnesium; zinc; selenium; and iodine. The report should provide practical advice and recommendations which will constitute an authoritative source of information to all those from Member States who work in the areas of nutrition, agriculture, food production and distribution, and health promotion.
- Thirdly, the Consultation was asked to identify key issues for future research concerning each vitamin and mineral under review and to make preliminary recommendations on that research.

The present report presents the outcome of the Consultation combined with up-to-date evidence that has since become available to answer a number of issues which remained unclear or controversial at the time of the Consultation. It was not originally thought that such an evidence-based consultation process would be so controversial, but the reality is that there are surprisingly few data on specific health status indicators on which to base conclusions, whereas there is a great deal of information relative to overt deficiency disease conditions. The defining of human nutrient requirements and recommended intakes are therefore largely based on expert interpretation and consensus on the best available scientific information.

When looking at recommended nutrient intakes (RNIs) in industrialized countries over the last 25 years, it is noticeable that for some micronutrients these have gradually increased. The question is whether this is the result of better scientific knowledge and understanding of the biochemical role of the nutrients, or whether the criteria for setting requirement levels have changed, or a combination of both. The scientific knowledge base has vastly expanded, but it appears that more rigorous criteria for defining recommended levels is also a key factor.

RNIs for vitamins and minerals were initially established on the understanding that they are meant to meet the basic nutritional needs of over 97% of the population. However, a fundamental criterion in industrialized countries has become one of the presumptive role that these nutrients play in "preventing" an increasing range of disease conditions that characterize affected populations. The latter approach implies trying to define the notion of "optimal nutrition", and this has been one of the factors nudging defined requirements to still higher levels.

This shift in the goal for setting RNIs is not without reason. The populations that are targeted for prevention through "optimal nutrition" are characterized by sedentary lifestyles and longer life expectancy. The populations in industrialized countries are ageing, and concern for the health of the older person has grown accordingly. In contrast, the micronutrient needs of population groups in developing countries are still viewed in terms of millions experiencing deficiency, and are then more appropriately defined as those that will satisfy basic nutritional needs of physically active younger populations. Nevertheless, one also needs to bear in mind the double burden of under- and overnutrition, which is growing rapidly in many developing countries.

Concern has been raised about possible differences in micronutrient needs of populations with different lifestyles for a very practical reason. The logic behind the establishment of micronutrient needs of industrialized nations has come about at the same time as a large and growing demand for a wide variety of supplements and fortificants, and manufacturers have responded quickly to meet this market. This phenomenon could easily skew national strategies for nutritional development, with an increased tendency to seek to resolve the micronutrient deficiency problems of developing countries by promoting supplements and fortification strategies, rather than through increasing the consumption of adequate and varied diets. Higher levels of RNIs often set in developed countries can easily be supported because they can be met with supplementation in addition to food which itself is often fortified. In contrast, it often becomes difficult to meet some of the micronutrient needs in some populations of developing countries by consuming locally available food, because foods are often seasonal, and neither supplementation nor fortification reach vulnerable population groups.

Among the nutrients of greatest concern is *calcium*; the RNI may be difficult to meet in the absence of dairy products. The recently revised United States/Canada dietary reference intakes (DRIs) propose only an acceptable intake (AI) for calcium instead of a recommended daily allowance (RDA) in recognition of the fact that intake data are out of step with the relatively high intake requirements observed with experimentally derived values.[1]

Another nutrient of concern is *iron*, particularly during pregnancy, where supplementation appears to be essential during the second half of pregnancy.

---

[1] Food and Nutrition Board. *Dietary reference intakes for calcium, phosphorus, magnesium, vitamin D, and fluoride.* Washington, DC. National Academy Press. 1997.

Folic acid requirements are doubled for women of childbearing age to prevent the incidence of neural tube defects in the fetus. Conversion factors for carotenoids are under review, with the pending conclusion that servings of green leafy vegetables needed to meet *vitamin A* requirements probably need to be at least doubled. In view of this uncertainty, only "recommended safe intakes" rather than RNIs are provided for this vitamin.

Selenium is the subject of growing interest because of its properties as an antioxidant. The RNIs recommended herein for this micronutrient are generally lower than those derived by the United States Food and Nutrition Board because the latter are calculated on a cellular basis, whereas the present report relies on more traditional whole-body estimates.[1]

Are these "developments" or "new understandings" appropriate for and applicable in developing countries? The scientific evidence for answering this question is still emerging, but the time may be near when RNIs may need to be defined differently, taking into account the perspective of developing countries based on developing country data. There may be a need to identify some biomarkers that are specific to conditions in each developing country. There is therefore a continuing urgent need for research to be carried out in developing countries about their specific nutrient needs. The current situation also implies that the RNIs for the micronutrients of concern discussed above will need to be re-evaluated as soon as significant additional data are available.

Kraisid Tontisirin
Director
Division of Food and Nutrition
Food and Agriculture Organization
of the United Nations

Graeme Clugston
Director
Department of Nutrition for
Health and Development
World Health Organization

---

[1] Food and Nutrition Board. *Dietary reference intakes for vitamin C, vitamin E, selenium and carotenoids. A report of the Panel on Dietary Antioxidants and Related Compounds.* Washington, DC, National Academy Press, 2000.

Acknowledgements

We wish to thank the authors of the background papers: Leif Hallberg, Department of Clinical Nutrition, Göteborg University, Annedalsklinikerna, Sahlgrenska University Hospital, Göteborg, Sweden; Glenville Jones, Department of Biochemistry—Medicine, Queen's University, Kingston, Ontario, Canada; Madhu Karmarkar, Senior Adviser, International Council for Control of Iodine Deficiency Disorders, New Delhi, India; Mark Levine, National Institute of Diabetes & Digestive & Kidney Diseases, National Institute of Health, Bethesda, MD, USA; Donald McCormick, Department of Biochemistry, Emory University School of Medicine, Atlanta, GA, USA; Colin Mills, Director, Postgraduate Studies, Rowett Research Institute, Bucksburn, Scotland; Christopher Nordin, Institute of Medical and Veterinary Sciences, Clinical Biochemistry Division, Adelaide, Australia; Maria Theresa Oyarzum, Institute of Nutrition and Food Technology (INTA), University of Chile, Santiago, Chile; Chandrakant Pandav, Regional Coordinator, South-Asia and Pacific International Council for Control of Iodine Deficiency Disorders; and Additional Professor, Center for Community Medicine, All India Institute of Medical Sciences, New Delhi, India; Brittmarie Sandström,[1] Research Department of Human Nutrition, The Royal Veterinary and Agricultural University, Frederiksberg, Denmark; John Scott, Department of Biochemistry, Trinity College, Dublin, Ireland; Martin Shearer, Vitamin K Research Unit of the Haemophilia Centre, The Rayne Institute, St Thomas's Hospital, London, England; Ajay Sood, Department of Endocrinology and Metabolism, All India Institute of Medical Sciences, New Delhi, India; David Thurnham, Howard Professor of Human Nutrition, School of Biomedical Sciences, Northern Ireland Centre for Diet and Health, University of Ulster, Londonderry, Northern Ireland; Maret Traber, Linus Pauling Institute, Department of Nutrition and Food Management, Oregon State University, Corvallis, OR, USA; Ricardo Uauy, Director, Institute of Nutrition and Food Technology (INTA), University of Chile, Santiago,

---

[1] Deceased.

Chile; Barbara Underwood, formerly Scholar-in-Residence, Food and Nutrition Board, Institute of Medicine, National Academy of Sciences, Washington, DC, USA; and Cees Vermeer, Faculteit der Geneeskunde Biochemie, Department of Biochemistry, University of Maastricht, Maastricht, Netherlands.

A special acknowledgement is made to the following individuals for their valuable contributions to, and useful comments on, the background documents: Christopher Bates, Medical Research Council, Human Nutrition Research, Cambridge, England; Robert E. Black, Department of International Health, Johns Hopkins School of Hygiene and Public Health, Baltimore, MD, USA; James Blanchard, Pharmaceutical Sciences, Department of Pharmacology and Toxicology, University of Arizona, Tucson, AZ, USA; Thomas Bothwell, Faculty of Medicine, University of the Witwatersrand, Witwatersrand, South Africa; Chen Chunming, Senior Adviser, Chinese Academy of Preventive Medicine, Beijing, China; William Cohn, F. Hoffman-La Roche Ltd, Division of Vitamins, Research and Technology Development, Basel, Switzerland; François Delange, International Council for Control of Iodine Deficieny Disorders, Brussels, Belgium; C. Gopalan, President, Nutrition Foundation of India, New Delhi, India; Robert P. Heaney, Creighton University Medical Center, Omaha, NE, USA; Basil Hetzel, Children's Health Development Foundation, Women's and Children's Hospital, North Adelaide, Australia; Glenville Jones, Department of Biochemistry—Medicine, Queen's University, Kingston, Ontario, Canada; Walter Mertz,[1] Rockville, MD, USA; Ruth Oniang'o, Jomo Kenyatta University of Agriculture and Technology, Nairobi, Kenya; Robert Parker, Division of Nutritional Sciences, Cornell University, Ithaca, NY, USA; Robert Russell, Professor of Medicine and Nutrition and Associate Director, Human Nutrition Research Center on Aging, Tufts University, United States Department of Agriculture Agricultural Research Service, Boston, MA, USA; Tatsuo Suda, Department of Biochemistry, Showa University School of Dentistry, Tokyo, Japan; John Suttie, Department of Biochemistry, University of Wisconsin-Madison, Madison, WI, USA; Henk van den Berg, TNO Nutrition and Food Research Institute, Zeist, Netherlands; Keith West Jr., Johns Hopkins School of Hygiene and Public Health, Division of Human Nutrition, Baltimore, MD, USA; and Parvin Zandi, Head, Department of Food Science and Technology, National Nutrition & Food Technology Research Institute, Tehran, Islamic Republic of Iran.

---

[1] Deceased.

Acknowledgements are also made to the members of the Secretariat: Ratko Buzina, formerly Programme of Nutrition, WHO, Geneva, Switzerland; Joan Marie Conway, Consultant, FAO, Rome, Italy; Richard Dawson, Consultant, Food and Nutrition Division, FAO, Rome, Italy; Sultana Khanum, Programme of Nutrition, WHO, Geneva, Switzerland; John R. Lupien, formerly Director, Food and Nutrition Division, FAO, Rome, Italy; Blab Nandi, Senior Food and Nutrition Officer, FAO Regional Office for Asia and the Pacific, Bangkok, Thailand; Joanna Peden, Public Health Nutrition Unit, London School of Hygiene and Tropical Medicine, London, England; and Zeina Sifri, Consultant, Food and Nutrition Division, FAO, Rome, Italy.

Finally, we express our special appreciation to Guy Nantel who coordinated the FAO edition of the report, and to Bruno de Benoist who was responsible for the WHO edition in close collaboration with Maria Andersson. We also wish to thank Kai Lashley and Ann Morgan for their assistance in editing the document and Anna Wolter for her secretarial support.

1. Concepts, definitions and approaches used to define nutritional needs and recommendations

1.1 Introduction

The dietary requirement for a micronutrient is defined as an intake level which meets a specified criteria for adequacy, thereby minimizing risk of nutrient deficit or excess. These criteria cover a gradient of biological effects related to a range of nutrient intakes which, at the extremes, include the intake required to prevent death associated with nutrient deficit or excess. However, for nutrients where insufficient data on mortality are available, which is the case for most micronutrients discussed in this report, other biological responses must be defined. These include clinical disease as determined by signs and symptoms of nutrient deficiency, and subclinical conditions identified by specific biochemical and functional measures. Measures of nutrient stores or critical tissue pools may also be used to determine nutrient adequacy.

Functional assays are presently the most relevant indices of subclinical conditions related to vitamin and mineral intakes. Ideally, these biomarkers should be sensitive to changes in nutritional state while at the same time be specific to the nutrient responsible for the subclinical deficiency. Often, the most sensitive indicators are not the most specific; for example, plasma ferritin, a sensitive indicator of iron status, may change not only in response to iron supply, but also as a result of acute infection or chronic inflammatory processes. Similarly anaemia, the defining marker of dietary iron deficiency, may also result from, among other things, deficiencies in folate, vitamin B_{12} or copper.

The choice of criteria used to define requirements is of critical importance, since the recommended nutrient intake to meet the defined requirement will clearly vary, depending, among other factors, on the criterion used to define nutrient adequacy (*1, 2, 3*). Unfortunately, the information base to scientifically support the definition of nutritional needs across age ranges, sex and physiologic states is limited for many nutrients. Where relevant and possible, requirement estimates presented here include an allowance for variations in micronutrient bioavailability and utilization. The use of nutrient balance to define requirements has been avoided whenever possible, since it is now generally recognized that balance can be reached over a wide range of nutrient intakes. However, requirement levels defined using nutrient balance have been used if no other suitable data are available.

1.2 Definition of terms

The following definitions relate to the micronutrient intake from food and water required to promote optimal health, that is, prevent vitamin and mineral deficiency and avoid the consequences of excess. Upper limits of nutrient intake are defined for specific vitamins and minerals where there is a potential problem with excess either from food or from food in combination with nutrient supplements.

1.2.1 Estimated average requirement

Estimated average requirement (EAR) is the average daily nutrient intake level that meets the needs of 50% of the "healthy" individuals in a particular age and gender group. It is based on a given criteria of adequacy which will vary depending on the specified nutrient. Therefore, estimation of requirement starts by stating the criteria that will be used to define adequacy and then establishing the necessary corrections for physiological and dietary factors. Once a mean requirement value is obtained from a group of subjects, the nutrient intake is adjusted for interindividual variability to arrive at a recommendation (4, 5, 6).

1.2.2 Recommended nutrient intake

Recommended nutrient intake (RNI) is the daily intake, set at the EAR plus 2 standard deviations (SD), which meets the nutrient requirements of almost all apparently healthy individuals in an age- and sex-specific population group. If the distribution of requirement values is not known, a Gaussian or normal distribution can be assumed, and from this it is expected that the mean requirement plus 2 SD will cover the nutrient needs of 97.5% of the population. If the SD is not known, a value based on each nutrient's physiology can be used and in most cases a variation in the range of 10–12.5% can be assumed (exceptions are noted within relevant chapters). Because of the considerable daily variation in micronutrient intake, daily requirement refers to the average intake over a period of time. The cumulative risk function for deficiency and toxicity is defined in Figure 1.1, which illustrates that as nutrient intake increases the risk of deficit drops and at higher intakes the risk of toxicity increases. The definition of RNI used in this report is equivalent to that of the recommended dietary allowance (RDA) as used by the Food and Nutrition Board of the United States National Academy of Sciences (4, 5, 6).

FIGURE 1.1
Risk function of deficiency and excess for individuals in a population related to food intake, assuming a Gaussian distribution of requirements to prevent deficit and avoid excess

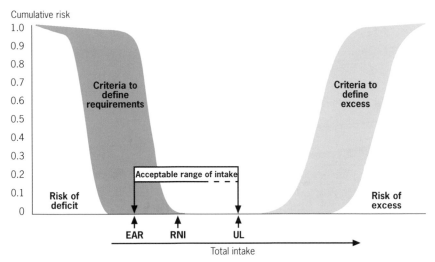

The shaded ranges correspond to different approaches to defining requirements to prevent deficit and excess, respectively. The estimated average requirement (EAR) is the average daily intake required to prevent deficit in half of the population. The recommended nutrient intake (RNI) is the amount necessary to meet the needs of most (97.5%) of the population, set as the EAR plus 2 standard deviations. The tolerable upper intake level (UL) is the level at which no evidence of toxicity is demonstrable.

1.2.3 Apparently healthy

The term, "apparently healthy" refers to the absence of disease based on clinical signs and symptoms of micronutrient deficiency or excess, and normal function as assessed by laboratory methods and physical evaluation.

1.2.4 Protective nutrient intake

The concept of protective nutrient intake has been introduced for some micronutrients to refer to an amount greater than the RNI which may be protective against a specified health or nutritional risk of public health relevance (e.g. vitamin C intake of 25 mg with each meal to enhance iron absorption and prevent anaemia) (7). When existing data provide justifiable differences between RNI values and protective intake levels comment to that effect is made in the appropriate chapter of this document. Protective intake levels are expressed either as a daily value or as an amount to be consumed with a meal.

3

1.2.5 Upper tolerable nutrient intake level

Upper limits (ULs) of nutrient intake have been set for some micronutrients and are defined as the maximum intake from food, water and supplements that is unlikely to pose risk of adverse health effects from excess in almost all (97.5%) apparently healthy individuals in an age- and sex-specific population group (see Figure 1.1). ULs should be based on long-term exposure to all foods, including fortified food products. For most nutrients no adverse effects are anticipated when they are consumed as foods because their absorption and/or excretion are regulated. The special situation of consumption of nutritional supplements which, when added to the nutrient intake from food, may result in a total intake in excess of the UL is addressed for specific micronutrients in subsequent chapters, as appropriate. The ULs as presented here do not meet the strict definition of the "no observed effect level" (NOEL) used in health risk assessment by toxicologists because in most cases, a dose–response curve for risk from exposure to a nutrient will not be available (8). For additional details on derivation of ULs, please refer to standard texts on this subject (9, 10).

The range of intakes between the RNI and UL should be considered sufficient to prevent deficiency while avoiding toxicity. If no UL can be derived from experimental or observational data in humans, the UL can be defined from available data on the range of observed dietary intake of apparently healthy populations. In the absence of known adverse effects a default value for the UL of 10 times the RNI is frequently used (5, 10, 11).

1.2.6 Nutrient excess

Traditional toxicology-based approaches to assessing adverse health effects from nutrient excess start by defining either the highest intake level at which no observed adverse effects of biological significance are found (i.e. the no observed adverse effect level (NOAEL)), or the lowest intake level at which adverse effects are observed (i.e. the lowest observed adverse effect level that are (LOAEL)). Uncertainty or modifying factors are then used to adjust a known NOAEL or LOAEL to define reference doses which represent chronic intake levels that are considered safe, or of no significant health risk, for humans. The nature of the adjustment used to modify the acceptable intake indicated by the NOAEL or LOAEL is based on the type and quality of the available data and its applicability to human populations (5, 9, 11).

Uncertainty factors are used in several circumstances: when the experimental data on toxicity is obtained from animal studies; when the data from humans are insufficient to fully account for variability of populations or special sensitivity subgroups of the general population; when the NOAEL has been obtained in studies of insufficient duration to assure chronic safety; when the database which supports the NOAEL is incomplete; or when the experimental data provide a LOAEL instead of a true NOAEL. The usual value for each uncertainty factor is 10, leading to a 10-fold reduction in the acceptable intake level for each of the considerations listed above. The reductions may be used in isolation or in combination depending on the specific micronutrient being assessed.

Modifying factors are additional uncertainty factors which have a value of 1 or more but less than 10, and are based on expert judgement of the overall quality of the data available. Given the paucity of human data, the limitations of animal models and uncertainties of interpretation, the traditional toxicological approach to determining limits for intake, as summarized here, may in fact lead to the definition of intakes which promote or even induce deficiency if followed by a population. This has recently been recognized by the WHO International Programme on Chemical Safety, and a special risk assessment model has been derived for elements that are both essential and have potential toxicity (5, 9).

1.2.7 Use of nutrient intake recommendations in population assessment

Recommendations given in this report are generally presented as population RNIs with a corresponding UL where appropriate. They are not intended to define the daily requirements of an individual. However "healthy" individuals consuming within the range of the RNI and the UL can expect to minimize their risk of micronutrient deficit and excess. Health professionals caring for special population groups that do not meet the defined characterization of "healthy" should, where possible, adjust these nutrient-based recommendations to the special needs imposed by disease conditions and/or environmental situations.

The use of dietary recommendations in assessing the adequacy of nutrient intakes of populations requires good quantitative information about the distribution of usual nutrient intakes as well as knowledge of the distribution of requirements. The assessment of intake should include all sources of intake, that is, food, water and supplements; appropriate dietary and food composition data are thus essential to achieve a valid estimate of intakes. The day-to-day variation in individual intake can be minimized by collecting intake data over several days. There are several statistical approaches that can be used to estimate the prevalence of inadequate intakes from the distribution of intakes and requirements. One such approach the EAR cut-point method which defines the fraction of a population that consumes less than the EAR for a given nutrient. It assumes that the variability of individual intakes is at least as large as the variability in requirements and that the distribution of intakes and requirements are independent of each other. The latter is most likely to be true in the case of vitamins and minerals, but clearly not for energy. The EAR cut-point method requires a single population with a symmetrical distribution around the mean. If these conditions are met, the prevalence of inadequate intakes corresponds to the proportion of intakes that fall below the EAR. It is clearly inappropriate to examine mean values of population intake and RNI to define the population at risk of inadequacy. The relevant information is the proportion of intakes in a population group that is below the EAR, not below the RNI (4, 5).

Figure 1.2 serves to illustrate the use of nutrient intake recommendations in risk assessment considering the model presented in Figure 1.1; the distributions of nutrient intakes for a population have been added to explore risk of excess or deficit (2, 4, 5). Figure 1.2a presents the case of a single population with intakes ranging from below the EAR to the UL with a mean intake close to the RNI. The fraction of the population that is below the EAR represents the prevalence of deficit; as depicted in the figure this is a sizeable group despite the fact that the mean intake for the population is close to the RNI. Figure 1.2b presents the case of a bimodal distribution of population intakes where the conditions to use the EAR cut-point method are not met. In this case it is clear that a targeted intervention to increase the intake of one group but not the other is needed. For example, if we examine the iron intake of a population we may find that vegetarians may be well below the recommended intake while those who consume meat may be getting sufficient iron. To achieve adequacy in this case we need to increase iron intake in the former but not the latter group (2, 12).

1.3 Approaches used in estimating nutrient intakes for optimal health

The methods used to estimate nutritional requirements have changed over time. Four currently used approaches are briefly outlined below: the clinical approach, nutrient balance, functional indicators of nutritional sufficiency (biochemical, physiological, molecular), and optimal nutrient intake. A detailed analysis of the relative merits of these approaches is beyond the scope of this chapter, but additional information on each can be found in subsequent chapters of this report. When no information is available the default approach to define a recommended intake based on the range of observed intakes of "healthy" populations is used.

FIGURE 1.2
Distribution of population intakes and risk of deficit and excess

(a)

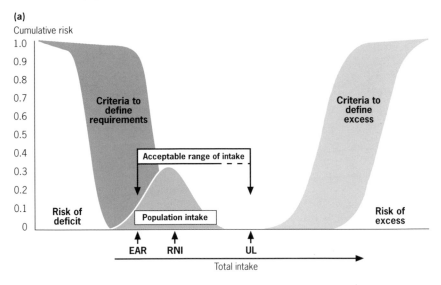

(b)

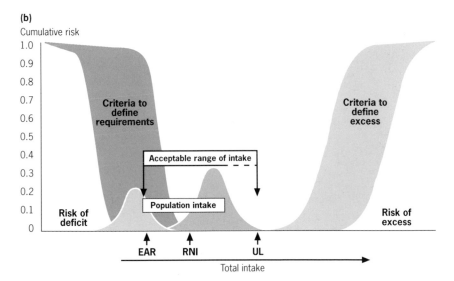

a) Examines the risk of inadequacy for a given distribution of intakes as shown by the shaded bell-shaped area. In this example, the proportion of individuals that have intakes below the EAR are at risk of deficiency (see text for details).

b) Illustrates the need to examine whether there is more than one group within the population distribution of intakes. In this case, the overall mean intake is above the RNI, suggesting a low risk of deficit. However, while a large proportion of the population (represented by the right-hand bell-shaped area) is over the RNI, there is in fact a significant proportion of the population (represented by the left-hand bell-shaped area) below the EAR, and thus at risk of deficiency. The intervention here should be targeted to increase the intake for the group on the left but not for the one on the right; the right-hand group may exceed the UL and be at risk for excess if their intake is increased.

7

1.3.1 The clinical approach

The traditional criteria to define essentiality of nutrients for human health require that a) a disease state, or functional or structural abnormality is present if the nutrient is absent or deficient in the diet and, b) that the abnormalities are related to, or a consequence of, specific biochemical or functional changes that can be reversed by the presence of the essential dietary component. End-points considered in recent investigations of essentiality of nutrients in experimental animals and humans include: reductions in ponderal or linear growth rates, altered body composition, compromised host defense systems, impairment of gastrointestinal or immune function, abnormal cognitive performance, increased susceptibility to disease, increased morbidity and changes in biochemical measures of nutrient status. To establish such criteria for particular vitamins and minerals requires a solid understanding of the biological effects of specific nutrients, as well as sensitive instrumentation to measure the effects, and a full and precise knowledge of the amount and chemical form of nutrients supplied by various foods and their interactions (2, 12).

1.3.2 Nutrient balance

Nutrient balance calculations typically involve assessing input and output and establishing requirement at the point of equilibrium (except in the case of childhood, pregnancy and lactation where the additional needs for growth, tissue deposition and milk secretion are considered). However, in most cases, balance based on input–output measurements is greatly influenced by prior level of intake, that is, subjects adjust to high intakes by increasing output and, conversely, they lower output when intake is low. Thus, if sufficient time is provided to accommodate to a given level of intake, balance can be achieved, and for this reason, the exclusive use of nutrient balance to define requirements should be avoided whenever possible (1, 5, 13).

In the absence of alternative sources of data, a starting point in defining nutritional requirements using the balance methodology is the use of factorial estimates of nutritional need. The "factorial model" is based on measuring the components that must be replaced when the intake of a specific nutrient is minimal or nil. This is the minimum possible requirement value and encompasses a) replacement of losses from excretion and utilization at low or no intake, b) the need to maintain body stores and, c) an intake that is usually sufficient to prevent clinical deficiency (6). Factorial methods should be used only as a first approximation for the assessment of individual requirements, or when functional clinical or biochemical criteria of adequacy have not been established. Furthermore, although nutrient balance studies may be of help in defining mineral needs, they are of little use for defining vitamin requirements (*14, 15*). This is because the carbon dioxide formed on the oxidation of vitamins is lost in expired air or hard to quantify, since it becomes part of the body pool and cannot be traced to its origin unless the vitamin is provided in an isotopically labelled form (*15*).

1.3.3 Functional responses

Various biomarkers are presently being evaluated for their specificity and sensitivity to assess nutrient-related organ function and thus predict deficiency or toxicity.

In terms of defining nutrient needs for optimal function, recent efforts have focused on the assessment of:

- *Neurodevelopment*: monitoring electro-physiologic responses to defined sensory stimuli; sleep–wake cycle organization; and neurobehavioural tests (*16, 17, 18*).
- *Bone health*: measuring bone mineral density by X-ray absorptiometry; markers of collagen synthesis and turnover; and hormonal responses associated with bone anabolism and catabolism (*19, 20*).
- *Biochemical normalcy*: measuring plasma and tissue concentrations of substrates or nutrient responsive enzymes, hormones or other indices of anabolic and catabolic activity; and plasma concentrations and tissue retention in response to a fixed nutrient load (*21, 22*).
- *Immune function*: measuring humoral and cellular response to antigens and mitogens in vitro or in vivo; antibody response to weak antigens such as immunizations; T-cell populations; cytokine responses; and mediators of inflammation related to tissue protection and damage (*23, 24*).
- *Body composition and tissue metabolic status*: using stable isotope assessment of body compartments (e.g. body water, lean and fat mass); radiation-determined body compartments measured by dual energy X-ray absorptiometry (DEXA) and computerized tomography; electrical impedance and conductivity to determine body compartments; and finally, magnetic resonance imaging and spectroscopy of body and organ compartments (i.e. brain and muscle high energy phosphate content) (*25, 26*).
- *Bioavailability*: evaluating stable and radioactive isotopes of mineral and vitamin absorption and utilization (*7, 27*).
- *Gene expression*: assessing the expression of multiple human mRNA with specific fluorescent cDNAs probes (which currently evaluate from 10 000–15 000 genes at a time and will soon be able to assess the expression of the full genome); and laser detection of hybridized genes to reveal mRNA abundance in relation to a given nutrient intake level. These novel

tools provide a powerful means of assessing the amount of nutrient required to trigger a specific mRNA response in a given tissue. These are in fact the best criteria for defining selenium needs without having to measure the key selenium dependent enzymes (i.e. liver or red blood cell glutathione peroxidase [GSHPx]) (28). In this case the measurement of sufficiency is based on the GSHPx–mRNA response to selenium supply rather than measuring the enzymatic activity of the corresponding protein. Micro-array systems tailored to evaluate nutrient modulated expression of key genes may become the most effective way of assessing human nutritional requirements in the future (29).

1.3.4 Optimal intake

Optimal intake is a relatively new approach to deriving nutrient requirements. The question "Optimal intake for what?" is usually answered with the suggestion that a balanced diet or specific nutrients can improve physical and mental performance, enhance immunity, prevent cancer, or add healthy years to our life. This response is unfortunately often used too generally, and is usually unsupported by appropriate population-based controlled randomized studies (15). The preferred approach to define optimal intake is to clearly establish the function of interest and the level of desired function (30). The selected function should be related in a plausible manner to the specific nutrient or food and serve to promote health or prevent disease.

If there is insufficient information from which to derive recommendations based on actual data using any of the approaches described above, the customary intake (based on an appropriate knowledge of food composition and food consumption) of healthy populations becomes a reasonable default approach. Indeed, the presently recommended nutrient intakes for term infants of several vitamins and minerals are based on this paradigm. Thus, the nutrient intake of the breast-fed infant becomes the relevant criteria since it is assumed that human milk is the optimal food for human growth and development. In this case, all other criteria are subservient to the estimate obtained from assessment of the range of documented intake observed in the full term breast-fed infant. Precise knowledge of human milk composition and volume of intake for postnatal age allows for the definition of the range of intakes typical for breast-fed infants. A notable exception, however, is the requirement for vitamin K at birth, since breast milk contains little vitamin K, and the sterile colon does not provide the vitamin K formed by colonic microorganisms.

Planners using RNIs are often faced with different, sometimes conflicting numbers, recommended by respectable national scientific bodies that have used varying approaches to define them (*31, 32*). In order to select the most appropriate for a given population, national planners should consider the information base and the criteria that led to the numerical derivation before determining which correspond more closely with the setting for which the food-based dietary guidelines are intended. The quantified RNI estimates derived from these various approaches may differ for one or more specific nutrients, but the effect of these numeric differences in establishing food-based dietary guidelines for the general population is often of a lesser significance (*2, 12, 33*). Selected examples of how various criteria are used to define numerical estimates of nutritional requirements are given below. More detail is provided in the respective chapters on individual micronutrients that follow.

Calcium

Adequate calcium intake levels suggested for the United States of America are higher than those accepted internationally, and extend the increased needs of adolescents to young adults (i.e. those aged < 24 years) on the basis of evidence that peak bone mass continues to increase until that age is reached (see Chapter 4). Results of bone density measurements support the need for calcium intake beyond that required for calcium balance and retention for growth. However, the situation in most Asian countries suggests that their populations may have sufficient calcium retention and bone mass despite lower levels of intake. This report acknowledges these differences and suggests that calcium intake may need to be adjusted for dietary factors (e.g. observed animal protein, sodium intake, vitamin D intake) and for sun exposure (which is related to geographic location/latitude, air pollution and other environmental conditions), since both affect calcium retention.

Iron

In the case of iron, the differences in quantification of obligatory losses made by various expert groups is possibly explained by differences in environmental sanitation and the prevalence of diarrhoea (*34*). In addition, the concern about iron excess may be greater in places where anaemia is no longer an issue, such as in northern Europe, while in other areas iron deficiency is of paramount significance. The use of different bioavailability adjustment factors in the definition of iron RNIs is a useful concept because the presence of dietary components that affect bioavailability differs between and within a given ecological setting. The present Expert Consultation established a recommendation based on absorbed iron; the RNI thus varies according to the bioavailability of iron in the diet. Recommended RNIs are provided for four bioavailability factors, 5%, 10%, 12% and 15%, depending on the composition of the typical local diet (see Chapter 13).

Folate

Food fortification or supplementation strategies will commonly be needed to satisfy the 400 µg/day folate recommended for adolescents and adults in this report (based on the intake required before conception and during early pregnancy to prevent neural tube defects) (35). Consumption from traditional food sources is not sufficient to meet this goal; however, food fortification and the advent of novel foods developed by traditional breeding or by genetic modification may eventually make it possible to meet the RNI with food-based approaches.

1.4 Conclusions

The quantitative definition of nutrient needs and their expression as recommended nutrient intakes have been important components of food and nutrition policy and programme implementation. RNIs provide the firm scientific basis necessary to satisfy the requirements of a group of healthy individuals and define adequacy of diets. Yet, by themselves, they are not sufficient as instruments of nutrition policy and programmes. In fact, single nutrient-based approaches have been of limited use in the establishment of nutritional and dietary priorities consistent with broad public health interests at the national and international levels (36).

In contrast to RNIs, food-based dietary guidelines (FBDGs) as instruments of policy are more closely linked to diet–health relationships of relevance to a particular country or region (12). FBDGs provide a broad perspective that examines the totality of the effects of a given dietary pattern in a given ecological setting, considering socioeconomic and cultural factors, and the biological and physical environment, all of which affect the health and nutrition of a given population or community (2, 5). Defining the relevant public health problems related to diet is an essential first step in developing nutrient intake goals in order to promote overall health and reduce health risks in view of the multifactorial nature of disease. Thus, FBDGs take into account the customary dietary pattern, the foods available, and the factors that determine the consumption of foods and indicate what aspects should be modified.

By utilizing the two approaches of FBDGs and RNIs, broad public health interests are supported by the use of empirically defined nutrient requirements. The role of RNIs in the development and formulation of FBDGs is summarized in Figure 1.3. The multiple final users and applications of these

FIGURE 1.3
Schematic representation of the process of applying nutritional requirements and recommendations in the definition of nutrient intake goals leading to the formulation of food-based dietary guidelines

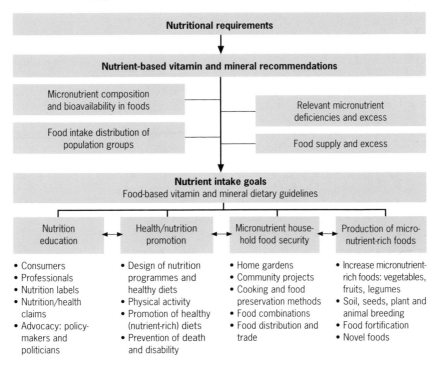

The boxes at the bottom of the scheme exemplify the multiple final users of this knowledge and the implications for policy and programmes.

concepts are exemplified in the lower part of the scheme. Nutrition education, health and nutrition promotion, household food security and the production of micronutrient-rich foods all require nutritional requirements based on the best available scientific information. As the science base for nutrition evolves, so too will the estimates of nutritional requirements, which, when combined with FBDGs, will lead to greater accuracy with respect to applications and policy-making and will enhance the health of final users.

We have gone beyond the era of requirements to prevent deficiency and excess to the present goal of preserving micronutrient-related functions. The next step in this evolution will surely be the incorporation of the knowledge and necessary tools to assess genetic diversity in the redefinition of nutritional requirements for optimal health throughout the life course. The goal in this case will be to meet the nutritional needs of population groups, while accounting for genetic heterogeneity within populations (*37*). Though this may lead

13

to the apparent contradiction of attempting to meet the requirements of populations based on the diverse and heterogeneous needs of individuals, it is in fact, a necessary step in providing optimal health—a long life, free of physical and mental disability—to all individuals.

References

1. Young VR. W.O. Atwater Memorial Lecture and the 2001 ASNS President's Lecture. Human nutrient requirements: the challenge of the post-genome era. *Journal of Nutrition*, 2002, 132:621–629.
2. Uauy R, Hertrampf E. Food-based dietary recommendations: possibilities and limitations. In: Bowman B, Russell R, eds. *Present knowledge in nutrition*, 8th ed. Washington, DC, International Life Sciences Institute Press, 2001:636–649.
3. Aggett PJ et al. Recommended dietary allowances (RDAs), recommended dietary intakes (RDIs), recommended nutrient intakes (RNIs), and population reference intakes (PRIs) are not "recommended intakes". *Journal of Pediatric and Gastroenterology Nutrition*, 1997, 25:236–241.
4. Food and Nutrition Board. *Dietary reference intakes: applications in dietary assessment*. Washington, DC, National Academy Press, 2001.
5. *Trace elements in human nutrition and health*. Geneva, World Health Organization, 1996.
6. *Energy and protein requirements. Report of a Joint FAO/WHO/UNU Expert Consultation*. Geneva, World Health Organization, 1985 (WHO Technical Report Series, No. 724; http://whqlibdoc.who.int/trs/WHO_TRS_724_ (chp1--chp6).pdf, accessed 26 June 2004; http://whqlibdoc.who.int/trs/ WHO_TRS_724_(chp7–chp13).pdf, accessed 26 June 2004).
7. Cook JD, Reddy MB. Effect of ascorbic acid intake on nonheme-iron absorption from a complete diet. *American Journal of Clinical Nutrition*, 2001, 73:93–98.
8. Olivares M, Araya M, Uauy R. Copper homeostasis in infant nutrition: deficit and excess. *Journal of Pediatric and Gastroenterology Nutrition*, 2000, 31: 102–111.
9. *Principles and methods for the assessment of risk from essential trace elements*. Geneva, World Health Organization, 2002 (Environmental Health Criteria, No. 228).
10. Food and Nutrition Board. *Dietary reference intakes. A risk assessment model for establishing upper intake levels for nutrients*. Washington, DC, National Academy Press, 1999.
11. *Assessing human health risks of chemicals: derivation of guidance values for health-based exposure limits*. Geneva, World Health Organization, 1994 (Environmental Health Criteria, No. 170).
12. *Preparation and use of food-based dietary guidelines. Report of a Joint FAO/WHO Consultation*. Geneva, World Health Organization, 1996 (WHO Technical Report Series, No. 880).
13. Hegsted M, Linkswiler HM. Long-term effects of level of protein intake on calcium metabolism in young adult women. *Journal of Nutrition*, 1981, 111:244–251.
14. Food and Nutrition Board. *Dietary reference intakes for vitamin A, vitamin K, arsenic, boron, chromium, copper, iodine, iron, manganese, molybdenum, nickel, silicon, vanadium, and zinc*. Washington, DC, National Academy Press, 2002.

15. Food and Nutrition Board. *Dietary reference intakes for vitamin C, vitamin E, selenium, and carotenoids.* Washington, DC, National Academy Press, 2000.
16. Fenstrom J, Uauy R, Arroyo P, eds. *Nutrition and brain.* Basel, Karger AG, 2001.
17. Lozoff B. Perinatal iron deficiency and the developing brain. *Pediatric Research*, 2000, 48:137–139.
18. Carlson SE, Neuringer M. Polyunsaturated fatty acid status and neuro-development: a summary and critical analysis of the literature. *Lipids*, 1999, 34:171–178.
19. Flohr F et al. Bone mineral density and quantitative ultrasound in adults with cystic fibrosis. *European Journal of Endocrinology*, 2002, 146:531–536.
20. Black AJ et al. A detailed assessment of alterations in bone turnover, calcium homeostasis, and bone density in normal pregnancy. *Journal of Bone and Mineral Research*, 2000, 15:557–563.
21. Prohaska JR, Brokate B. Lower copper, zinc-superoxide dismutase protein but not mRNA in organs of copper-deficient rats. *Archives of Biochemistry and Biophysics*, 2001, 393:170–176.
22. Mize CE et al. Effect of phosphorus supply on mineral balance at high calcium intakes in very low birth weight infants. *American Journal of Clinical Nutrition*, 1995, 62:385–391.
23. Chandra RK. Nutrition and the immune system from birth to old age. *European Journal of Clinical Nutrition*, 2002, 56(Suppl. 3):S73–S76.
24. Sandstrom B et al. Acrodermatitis enteropathica, zinc metabolism, copper status, and immune function. *Archives of Pediatrics and Adolescent Medicine*, 1994, 148:980–985.
25. Bertocci LA, Mize CE, Uauy R. Muscle phosphorus energy state in very-low-birth-weight infants: effect of exercise. *American Journal of Physiology*, 1992, 262:E289–E294.
26. Mayfield SR, Uauy R, Waidelich D. Body composition of low-birth-weight infants determined by using bioelectrical resistance and reactance. *American Journal of Clinical Nutrition*, 1991, 54:296–303.
27. Lonnerdal B. Bioavailability of copper. *American Journal of Clinical Nutrition*, 1996, 63(Suppl.):S821–S829.
28. Weiss Sachdev S, Sunde RA. Selenium regulation of transcript abundance and translational efficiency of glutathione peroxidase-1 and -4 in rat liver. *Biochemical Journal*, 2001, 357:851–858.
29. Endo Y et al. Dietary protein quantity and quality affect rat hepatic gene expression. *Journal of Nutrition*, 2002, 132:3632–3637.
30. Koletzko B et al. Growth, development and differentiation: a functional food science approach. *British Journal of Nutrition*, 1998, 80(Suppl. 1):S5–S45.
31. Howson CP, Kennedy ET, Horwitz A, eds. *Prevention of micronutrient deficiencies. Tools for policymakers and public health workers.* Washington, DC, National Academy Press, 1998.
32. *Preventing iron deficiency in women and children: technical consensus on key issues.* Boston, The International Nutrition Foundation, and Ottawa, The Micronutrient Initiative, 1999 (http://www.micronutrient.org/resources/publications/nvironbk.pdf, accessed 24 June 2004).
33. *Nutrition and your health: dietary guidelines for Americans*, 5th ed. Washington, DC, United States Department of Health and Human Services, and

United States Department of Agriculture, 2000 (http://www.health.gov/ dietaryguidelines/dga2000/document/frontcover.htm, accessed 24 June 2004).

34. Albonico M et al. Epidemiological evidence for a differential effect of hookworm species, *Ancylostoma duodenale* or *Necator americanus*, on iron status of children. *International Journal of Epidemiology*, 1998, 27:530–537.

35. Oakley GP, Adams MJ, Dickinson CM. More folic acid for everyone, now. *Journal of Nutrition*, 1996, 126(Suppl.):S751–S755.

36. *International Conference on Nutrition. World declaration and plan of action for nutrition, 1992.* Rome, Food and Agriculture Organization of the United Nations, 1992.

37. Ames BN, Elson-Schwab I, Silver EA. High-dose vitamin therapy stimulates variant enzymes with decreased coenzyme binding affinity (increased K(m)): relevance to genetic disease and polymorphisms. *American Journal of Clinical Nutrition*, 2002, 75:616–658.

2. Vitamin A

2.1 Role of vitamin A in human metabolic processes

Vitamin A (retinol) is an essential nutrient needed in small amounts by humans for the normal functioning of the visual system; growth and development; and maintenance of epithelial cellular integrity, immune function, and reproduction. These dietary needs for vitamin A are normally provided for as preformed retinol (mainly as retinyl ester) and provitamin A carotenoids.

2.1.1 Overview of vitamin A metabolism

Preformed vitamin A in animal foods occurs as retinyl esters of fatty acids in association with membrane-bound cellular lipid and fat-containing storage cells. Provitamin A carotenoids in foods of vegetable origin are also associated with cellular lipids but are embedded in complex cellular structures such as the cellulose-containing matrix of chloroplasts or the pigment-containing portion of chromoplasts. Normal digestive processes free vitamin A and carotenoids from food matrices, which is a more efficient process from animal than from vegetable tissues. Retinyl esters are hydrolysed and the retinol and freed carotenoids are incorporated into lipid-containing, water-miscible micellar solutions. Products of fat digestion (e.g. fatty acids, monoglycerides, cholesterol, and phospholipids) and secretions in bile (e.g. bile salts and hydrolytic enzymes) are essential for the efficient solubilization of retinol and especially for solubilization of the very lipophilic carotenoids (e.g. α- and β-carotene, β-cryptoxanthin, and lycopene) in the aqueous intestinal milieu. Micellar solubilization is a prerequisite to their efficient passage into the lipid-rich membrane of intestinal mucosal cells (i.e. enterocytes) (1–3). Diets critically low in dietary fat (under about 5–10 g daily) (4) or disease conditions that interfere with normal digestion and absorption leading to steatorrhoea (e.g. pancreatic and liver diseases and frequent gastroenteritis) can therefore impede the efficient absorption of retinol and carotenoids. Retinol and some carotenoids enter the intestinal mucosal brush border by diffusion in accord with the concentration gradient between the micelle and plasma membrane of enterocytes. Some carotenoids pass into the enterocyte and are solubilized into chylomicrons without further change whereas some of the provitamin A carotenoids are converted to retinol by a cleavage enzyme in the brush border (*3*). Retinol is trapped intracellularly by re-esterification or binding to specific intracellular binding proteins. Retinyl esters and unconverted carotenoids together with other lipids are incorporated into chylomicrons, excreted into intestinal lymphatic channels, and delivered to the blood through the thoracic duct (*2*).

Tissues extract most lipids and some carotenoids from circulating chylomicrons, but most retinyl esters are stripped from the chylomicron remnant, hydrolysed, and taken up primarily by parenchymal liver cells. If not immediately needed, retinol is re-esterified and retained in the fat-storing cells of the liver (variously called adipocytes, stellate cells, or Ito cells). The liver parenchymal cells also take in substantial amounts of carotenoids. Whereas most of the body's vitamin A reserve remains in the liver, carotenoids are also deposited elsewhere in fatty tissues throughout the body (*1*). Usually, turnover of carotenoids in tissues is relatively slow, but in times of low dietary carotenoid intake, stored carotenoids are mobilized. A recent study in one subject using stable isotopes suggests that retinol can be derived not only from conversion of dietary provitamin carotenoids in enterocytes—the major site of bioconversion—but also from hepatic conversion of circulating provitamin carotenoids (*5*). The quantitative contribution to vitamin A requirements of carotenoid converted to retinoids beyond the enterocyte is unknown.

Following hydrolysis of stored retinyl esters, retinol combines with a plasma-specific transport protein, retinol-binding protein (RBP). This process, including synthesis of the unoccupied RBP (apo-RBP), occurs to the greatest extent within liver cells but it may also occur in some peripheral tissues. The RBP-retinol complex (holo-RBP) is secreted into the blood where it associates with another hepatically synthesized and excreted larger protein, transthyretin. The transthyretin-RBP-retinol complex circulates in the blood, delivering the lipophilic retinol to tissues; its large size prevents its loss through kidney filtration (*1*). Dietary restriction in energy, proteins, and some micronutrients can limit hepatic synthesis of proteins specific to mobilization and transport of vitamin A. Altered kidney functions or fever associated with infections (e.g. respiratory infections (*6*) or diarrhoea [*7*]) can increase urinary vitamin A loss.

Holo-RBP transiently associates with target tissue membranes, and specific intracellular binding proteins then extract the retinol. Some of the transiently sequestered retinol is released into the blood unchanged and is recycled (i.e. conserved) (*1*, *8*). A limited reserve of intracellular retinyl esters is formed that subsequently can provide functionally active retinol and its oxidation products (i.e. isomers of retinoic acid) as needed intracellularly. These biologically active forms of vitamin A are associated with specific cellular proteins which bind with retinoids within cells during metabolism and with nuclear receptors that mediate retinoid action on the genome (9). Retinoids modulate the transcription of several hundreds of genes (10–12). In addition to the latter role of retinoic acid, retinol is the form required for functions in the visual (13) and reproductive systems (14) and during embryonic development (15).

Holo-RBP is filtered into the glomerulus but recovered from the kidney tubule and recycled. Normally vitamin A leaves the body in urine only as inactive metabolites resulting from tissue utilization and in bile secretions as potentially recyclable active glucuronide conjugates of retinol (8). No single urinary metabolite has been identified which accurately reflects tissue levels of vitamin A or its rate of utilization. Hence, at this time urine is not a useful biological fluid for assessment of vitamin A nutriture.

2.1.2 Biochemical mechanisms for vitamin A functions

Vitamin A functions at two levels in the body: the first is in the visual cycle in the retina of the eye; the second is in all body tissues where it systemically maintains the growth and soundness of cells. In the visual system, carrier-bound retinol is transported to ocular tissue and to the retina by intracellular binding and transport proteins. Rhodopsin, the visual pigment critical to dim-light vision, is formed in rod cells after conversion of all-*trans*-retinol to retinaldehyde, isomerization to the 11-*cis*-form, and binding to opsin. Alteration of rhodopsin through a cascade of photochemical reactions results in the ability to see objects in dim light (13). The speed at which rhodopsin is regenerated is related to the availability of retinol. Night blindness is usually an indicator of inadequate available retinol, but it can also be due to a deficit of other nutrients that are critical to the regeneration of rhodopsin, such as protein and zinc, and to some inherited diseases, such as retinitis pigmentosa.

The growth and differentiation of epithelial cells throughout the body are especially affected by vitamin A deficiency (VAD). In addition, goblet cell numbers are reduced in epithelial tissues and as a consequence, mucous secretions (with their antimicrobial components) diminish. Cells lining protective tissue surfaces fail to regenerate and differentiate, hence they flatten and accumulate keratin. Both factors—the decline in mucous secretions and loss of cellular integrity—reduce the body's ability to resist invasion from potentially pathogenic organisms. Pathogens can also compromise the immune system by directly interfering with the production of some types of protective secretions and cells (*11*). Classical symptoms of xerosis (drying or non-wetability) and desquamation of dead surface cells as seen in ocular tissue (i.e. xerophthalmia) are the external evidence of the changes also occurring to various degrees in internal epithelial tissues.

Current understanding of the mechanism of vitamin A action within cells outside the visual cycle is that cellular functions are mediated through specific nuclear receptors. Binding with specific isomers of retinoic acid (i.e. all-*trans*- and 9-*cis*-retinoic acid) activates these receptors. Activated receptors bind to DNA response elements located upstream of specific genes to regulate the level of expression of those genes (*12*). These retinoid-activated genes regulate the synthesis of a large number of proteins vital to maintaining normal physiologic functions. There may, however, be other mechanisms of action that are as yet undiscovered (*10*).

2.2 Populations at risk for, and consequences of, vitamin A deficiency

2.2.1 Definition of vitamin A deficiency

VAD is not easily defined. WHO defines it as tissue concentrations of vitamin A low enough to have adverse health consequences even if there is no evidence of clinical xerophthalmia (*16*). In addition to the specific signs and symptoms of xerophthalmia and the risk of irreversible blindness, non-specific symptoms include increased morbidity and mortality, poor reproductive health, increased risk of anaemia, and contributions to slowed growth and development. However, these nonspecific adverse effects may be caused by other nutrient deficits as well, making it difficult to attribute non-ocular symptoms specifically to VAD in the absence of biochemical measurements reflective of vitamin A status.

2.2.2 Geographic distribution and magnitude

In 1995, WHO estimated the global distribution of VAD (Table 2.1) and categorized countries according to the seriousness of VAD as a public health problem on the basis of both clinical and moderate and severe subclinical (prevalence of low blood levels of retinol) indicators of deficiency (*16, 17*). It was estimated that about 3 million children have some form of xerophthalmia and, on the basis of blood levels, another 250 million are subclinically deficient (*17*). The magnitude of the subclinical estimate is currently being re-evaluated to establish quantitatively a benchmark for measuring prevalence trends. The actual number of subclinical deficiencies based on the prevalence of low serum levels of retinol, however, remains uncertain because

TABLE 2.1
Estimates of clinical and subclinical vitamin A deficiency in preschool children, by WHO region[a]

Region	Clinical (millions)	Subclinical (severe and moderate) (millions)	Prevalence (%)
Africa	1.04	52	49
The Americas	0.06	16	20
South-East Asia	1.45	125	69
Europe	NA	NA	NA
Eastern Mediterranean	0.12	16	22
Western Pacific	0.13	42	27
Subtotal	2.80	251	
Total		254	

NA, not applicable.
[a] Based on a projection for 1994 from those countries in each region where data were available.
Source: adapted from reference (17).

of the confounding and poorly quantified role of infections (see section 2.2.5).

Epidemiological studies repeatedly report clustering of VAD, presumably resulting from concurrent occurrences of several risk factors. This clustering may occur among both neighbourhoods and households (18).

2.2.3 Age and sex

VAD can occur in individuals of any age. However, it is a disabling and potentially fatal public health problem for children under 6 years of age. VAD-related blindness is most prevalent in children under 3 years of age (19). This period of life is characterized by high requirements for vitamin A to support rapid growth, and the transition from breastfeeding to dependence on other dietary sources of the vitamin. In addition, adequate intake of vitamin A reduces the risk of catching respiratory and gastrointestinal infections. The increased mortality risk from concurrent infections extends at least to 6 years of age and is associated with both clinical and subclinical VAD (20). There is little information regarding the health consequences of VAD in school-age children. The prevalence of Bitot's spots (i.e. white foamy patches on the conjunctiva) may be highest in this age group but their occurrence may reflect past more than current history of VAD (21). Women of reproductive age are also thought to be vulnerable to VAD during pregnancy and lactation because they often report night blindness (22, 23) and because their breast milk is frequently low in vitamin A (*24, 25*). Not all night blindness in pregnant women, however, responds to vitamin A treatment (*23*).

There is no consistent, clear indication in humans of a sex differential in vitamin A requirements during childhood. Growth rates, and presumably the need for vitamin A, from birth to 10 years for boys are consistently higher than those for girls (*26*). In the context of varied cultural and community settings, however, variations in gender-specific child-feeding and care practices are likely to subsume a small sex differential in requirements to account for reported sex differences in the prevalence of xerophthalmia. Pregnant and lactating women require additional vitamin A to support maternal and fetal tissue growth and lactation losses, additional vitamin A which is not needed by other post-adolescent adults (*27*).

2.2.4 Risk factors

VAD is most common in populations consuming most of their vitamin A needs from provitamin carotenoid sources and where minimal dietary fat is available (*28*). About 90% of ingested preformed vitamin A is absorbed, whereas the absorption efficiency of provitamin A carotenoids varies widely, depending on the type of plant source and the fat content of the accompanying meal (*29*). Where possible, an increased intake of dietary fat is likely to improve the absorption of vitamin A in the body.

In areas with endemic VAD, fluctuations in the incidence of VAD throughout the year reflect the balance between intake and need. Periods of general food shortage (and specific shortages in vitamin A-rich foods) coincide with peak incidence of VAD and common childhood infectious diseases (e.g. diarrhoea, respiratory infections, and measles). Seasonal food availability influences VAD prevalence directly by influencing access to provitamin A sources; for example, the scarcity of mangoes in hot arid months followed by the glutting of the market with mangoes during harvest seasons (*30*). Seasonal growth spurts in children, which frequently follow seasonal post-harvest increases in energy and macronutrient intakes, can also affect the balance. These increases are usually obtained from staple grains (e.g. rice) and tubers (e.g. light-coloured yams) that are not, however, good sources of some micronutrients (e.g. vitamin A) to support the growth spurt (*31*).

Food habits and taboos often restrict consumption of potentially good food sources of vitamin A (e.g. mangoes and green leafy vegetables). Culture-specific factors for feeding children, adolescents, and pregnant and lactating women are common (*28, 32–34*). Illness- and childbirth-related proscriptions of the use of specific foods pervade many traditional cultures (*35*). Such influences alter short- and long-term food distribution within families. However, some cultural practices can be protective of vitamin A status and they need to be identified and reinforced.

2.2.5 Morbidity and mortality

The consequences of VAD are manifested differently in different tissues. In the eye, the symptoms and signs, together referred to as xerophthalmia, have a long, well-recognized history and have until recently been the basis for estimating the global burden from the disease (19). Although ocular symptoms and signs are the most specific indicators of VAD, they occur only after other tissues have impaired functions that are less specific and less easily assessed.

The prevalence of ocular manifestations (i.e. xerophthalmia or clinical VAD) is now recognized to far underestimate the magnitude of the problem of functionally significant VAD. Many more preschool-age children, and perhaps older children and women who are pregnant or lactating, have their health compromised when they are subclinically deficient. In young children, subclinical deficiency, like clinical deficiency, increases the severity of some infections, particularly diarrhoea and measles, and increases the risk of death (20, 36). Moreover, the incidence (37) and prevalence (38) of diarrhoea may also increase with subclinical VAD. Meta-analyses conducted by three independent groups using data from several randomized trials provide convincing evidence that community-based improvement of the vitamin A status of deficient children aged 6 months to 6 years reduces their risk of dying by 20–30% on average (20, 39, 40). Mortality in children who are blind from keratomalacia or who have corneal disease is reported to be from 50% to 90% (19, 41), and measles mortality associated with VAD is increased by up to 50% (42). Limited data are available from controlled studies of the possible link between morbidity history and vitamin A status of pregnant and lactating women (43).

There are discrepancies in the link between incidence and severity of infectious morbidity of various etiologies and vitamin A status. A great deal of evidence supports an association of VAD with severity of an infection once acquired, except for respiratory diseases, which are non-responsive to treatment (16, 36–38, 44). The severity of pneumonia associated with measles, however, is an exception because it decreases with the treatment of vitamin A supplementation (42, 45).

Infectious diseases depress circulating retinol and contribute to vitamin A depletion. Enteric infections may alter the absorptive surface area, compete for absorption-binding sites, and increase urinary loss (7, 46, 47). Febrile systemic infections also increase urinary loss (6, 48) and metabolic utilization rates and may reduce apparent retinol stores if fever occurs frequently (*49*). In the presence of latent deficiency, disease occurrence is often associated with precipitating ocular signs (*50, 51*). Measles virus infection is especially devastating to vitamin A metabolism, adversely interfering with both efficiencies of utilization and conservation (*42, 51, 52*). Severe protein–energy malnutrition affects many aspects of vitamin A metabolism, and even when some retinyl ester stores are still present, malnutrition—often coupled with infection—can prevent transport-protein synthesis, resulting in immobilization of existing vitamin A stores (*53*).

The compromised integrity of the epithelium, together with the possible alteration in hormonal balance at severe levels of deficiency, impairs normal reproductive functions in animals (*9, 14, 15, 24, 54, 55*). Controlled human studies are, of course, lacking. In animals and humans, congenital anomalies can result if the fetus is exposed to severe deficiency or large excesses of vitamin A at critical periods early in gestation (first trimester) when fetal organs are being formed (*24, 56*). Reproductive performance, as measured by infant outcomes, in one community-based clinical intervention trial, however, was not influenced by vitamin A status (*43*).

The growth of children may be impaired by VAD. Interventions with vitamin A only have not consistently demonstrated improved growth in community studies because VAD seldom occurs in isolation from other nutrient deficiencies that also affect growth and may be more limiting (*57*).

A lack of vitamin A can affect iron metabolism when deficiencies of both nutrients coexist and particularly in environments that favour frequent infections (*58*). Maximum haemoglobin response occurs when iron and vitamin A deficiencies are corrected together (*59*). VAD appears to influence the availability of storage iron for use by haematopoietic tissue (*59, 60*). However, additional research is needed to clarify the mechanisms of the apparent interaction.

2.3 Units of expression

In blood, tissues, and human milk, vitamin A levels are conventionally expressed in μg/dl or μmol/l of all-*trans*-retinol. Except for postprandial conditions, most of the circulating vitamin A is retinol whereas in most tissues (such as the liver), secretions (such as human milk), and other animal food sources, it exists mainly as retinyl esters, which are frequently hydrolysed before analytical detection.

To express the vitamin A activity of carotenoids in diets on a common basis, a Joint FAO/WHO Expert Group (*61*) in 1967 introduced the concept of the retinol equivalent (RE) and established the following relationships among food sources of vitamin A:

1 µg retinol	= 1 RE
1 µg β-carotene	= 0.167 µg RE
1 µg other provitamin A carotenoids	= 0.084 µg RE.

These equivalencies were derived from balance studies to account for the less efficient absorption of carotenoids (at that time thought to be about one third that of retinol) and their bioconversion to vitamin A (one half for β-carotene and one fourth for other provitamin A carotenoids). It was recognized at the time that the recommended conversion factors (i.e. 1:6 for vitamin A:β-carotene and 1:12 for vitamin A:all other provitamin carotenoids) were only best approximations for a mixed diet, which could under- or overestimate bioavailability depending not only on the quantity and source of carotenoids in the diet, but also on how the foods were processed and served (e.g. cooked or raw, whole or puréed, with or without fat). In 1988, a Joint FAO/WHO Expert Consultation (62) confirmed these conversion factors for operational application in evaluating mixed diets. In reaching its conclusion, the Consultation noted the controlled depletion–repletion studies in adult men using a dark adaptation endpoint that reported a 2:1 equivalency of supplemental β-carotene to retinol (63), and the range of factors that could alter the equivalency ratio when dietary carotenoids replaced supplements.

Recently there has been renewed interest in re-examining conventional conversion factors by using more quantitative stable isotope techniques for measuring whole-body stores in response to controlled intakes (64–66) and by following post-absorption carotenoids in the triacylglycerol-rich lipoprotein fraction (67–70). The data are inconsistent but suggest that revision toward lower absorbability of provitamin A carotenoids is warranted (64, 68, 69). These studies indicate that the conditions that limit carotenoids from entering enterocytes rather than conversion once in the enterocyte are more significant than previously thought (71).

Other evidence questions the validity of factors used earlier, which suggests that 6 µg of food-sourced β-carotene is equivalent to 2 µg pure β-carotene in oil, and equivalent to 1 µg dietary retinol. Currently, however, only one study has used post-absorptive serum carotenoids to directly compare, in healthy, adequately nourished adult humans in Holland, the absorption of carotene in oil with that of dietary β-carotene from a mixed diet predominately containing vegetables (72). The investigators reported that about 7 μg of β-carotene from the mixed predominately vegetable diet is equivalent to 1 μg pure β-carotene when it is provided in oil. Assuming that 2 μg β-carotene in the enterocyte is equivalent to 1 μg retinol, the conversion factor would be 1:14 for β-carotene and 1:28 for other provitamin A carotenoids. Other researchers using a similar methodology have reported factors from a variety of specific food sources that fall within this range. Lowest bioavailability is reported for leafy green vegetables and raw carrots and highest for fruit/tuber diets (68, 73–75). In view of the data available to date, conversion factors from usual mixed vegetable diets of 1:14 for β-carotene and 1:28 for other provitamin A carotenoids as suggested by Van het Hof et al. (72) are recommended. Where green leafy vegetables or fruits are more prominent than in the usual diet in Holland, adjustment to higher or lower conversion factors could be considered. For example, in the United States of America where fruits constitute a larger portion of the diet, the Food and Nutrition Board of the Institute of Medicine suggests retinol activity equivalency (RAE) factors of 12:1 for β-carotene and 24:1 for other provitamin A carotenoids (76).

Retinol equivalents in a diet are calculated as the sum of the weight of the retinol portion of preformed vitamin A plus the weight of β-carotene divided by its conversion factor, plus the weight of other provitamin A carotenoids divided by their conversion factor (62). Most recent food composition tables report β-carotene and, sometimes, other provitamin A carotenoids as μg/g edible portion. However, older food composition tables frequently report vitamin A as international units (IUs). The following conversion factors can be used to calculate comparable values as μg:

$$1 \text{ IU retinol} = 0.3 \text{ μg retinol}$$
$$1 \text{ IU β-carotene} = 0.6 \text{ μg β-carotene}$$
$$1 \text{ IU retinol} = 3 \text{ IU β-carotene.}$$

It is strongly recommended that weight or molar units replace the use of IUs to decrease confusion and overcome limitations in the non-equivalence of the IU values for retinol and β-carotene. For example, after converting all values from food composition tables to weight units, the vitamin A equivalency of a mixed diet should be determined by dividing the weight by the recommended weight equivalency value for preformed and specific provitamin A carotenoids. Hence, if a diet contained 150 μg retinol, 1550 μg β-carotene, and 1200 μg other provitamin A carotenoids, the vitamin A equivalency of the diet would be:

$$150 \text{ μg} + (1550 \text{ μg} \div 14) + (1200 \text{ μg} \div 28) = 304 \text{ μg retinol equivalency.}$$

2.4 Sources and supply patterns of vitamin A

2.4.1 Dietary sources

Preformed vitamin A is found almost exclusively in animal products, such as human milk, glandular meats, liver and fish liver oils (especially), egg yolk, whole milk, and other dairy products. Preformed vitamin A is also used to fortify processed foods, which may include sugar, cereals, condiments, fats, and oils (77). Provitamin A carotenoids are found in green leafy vegetables (e.g. spinach, amaranth, and young leaves from various sources), yellow vegetables (e.g. pumpkins, squash, and carrots), and yellow and orange non-citrus fruits (e.g. mangoes, apricots, and papayas). Red palm oil produced in several countries worldwide is especially rich in provitamin A (78). Some other indigenous plants also may be unusually rich sources of provitamin A. Such examples are the palm fruit known in Brazil as *buriti*, found in areas along the Amazon River (as well as elsewhere in Latin America) (79), and the fruit known as *gac* in Viet Nam, which is used to colour rice, particularly on ceremonial occasions (80). Foods containing provitamin A carotenoids tend to have less biologically available vitamin A but are more affordable than animal products. It is mainly for this reason that carotenoids provide most of the vitamin A activity in the diets of economically deprived populations.

2.4.2 Dietary intake and patterns

Although vitamin A status cannot be assessed from dietary intake alone, dietary intake assessment can provide evidence of risk of an inadequate status. However, quantitative collection of dietary information is fraught with measurement problems. These problems arise both from obtaining representative quantitative dietary histories from individuals, communities, or both, and from interpreting these data while accounting for differences in bioavailability, preparation losses, and variations in food composition data among population groups (77). This is especially difficult in populations consuming most of their dietary vitamin A from provitamin carotenoid sources. Simplified guidelines have been developed recently in an effort to improve the collection of reliable dietary intake information from individuals and communities (69, 81).

2.4.3 World and regional supply and patterns

In theory, the world's food supply is sufficient to meet global requirements for vitamin A. Great differences exist, however, in the availability of sources (animal and vegetable) and in per capita consumption of the vitamin among different countries, age categories, and socioeconomic groups. VAD as a global public health problem is therefore largely due to inequitable food distribution among and within countries and households in relation to the need for ample bioavailable vitamin A sources (82, 83).

FAO global estimates for 1984 indicate that preformed vitamin A constituted about one third of total dietary vitamin A activity (62). World availability of vitamin A for human consumption at that time was approximately 220 µg of preformed retinol per capita per day and 560 µg RE from provitamin carotenoids (about 3400 µg carotenoids for a 1:6 conversion factor) per person per day, a total of about 790 µg RE. These values are based on supply estimates and not consumption estimates. Losses commonly occur during food storage and processing, both industrially and in the home (77).

The estimated available regional supply of vitamin A from a more recent global evaluation shown in Table 2.2 illustrates the variability in amounts and sources of vitamin A. This variability is linked to access to the available supply of foods containing vitamin A, which varies with household income, with poverty being a yardstick for risk of VAD. VAD is most prevalent in South-East Asia, Africa, and the Western Pacific (Table 2.1), where vegetable sources contribute nearly 80% or more of the available supply of retinol equivalents. Furthermore, in South-East Asia the total available supply is about half of that of most other regions and is particularly low in animal sources. In contrast, the Americas, Eastern Mediterranean, and Europe have a supply ranging from 700 to 1000 µg RE/day, one third of which comes from animal sources. Based on national data from the United States Continuing Survey of Food Consumption (84) and the third National Health and Nutrition Examination Survey (85) mean dietary intakes of children aged 0–6 years were estimated to be 864 ± 497 and 921 ± 444 µg RE per day, respectively. In the Dietary and Nutritional Survey of British Adults (86), the median intake of men and women aged 35–49 years was 1118 µg RE and 926 µg RE, respectively, which corresponded to serum retinol concentrations of 2.3 µmol/l and 1.8 µmol/l, respectively. In a smaller scale survey in the United Kingdom, median intakes for non-pregnant women who did not consume liver or liver products during the survey week were reported to be 686 µg RE per day (87).

The available world supply figures in Table 2.2 were recently recalculated using a bioavailability ratio of 1:30 for retinol to other provitamin A carotenoids (88). This conversion factor was justified on the basis of one published controlled intervention study conducted in Indonesia (89) and a limited number of other studies not yet published in full. Applying the unconfirmed conversion factor to the values in Table 2.2 would lead to the conclusion that regional and country needs for vitamin A could not be met from predominantly vegetarian diets. However, this is inconsistent with the preponderance of epidemiological evidence. Most studies report a positive response when

TABLE 2.2
Available supply of vitamin A, by WHO region

Region	Animal sources (μg RE/day)	Vegetable sources (μg RE/day)	Total (μg RE/day)
Africa	122	654 (84)[a]	776
The Americas	295	519 (64)	814
South-East Asia	53	378 (90)	431
Europe	271	467 (63)	738
Eastern Mediterranean	345	591 (63)	936
Western Pacific	216	781 (78)	997
Total	212	565 (72)	777

[a] Numbers in parentheses indicate the percentage of total retinol equivalents from carotenoid food sources.
Source: reference (20).

vegetable sources of provitamin A are given under controlled conditions to deficient subjects freed of confounding parasite loads and provided with sufficient dietary fat (90, 91). Emerging data are likely to justify a lower biological activity for provitamin A carotenoids because of the mix of total carotenoids found in food sources in a usual meal (67–69). The present Consultation concluded that the 1:6 bioconversion factor originally derived on the basis of balance studies should be retained until there is firm confirmation of more precise methodologies from ongoing studies.

2.5 Indicators of vitamin A deficiency

2.5.1 Clinical indicators of vitamin A deficiency

Ocular signs of VAD are assessed by clinical examination and history, and are quite specific in preschool-age children. However, these are rare occurrences that require examination of large populations in order to obtain incidence and prevalence data. Subclinical VAD being the more prevalent requires smaller sample sizes for valid prevalence estimates (16).

A full description of clinical indicators of VAD, with coloured illustrations for each, can be found in the WHO field guide (19). The most frequently occurring is night-blindness, which is the earliest manifestation of xerophthalmia. In its mild form it is generally noticeable after stress from a bright light that bleaches the rhodopsin (visual purple) found in the retina. VAD prolongs the time to regenerate rhodopsin, and thus delays adaptation time in dark environments. Night-blind young children tend to stumble when going from bright to dimly-lit areas and they, as well as night-blind mothers, tend to remain inactive at dusk and at night (92).

No field-applicable objective tool is currently available for measuring night-blindness in children under about 3 years of age. However, it can be measured by history in certain cultures (*93*). In areas where night-blindness is prevalent, many cultures coin a word descriptive of the characteristic symptom that they can reliably recall on questioning, making this a useful tool for assessing the prevalence of VAD (*94*). It must be noted that questioning for night-blindness is not always a reliable assessment measure where a local term is absent. In addition, there is no clearly defined blood retinol level that is directly associated with occurrence of the symptom, such that could be used in conjunction with questioning. Vitamin A-related night-blindness, however, responds rapidly (usually within 1–2 days) to administration of vitamin A.

2.5.2 Subclinical indicators of vitamin A deficiency

Direct measurement of concentrations of vitamin A in the liver (where it is stored) or in the total body pool relative to known specific vitamin A-related conditions (e.g. night-blindness) would be the indicator of choice for determining requirements. This cannot be done with the methodology currently available for population use. There are several more practical biochemical methods for estimating subclinical vitamin A status but all have limitations (*16, 93, 95, 96*). Each method is useful for identifying deficient populations, but not one of these indicators is definitive or directly related quantitatively to disease occurrence. The indicators of choice are listed in Table 2.3. These indicators are less specific to VAD than clinical signs of the eye and less sensitive than direct measurements for evaluating subclinical vitamin A status. WHO recommends that where feasible at least two subclinical biochemical indicators, or one biochemical and a composite of non-biochemical risk factors, should be measured and that both types of indicators should point to deficiency in order to identify populations at high risk of VAD (*16*). Cut-off points given in Table 2.3 represent the consensus gained from practical experience in comparing populations with some evidence of VAD with those without VAD. There are no field studies that quantitatively relate the prevalence of adverse health symptoms (e.g. incidence or prevalence of severe diarrhoeal disease) and relative levels of biologic indicator cut-off values. Furthermore, each of the biochemical indicators listed is subject to confounding factors which may be unrelated to vitamin A status (e.g. infections).

Although all biochemical indicators currently available have limitations, the preferred biochemical indicator for population assessment is the distribution of serum levels of vitamin A (serum retinol). Only at very low blood levels (<0.35 μmol/l) is there an association with corneal disease prevalence (*97*). Blood levels between 0.35 and 0.70 μmol/l are likely to characterize subclinical deficiency (*98*), but subclinical deficiency may still be present at levels

TABLE 2.3
Indicators of subclinical VAD in mothers and in children aged 6–71 months

Indicator	Cut-off to indicate deficiency
Night-blindness (24–71 months)	≥1% report a history of night-blindness
Biochemical	
Breast-milk retinol	≤1.05 μmol/l (≤8 μg/g milk fat)
Serum retinol	≤0.70 μmol/l
Relative dose response	≥20%
Modified relative dose response	Ratio ≥0.06

Source: adapted from reference (16).

between 0.70 and 1.05 μmol/l and occasionally above 1.05 μmol/l (99). The prevalence of values below 0.70 μmol/l is a generally accepted population cut-off for preschool-age children to indicate risk of inadequate vitamin A status (16) and above 1.05 μmol/l to indicate an adequate status (100, 101). As noted elsewhere, clinical and subclinical infections can lower serum levels of vitamin A on average by as much as 25%, independently of vitamin A intake (102, 103). Therefore, at levels between about 0.5 and 1.05 μmol/l, the relative dose response or the modified relative dose response test on a subsample of the population can be useful for identifying the prevalence of critically depleted body stores when interpreting the left portion of serum retinol distribution curves.

2.6 Evidence used for making recommendations

Requirements and safe levels of intake for vitamin A recommended in this report do not differ significantly from those proposed by the 1988 Joint FAO/WHO Expert Consultation (62) except to the extent that they have been adapted to the age, pregnancy, and lactation categories defined by the present Expert Consultation. The term "safe level of intake" used in the 1988 report is retained because the intake levels do not strictly correspond to the definition of a recommended nutrient intake recommended here (see section 1.2).

The mean requirement for an individual is defined as the minimum daily intake of vitamin A, expressed as μg retinol equivalents (μg RE), to prevent xerophthalmia in the absence of clinical or subclinical infection. This intake should account for the proportionate bioavailability of preformed vitamin A (about 90%) and provitamin A carotenoids from a diet that contains sufficient fat (e.g. at least 10 g daily). The required level of intake is set to prevent clinical signs of deficiency, allow for normal growth, and reduce the risk of vitamin A-related severe morbidity and mortality within any given population. It does not allow for frequent or prolonged periods of infections or other stresses.

The safe level of intake for an individual is defined as the average continuing intake of vitamin A required to permit adequate growth and other vitamin A-dependent functions and to maintain an acceptable total body reserve of the vitamin. This reserve helps offset periods of low intake or increased need resulting from infections and other stresses. Useful indicators include a plasma retinol concentration above 0.70 μmol/l, which is associated with a relative dose response below 20%, or a modified relative dose response below 0.06. For lactating women, breast-milk retinol levels above 1.05 μmol/l (or above 8 μg/g milk fat) are considered to reflect minimal maternal stores because levels above 1.05 μmol/l are common in populations known to be healthy and without evidence of insufficient dietary vitamin A (24, 25).

2.6.1 Infants and children

Vitamin A requirements for infants are calculated from the vitamin A provided in human milk. During at least the first 6 months of life, exclusive breastfeeding can provide sufficient vitamin A to maintain health, permit normal growth, and maintain sufficient stores in the liver (104).

Reported retinol concentrations in human milk vary widely from country to country (0.70–2.45 μmol/l). In some developing countries, the vitamin A intake of breast-fed infants who grow well and do not show signs of deficiency ranges from 120 to 170 μg RE/day (25, 104). Such intakes are considered adequate to cover infant requirements if the infant's weight is assumed to be at least at the 10th percentile according to WHO standards (62). However, this intake is unlikely to build adequate body stores, given that xerophthalmia is common in preschool-age children in the same communities with somewhat lower intakes. Because of the need for vitamin A to support the growth rate of infancy, which can vary considerably, a requirement estimate of 180 μg RE/day seems appropriate.

The safe level for infants up to 6 months of age is based on observations of breast-fed infants in communities in which good nutrition is the norm. Average consumption of human milk by such infants is about 750 ml/day during the first 6 months (104). Assuming an average concentration of vitamin A in human milk of about 1.75 μmol/l, the mean daily intake would be about 375 μg RE, which is therefore the recommended safe level. From 7–12 months, human milk intake averages 650 ml/day, which would provide 325 μg of vitamin A daily. Because breast-fed infants in endemic vitamin A-deficient

populations are at increased risk of death from 6 months onward, the requirement and recommended safe intake levels are increased to 190 µg RE/day and
400 µg RE/day, respectively.

The requirement (with allowance for variability) and the recommended
safe intake for older children may be estimated from those derived for late
infancy (i.e. 20 and 39 µg RE/kg body weight/day) (62). On this basis, and
including allowances for storage requirements and variability, requirements
for preschool-age children would be in the range of 200–400 µg RE daily. In
poor communities where children 1–6 years old are reported to have intakes
of about 100–200 µg RE/day, signs of VAD do occur; in southern India these
signs were relieved and risk of mortality was reduced when the equivalent of
350–400 µg RE/day was given to children weekly (105). In the United States,
most preschool-age children maintain serum retinol levels of 0.70 µmol/l or
higher while consuming diets providing 300–400 µg RE/day (from the data-
bank for the third National Health and Nutrition Examination Survey
[http://www.cdc.gov/nchs/nhanes.htm]).

2.6.2 Adults

Estimates for the requirements and recommended safe intakes for adults are
also extrapolated from those derived for late infancy, i.e. 4.8 and 9.3 µg RE/kg
body weight/day (62). Detailed account of how the requirement for vitamin
A is arrived at is provided in the FAO/WHO report of 1988 (62) and is not
repeated here because no new studies have been published that indicate a need
to revise the assumptions on which those calculations were based. The safe
intakes recommended are consistent with the per capita vitamin A content in
the food supply of countries that show adequate vitamin A status in all sectors
of the population. Additional evidence that the existing safe level of intake is
adequate for adults on a population basis is provided by an analysis of dietary
data from the 1990 survey of British adults in whom there was no evidence
of VAD (86). In another survey in the United Kingdom, the median intake of
vitamin A among non-pregnant women who did not consume liver or liver
products during the survey week was 686 µg RE/day (87). This value is substantially above the estimated mean requirement for pregnant women and falls
quite short of the amount at which teratology risk is reported (106–108).
About one third of the calculated retinol equivalents consumed by the British
women came from provitamin A sources (20% from carrots).

2.6.3 Pregnant women

During pregnancy, women need additional vitamin A to sustain the
growth of the fetus and to provide a limited reserve in the fetal liver, as

well as to maintain their own tissue growth. Currently, there are no reliable figures available for the specific vitamin A requirements for these processes (27).

Newborn infants need around 100 µg of retinol daily to meet their needs for growth. During the third trimester the fetus grows rapidly and, although obviously smaller in size than the infant born full term, the fetus presumably has similar needs. Incremental maternal needs associated with pregnancy are assumed to be provided from maternal reserves in populations of adequately nourished healthy mothers. In populations consuming vitamin A at the basal requirement, an additional increment of 100 µg/day during the full gestation period should enhance maternal storage during early pregnancy and allow for adequate amounts of vitamin A to be available for the rapidly growing fetus in late pregnancy. However, this increment may be minimal for women who normally ingest only the basal requirement of vitamin A, inasmuch as the needs and growth rate of the fetus will not be affected by the mother's initial vitamin A reserves.

A recent study in Nepal (43), where night-blindness is prevalent in pregnant women, provided 7000 µg RE (about 23 300 IU) weekly to pregnant and lactating women (equivalent to 1000 µg RE/day). This level of intake normalized serum levels of vitamin A and was associated with a decrease in prevalence of night-blindness and a decrease in maternal mortality. However, the findings of this study need to be confirmed. In the interim period it seems prudent, recognizing that a large portion of the world's population of pregnant women live under conditions of deprivation, to increase by 200 µg RE the recommended safe level to ensure adequacy of intake during pregnancy. Because therapeutic levels of vitamin A are generally higher than preventive levels, the safe intake level recommended during pregnancy is 800 µg RE/day. Women who are or who might become pregnant should carefully limit their total daily vitamin A intake to a maximum of 3000 µg RE (10 000 IU) to minimize risk of fetal toxicity (109).

2.6.4 Lactating women

If the amount of vitamin A recommended for infants is supplied by human milk, mothers who are breastfeeding should intake at least as much vitamin A in their diets as is needed to replace the amount lost through breastfeeding. Thus, the increments in basal and safe recommended intakes during lactation are 180 µg RE and 350 µg RE, respectively. After the infant reaches the age of 6 months or when solid foods are introduced, the mother's need for additional amounts of vitamin A lessens.

2.6.5 Elderly

There is no indication that the vitamin A requirements of healthy elderly individuals differ from those of other adults. It should be remembered, however, that diseases that impede vitamin A absorption, storage, and transport might be more common in the elderly than in other age groups.

2.7 Recommendations for vitamin A requirements

Table 2.4 summarizes the estimated mean requirements for vitamin A and the recommended safe intakes, taking into account the age and sex differences in mean body weights. For most values the true mean and variance are not known. It should be noted that there are no adequate data available to derive mean requirements for any group and, therefore, a recommended nutrient intake cannot be calculated. However, information is available on cures achieved in a few vitamin A-deficient adult men and on the vitamin A status of groups receiving intakes that are low but nevertheless adequate to prevent the appearance of deficiency-related syndromes. The figures for mean dietary requirements are derived from these, with the understanding that the curative dose is higher than the preventive dose. They are at the upper limits of the range so as to cover the mean dietary requirements of 97.5% of the population (62).

TABLE 2.4
Estimated mean requirement and safe level of intake for vitamin A, by group

Group	Mean requirement (µg RE/day)	Recommended safe intake (µg RE/day)
Infants and children		
0–6 months	180	375
7–12 months	190	400
1–3 years	200	400
4–6 years	200	450
7–9 years	250	500
Adolescents,		
10–18 years	330–400	600
Adults		
Females,		
19–65 years	270	500
65+ years	300	600
Males,		
19–65 years	300	600
65+ years	300	600
Pregnant women	370	800
Lactating women	450	850

Source: adapted from reference (62).

In calculating the safe intake, a normative storage requirement was calculated as a mean for adults equivalent to 434 μg RE/day, and the recommended safe intake was derived in part by using this value plus 2 standard deviations. It is doubtful that this value can be applied to growing children. The safe intake for children was compared with the distribution of intakes and comparable serum vitamin A levels reported for children 0–6 years of age from the United States and with distributions of serum levels of vitamin A of children aged 9–62 months in Australia (*110*), where evidence of VAD is rare.

2.8 Toxicity

Because vitamin A is fat soluble and can be stored, primarily in the liver, routine consumption of large amounts of vitamin A over a period of time can result in toxic symptoms, including liver damage, bone abnormalities and joint pain, alopecia, headaches, vomiting, and skin desquamation. Hypervitaminosis A appears to be due to abnormal transport and distribution of vitamin A and retinoids caused by overloading of the plasma transport mechanisms (*111*).

The smallest daily supplement associated with liver cirrhosis that has been reported is 7500 μg taken for 6 years (*107, 108*). Very high single doses can also cause transient acute toxic symptoms that may include bulging fontanelles in infants; headaches in older children and adults; and vomiting, diarrhoea, loss of appetite, and irritability in all age groups. Rarely does toxicity occur from ingestion of food sources of preformed vitamin A. When this occurs, it usually results from very frequent consumption of liver products. Toxicity from food sources of provitamin A carotenoids is not reported, except for the cosmetic yellowing of skin.

Infants, including neonates (*112*), administered single doses equivalent to 15 000–30 000 μg retinol (50 000–100 000 IU) in oil generally show no adverse symptoms. However, daily prophylactic or therapeutic doses should not exceed 900 μg, which is well above the mean requirement of about 200 μg/day for infants. An increase in bulging fontanelles occurred in infants under 6 months of age in one endemically deficient population given two or more doses of 7500 μg or 15 000 μg preformed vitamin A in oil (*113, 114*), but other large-scale controlled clinical trials have not reported increased bulging after three doses of 7500 μg given with diphtheria-pertussis-tetanus immunizations at about 6, 10, and 14 weeks of age (*115*). No effects were detected at 3 years of age that related to transient vitamin A-induced bulging that had occurred before 6 months of age (*112, 116*).

Most children aged 1–6 years tolerate single oral doses of 60 000 μg (200 000 IU) vitamin A in oil at intervals of 4–6 months without adverse symptoms (*107*). Occasionally diarrhoea or vomiting is reported but these symptoms are transient with no lasting sequelae. Older children seldom experience toxic symptoms unless they habitually ingest vitamin A in excess of 7500 µg (25 000 IU) for prolonged periods of time (*107*).

When women take vitamin A at daily levels of more than 7500 µg (25 000 IU) during the early stages of gestation, fetal anomalies and poor reproductive outcomes are reported (*108*). One report suggests an increased risk of teratogenicity at intakes as low as 3000 µg (10 000 IU), but this is not confirmed by other studies (*108*). Women who are pregnant or might become pregnant should avoid taking excessive amounts of vitamin A. A careful review of the latest available information by a WHO Expert Group recommended that daily intakes in excess of 3000 µg (10 000 IU), or weekly intakes in excess of 7500 µg (25 000 IU) should not be taken at any period during gestation (*109*). High doses of vitamin A (60 000 µg, or 200 000 IU) can be safely given to breastfeeding mothers for up to 2 months postpartum and up to 6 weeks to mothers who are not breastfeeding.

2.9 Recommendations for future research

Further research is needed in the following areas:

- the interaction of vitamin A and iron with infections, as they relate to serum levels and disease incidence and prevalence;
- the relationship between vitamin A, iron, and zinc and their roles in the severity of infections;
- the nutritional role of 9-*cis* retinoic acid and the mechanism which regulates its endogenous production;
- the bioavailability of provitamin A carotenoids from different classes of leafy and other green and orange vegetables, tubers, and fruits as typically provided in diets (e.g. relative to the level of fat in the diet or meal);
- identification of a reliable indicator of vitamin A status for use in direct quantification of mean requirements and for relating status to functions.

References

1. Blomhoff R et al. Vitamin A metabolism: new perspectives on absorption, transport, and storage. *Physiological Reviews*, 1991, 71:951–990.
2. Ong DE. Absorption of vitamin A. In: Blomhoff R, ed. *Vitamin A in health and disease*. New York, NY, Marcel Dekker, 1994:37–72.
3. Parker RS. Absorption, metabolism, and transport of carotenoids. *FASEB Journal*, 1996, 10:542–551.
4. Jayarajan P, Reddy V, Mohanram M. Effect of dietary fat on absorption of

β-carotene from green leafy vegetables in children. *Indian Journal of Medical Research*, 1980, 71:53–56.

5. Novotny JA et al. Compartmental analysis of the dynamics of β-carotene metabolism in an adult volunteer. *Journal of Lipid Research*, 1995, 36: 1825–1838.

6. Stephensen CB et al. Vitamin A is excreted in the urine during acute infection. *American Journal of Clinical Nutrition*, 1994, 60:388–392.

7. Alvarez JO et al. Urinary excretion of retinol in children with acute diarrhea. *American Journal of Clinical Nutrition*, 1995, 61:1273–1276.

8. Green MH, Green JB. Dynamics and control of plasma retinol. In: Blomhoff R, ed. *Vitamin A in health and disease*. New York, NY, Marcel Dekker, 1994:119–133.

9. Ross C, Gardner EM. The function of vitamin A in cellular growth and differentiation, and its roles during pregnancy and lactation. In: Allen L, King J, Lönnerdal B, eds. *Nutrient regulation during pregnancy, lactation, and infant growth*. New York, NY, Plenum Press, 1994:187–200.

10. Chambon P. A decade of molecular biology of retinoic acid receptors. *FASEB Journal*, 1996, 10:940–954.

11. Ross AC, Stephensen CB. Vitamin A and retinoids in antiviral responses. *FASEB Journal*, 1996, 10:979–985.

12. Pemrick SM, Lucas DA, Grippo JF. The retinoid receptors. *Leukemia*, 1994, 8(Suppl. 3):S1–S10.

13. Rando RR. Retinoid isomerization reactions in the visual system. In: Blomhoff R, ed. *Vitamin A in health and disease*. New York, NY, Marcel Dekker, 1994:503–529.

14. Eskild LW, Hansson V. Vitamin A functions in the reproductive organs. In: Blomhoff R, ed. *Vitamin A in health and disease*. New York, NY, Marcel Dekker, 1994:531–559.

15. Morriss-Kay GM, Sokolova N. Embryonic development and pattern formation. *FASEB Journal*, 1996, 10:961–968.

16. *Indicators for assessing vitamin A deficiency and their application in monitoring and evaluating intervention programmes*. Geneva, World Health Organization, 1996 (WHO/NUT/96.10; http://whqlibdoc.who.int/hq/1996/WHO_NUT_96.10.pdf, accessed 24 June 2004).

17. *Global prevalence of vitamin A deficiency*. Geneva, World Health Organization, 1995 (WHO/NUT/95.3).

18. Katz J et al. Clustering of xerophthalmia within households and villages. *International Journal of Epidemiology*, 1993, 22:709–715.

19. Sommer A. *Vitamin A deficiency and its consequences: a field guide to detection and control*, 3rd ed. Geneva, World Health Organization, 1994.

20. Beaton GH et al. *Effectiveness of vitamin A supplementation in the control of young child morbidity and mortality in developing countries*. Geneva, United Nations Administrative Committee on Coordination/Subcommittee on Nutrition, 1993 (ACC/SCN State-of-the-art Series, Nutrition Policy Discussion Paper No. 13).

21. Sommer A, Emran N, Tjakrasudjatma S. Clinical characteristics of vitamin A responsive and nonresponsive Bitot's spots. *American Journal of Ophthalmology*, 1980, 90:160–171.

22. Bloem MW, Matzger H, Huq N. Vitamin A deficiency among women in the reproductive years: an ignored problem. In: *Report of the XVI IVACG*

Meeting. Washington, DC, International Vitamin A Consultative Group, ILSI Human Nutrition Institute, 1994.

23. Christian P et al. Night blindness of pregnancy in rural Nepal—nutritional and health risks. *International Journal of Epidemiology*, 1998, 27:231–237.

24. Wallingford JC, Underwood BA. Vitamin A deficiency in pregnancy, lactation, and the nursing child. In: Baurenfeind JC, ed. *Vitamin A deficiency and its control.* New York, NY, Academic Press, 1986:101–152.

25. Newman V. Vitamin A and breast-feeding: a comparison of data from developed and developing countries. *Food and Nutrition Bulletin*, 1994, 15:161–176.

26. *Physical status: the use and interpretation of anthropometry. Report of a WHO Expert Committee.* Geneva, World Health Organization, 1995 (WHO Technical Report Series, No. 854).

27. Committee on Nutritional Status During Pregnancy and Lactation. Vitamins A, E, and K. In: *Nutrition during pregnancy. Part II. Nutrient supplements.* Washington, DC, National Academy Press, 1990:336–350.

28. Mele L et al. Nutritional and household risk factors for xerophthalmia in Aceh, Indonesia: a case–control study. *American Journal of Clinical Nutrition*, 1991, 53:1460–1465.

29. Erdman J Jr. The physiologic chemistry of carotenes in man. *Clinical Nutrition*, 1988, 7:101–106.

30. Marsh RR et al. Improving food security through home gardening: a case study from Bangladesh. In: *Technology for rural homes: research and extension experiences.* Reading, The Agricultural Extension and Rural Development Department, University of Reading, 1995.

31. Sinha DP, Bang FB. Seasonal variation in signs of vitamin A deficiency in rural West Bengal children. *Lancet*, 1973, 2:228–231.

32. Johns T, Booth SL, Kuhnlein HV. Factors influencing vitamin A intake and programmes to improve vitamin A status. *Food and Nutrition Bulletin*, 1992, 14:20–33.

33. Tarwotjo I et al. Dietary practices and xerophthalmia among Indonesian children. *American Journal of Clinical Nutrition*, 1982, 35:574–581.

34. Zeitlan MF et al. Mothers' and children's intakes of vitamin A in rural Bangladesh. *American Journal of Clinical Nutrition*, 1992, 56:136–147.

35. Mahadevan I. Belief systems in food of the Telugu-speaking people of the Telengana region. *Indian Journal of Social Work*, 1961, 21:387–396.

36. Anonymous. Vitamin A supplementation in northern Ghana: effects on clinic attendance, hospital admissions, and child mortality. Ghana VAST Study Team. *Lancet*, 1993, 342:7–12.

37. Barreto ML et al. Effect of vitamin A supplementation on diarrhoea and acute lower-respiratory-tract infections in young children in Brazil. *Lancet*, 1994, 344:228–231.

38. Bhandari N, Bhan MK, Sazawal S. Impact of massive dose of vitamin A given to preschool children with acute-diarrhoea on subsequent respiratory and diarrhoeal morbidity. *British Medical Journal*, 1994, 309:1404–1407.

39. Fawzi WW et al. Vitamin A supplementation and child mortality. A meta-analysis. *Journal American Medical Association*, 1993, 269:898–903.

40. Glasziou PP, Mackerras DEM. Vitamin A supplementation in infectious diseases: a meta-analysis. *British Medical Journal*, 1993, 306:366–370.

41. Menon K, Vijayaraghavan K. Sequelae of severe xerophthalmia: a follow-up study. *American Journal of Clinical Nutrition*, 1979, 33:218–220.

42. Hussey GD, Klein M. A randomized controlled trial of vitamin A in children with severe measles. *New England Journal of Medicine*, 1990, 323:160–164.

43. West KP et al. Impact of weekly supplementation of women with vitamin A or beta-carotene on fetal, infant and maternal mortality in Nepal. In: *Report of the XVIII IVACG Meeting. Sustainable control of vitamin A deficiency*. Washington, DC, International Vitamin A Consultative Group, ILSI Human Nutrition Institute, 1997:86.

44. The Vitamin A and Pneumonia Working Group. Potential interventions for the prevention of childhood pneumonia in developing countries: a meta-analysis of data from field trials to assess the impact of vitamin A supplementation on pneumonia morbidity and mortality. *Bulletin of the World Health Organization*, 1995, 73:609–619.

45. Coutsoudis A, Broughton M, Coovadia HM. Vitamin A supplementation reduces measles morbidity in young African children: a randomized, placebo-controlled, double blind trial. *American Journal of Clinical Nutrition*, 1991, 54:890–895.

46. Solomons NW, Keusch GT. Nutritional implications of parasitic infections. *Nutrition Reviews*, 1981, 39:149–161.

47. Feachem RG. Vitamin A deficiency and diarrhoea: a review of interrelationships and their implications for the control of xerophthalmia and diarrhoea. *Tropical Disease Bulletin*, 1987, 84:R1–R16.

48. Thurnham DI, Singkamani R. The acute phase response and vitamin A status in malaria. *Transactions of the Royal Society of Tropical Medicine and Hygiene*, 1991, 85:194–199.

49. Campos FACS, Flores H, Underwood BA. Effect of an infection on vitamin A status of children as measured by the relative dose response (RDR). *American Journal of Clinical Nutrition*, 1987, 46:91–94.

50. Curtale F et al. Intestinal helminths and xerophthalmia in Nepal. *Journal of Tropical Pediatrics*, 1995, 41:334–337.

51. Sommer A, West KP Jr. Infectious morbidity. In: *Vitamin A deficiency, health, survival, and vision*. New York, NY, Oxford University Press, 1996:19–98.

52. Foster A, Yorston D. Corneal ulceration in Tanzanian children: relationship between measles and vitamin A deficiency. *Transactions of the Royal Society of Tropical Medicine and Hygiene*, 1992, 86:454–455.

53. Arroyave G et al. Serum and liver vitamin A and lipids in children with severe protein malnutrition. *American Journal of Clinical Nutrition*, 1961, 9:180–185.

54. Bates CJ. Vitamin A in pregnancy and lactation. *Proceedings of the Nutrition Society*, 1983, 42:65–79.

55. Takahashi Y et al. Vitamin A deficiency and fetal growth and development in the rat. *Journal of Nutrition*, 1975, 105:1299–1310.

56. Public Affairs Committee of the Teratology Society. Teratology Society Position Paper. Recommendations for vitamin A use during pregnancy. *Teratology*, 1987, 35:269–275.

57. Underwood BA. The role of vitamin A in child growth, development and survival. In: Allen L, King J, Lönnerdal B, eds. *Nutrient regulation during pregnancy, lactation, and infant growth*. New York, NY, Plenum Press, 1994: 195–202.

58. *IVACG Statement on vitamin A and iron interactions.* Washington, DC, International Vitamin A Consultative Group, ILSI Human Nutrition Institute, 1998 (http://ivacg.ilsi.org/publications/publist.cfm?publicationid=219, accessed 24 June 2004).

59. Suharno D et al. Supplementation with vitamin A and iron for nutritional anaemia in pregnant women in West Java, Indonesia. *Lancet*, 1993, 342:1325–1328.

60. Sijtsma KW et al. Iron status in rats fed on diets containing marginal amounts of vitamin A. *British Journal of Nutrition*, 1993, 70:777–785.

61. *Requirements of vitamin A, thiamine, riboflavin and niacin. Report of a Joint FAO/WHO Expert Group.* Geneva, World Health Organization, 1967 (WHO Technical Report Series, No. 362).

62. *Requirements of vitamin A, iron, folate and vitamin B₁₂. Report of a Joint FAO/WHO Expert Consultation.* Rome, Food and Agriculture Organization of the United Nations, 1988 (FAO Food and Nutrition Series, No. 23).

63. Sauberlich HE et al. Vitamin A metabolism and requirement in human subjects studied with the use of labeled retinol. *Vitamins and Hormones*, 1974, 32:251–275.

64. Tang G et al. Green and yellow vegetables can maintain body stores of vitamin A in Chinese children. *American Journal of Clinical Nutrition*, 1999, 70:1069–1076.

65. Furr HC et al. Vitamin A concentrations in liver determined by isotope dilution assay with tetradeuterated vitamin A and by biopsy in generally healthy adult humans. *American Journal of Clinical Nutrition*, 1989, 49:713–716.

66. Haskell MJ et al. Plasma kinetics of an oral dose of [²H₄] retinyl acetate in human subjects with estimated low or high total body stores of vitamin A. *American Journal of Clinical Nutrition*, 1998, 68:90–95.

67. van den Berg H, van Vliet T. Effect of simultaneous, single oral doses of β-carotene with lutein or lycopene on the β-carotene and retinyl ester responses in the triacylglycerol-rich lipoprotein fraction of men. *American Journal of Clinical Nutrition*, 1998, 68:82–89.

68. Castenmiller JJ, West CE. Bioavailability and bioconversion of carotenoids. *Annual Review of Nutrition*, 1998, 18:19–38.

69. Parker RS et al. Bioavailability of carotenoids in human subjects. *Proceedings of the Nutrition Society*, 1999, 58:1–8.

70. van Vliet T, Schreurs WH, van den Berg H. Intestinal β-carotene absorption and cleavage in men: response of β-carotene and retinyl esters in the triglyceride-rich lipoprotein fraction after a single oral dose of β-carotene. *American Journal Clinical Nutrition*, 1995, 62:110–116.

71. Edwards AJ et al. A novel extrinsic reference method for assessing the vitamin A value of plant foods. *American Journal of Clinical Nutrition*, 2001, 74:348–355.

72. Van het Hof KH et al. Bioavailability of lutein from vegetables is five times higher than that of β-carotene. *American Journal of Clinical Nutrition*, 1991, 70:261–268.

73. de Pee S et al. Orange fruit is more effective than dark-green, leafy vegetables in increasing serum concentrations of retinol and beta-carotene in schoolchildren in Indonesia. *American Journal of Clinical Nutrition*, 1998, 68:1058–1067.

74. Miccozzi MS et al. Plasma carotenoid response to chronic intake of selected

foods and β-carotene supplements in men. *American Journal of Clinical Nutrition*, 1992, 55:1120–1125.

75. Torronen R et al. Serum β-carotene response to supplementation with raw carrots, carrot juice or purified β-carotene in healthy non-smoking women. *Nutrition Reviews*, 1996, 16:565–575.

76. Food and Nutrition Board. *Dietary reference intakes for vitamin A, vitamin K, arsenic, boron, chromium, copper, iodine, iron, manganese, molybdenum, nickel, silicon, vanadium, and zinc.* Washington, DC, National Academy Press, 2002.

77. Rodriguez-Amaya DB. *Carotenoids and food preparation: the retention of provitamin A carotenoids in prepared, processed, and stored foods.* Arlington, VA, John Snow and Opportunities for Micronutrient Interventions Project, 1997 (http://www.mostproject.org/carrots2.pdf, accessed 24 June 2004).

78. Booth SL, Johns T, Kuhnlein HV. Natural food sources of vitamin A and provitamin A. *UNU Food and Nutrition Bulletin*, 1992, 14:6–19.

79. Advisory Committee on Technology Innovations. Burití palm. In: *Underexploited tropical plants with promising economic value. Report of an Ad Hoc Panel of the Advisory Committee on Technology Innovations, Board on Science and Technology for International Development, Commission on International Relations.* Washington, DC, National Academy of Sciences, 1975:133–137.

80. Vuong LT. An indigenous fruit of North Vietnam with an exceptionally high β-carotene content. *Sight and Life Newsletter*, 1997, 2:16–18.

81. *Report of the International Vitamin A Consultative Group. Guidelines for the development of a simplified dietary assessment to identify groups at risk for inadequate intake of vitamin A.* Washington, DC, International Life Sciences Institute, Nutrition Foundation, 1989.

82. Périssé J, Polacchi W. Geographical distribution and recent changes in world supply of vitamin A. *Food and Nutrition*, 1980, 6:21–27.

83. *Second report on the world nutrition situation. Volume 1. Global and regional results.* Washington, DC, United Nations Administrative Committee on Coordination/Subcommittee on Nutrition, 1992.

84. *Food and nutrient intakes by individuals in the United States, by sex and age, 1994–96.* Washington, DC, United States Department of Agriculture, Agricultural Research Service, 1998 (Nationwide Food Surveys Report, 96–2).

85. *National Health and Nutrition Examination Survey III, 1988–1994* [CD-ROM]. Hyatsville, MD, Centers for Disease Control and Prevention, 1998 (CD-ROM Series 11, No. 2A).

86. Gregory J et al. *The Dietary and Nutritional Survey of British Adults.* London, Her Majesty's Stationery Office, 1990.

87. Tyler HA, Day MJL, Rose HJ. Vitamin A and pregnancy. *Lancet*, 1991, 337:48–49.

88. Bloem MW, de Pee S, Darnton-Hill I. Vitamin A deficiency in India, Bangladesh and Nepal. In: Gillespie S, ed. *Malnutrition in South Asia. A regional profile.* Kathmandu, United Nations Children's Fund Regional Office for South Asia, 1997:125–144.

89. de Pee S et al. Lack of improvement in vitamin A status with increased consumption of dark-green leafy vegetables. *Lancet*, 1995, 346:75–81.

90. Yin S et al. Green and yellow vegetables rich in provitamin A carotenoids can sustain vitamin A status in children. *FASEB Journal*, 1998, 12:A351.

91. Jalal F et al. Serum retinol concentrations in children are affected by food

sources of β-carotene, fat intake, and anthelmintic drug treatment. *American Journal of Clinical Nutrition*, 1998, 68:623–629.

92. Christian P et al. Working after the sun goes down. Exploring how night blindness impairs women's work activities in rural Nepal. *European Journal of Clinical Nutrition*, 1998, 52:519–524.

93. Underwood BA, Olson JA, eds. *A brief guide to current methods of assessing vitamin A status. A report of the International Vitamin A Consultative Group.* Washington, DC, International Life Sciences Institute, Nutrition Foundation, 1993.

94. Sommer A et al. History of night blindness: a simple tool for xerophthalmia screening. *American Journal of Clinical Nutrition*, 1980, 33:887–891.

95. Underwood BA. Biochemical and histological methodologies for assessing vitamin A status in human populations. In: Packer L, ed. *Methods in enzymology: retinoids, part B.* New York, NY, Academic Press, 1990:242–250.

96. Olson JA. Measurement of vitamin A status. *Voeding*, 1992, 53:163–167.

97. Sommer A, Muhilal H. Nutritional factors in corneal xerophthalmia and keratomalacia. *Archives of Ophthalmology*, 1982, 100:399–403.

98. Wachtmeister L et al. Attempts to define the minimal serum level of vitamin A required for normal visual function in a patient with severe fat malabsorption. *Acta Ophthalmologica*, 1988, 66:341–348.

99. Flores H et al. Assessment of marginal vitamin A deficiency in Brazilian children using the relative dose response procedure. *American Journal of Clinical Nutrition*, 1984, 40:1281–1289.

100. Flores H et al. Serum vitamin A distribution curve for children aged 2–6 y known to have adequate vitamin A status: a reference population. *American Journal of Clinical Nutrition*, 1991, 54:707–711.

101. Onlu Pilch SM. Analysis of vitamin A data from the health and nutrition examination surveys. *Journal of Nutrition*, 1987, 117:636–640.

102. Christian P et al. Hyporetinolemia, illness symptoms, and acute phase protein response in pregnant women with and without night blindness. *American Journal of Clinical Nutrition*, 1998, 67:1237–1243.

103. Filteau SM et al. Influence of morbidity on serum retinol of children in a community-based study in northern Ghana. *American Journal of Clinical Nutrition*, 1993, 58:192–197.

104. *Complementary feeding of young children in developing countries: a review of current scientific knowledge.* Geneva, World Health Organization, 1998 (WHO/NUT/98.1; http://www.who.int/child-adolescenthealth/publications/NUTRITION/WHO_NUT_98.1.htm, accessed 24 June 2004).

105. Rahmathullah L et al. Reduced mortality among children in Southern India receiving a small weekly dose of vitamin A. *New England Journal of Medicine*, 1990, 323:929–935.

106. Miller RK et al. Periconceptional vitamin A use: how much is teratogenic? *Reproductive Toxicology*, 1998, 12:75–88.

107. Hathcock JN et al. Evaluation of vitamin A toxicity. *American Journal of Clinical Nutrition*, 1990, 52:183–202.

108. Hathcock JN. Vitamins and minerals: efficacy and safety. *American Journal of Clinical Nutrition*, 1997, 66:427–437.

109. *Safe vitamin A dosage during pregnancy and lactation.* Geneva, World Health Organization, 1998 (WHO/NUT/98.4; http://whqlibdoc.who.int/hq/1998/WHO_NUT_98.4.pdf, accessed 24 June 2004).

110. Karr M et al. Age-specific reference intervals for plasma vitamin A, E and

beta-carotene and for serum zinc, retinol-binding protein and prealbumin for Sydney children aged 9–62 months. *International Journal of Vitamin and Nutrition Research,* 1997, 67:432–436.

111. Smith FR, Goodman DS. Vitamin A transport in human vitamin A toxicity. *New England Journal of Medicine,* 1976, 294:805–808.

112. Humphrey JH et al. Neonatal vitamin A supplementation: effect on development and growth at 3 y of age. *American Journal of Clinical Nutrition,* 1998, 68:109–117.

113. Baqui AH et al. Bulging fontanelle after supplementation with 25,000 IU vitamin A in infancy using immunization contacts. *Acta Paediatrica,* 1995, 84:863–866.

114. de Francisco A et al. Acute toxicity of vitamin A given with vaccines in infancy. *Lancet,* 1993, 342:526–527.

115. WHO/CHD Immunisation-linked Vitamin A Supplementation Study Group. Randomised trial to assess benefits and safety of vitamin A supplementation linked to immunisation in early infancy. *Lancet,* 1998, 352:1257–1263.

116. van Dillen J, de Francisco A, Ovenrweg-Plandsoen WCG. Long-term effect of vitamin A with vaccines. *Lancet,* 1996, 347:1705.

3. Vitamin D

3.1 Role of vitamin D in human metabolic processes

Vitamin D is required to maintain normal blood levels of calcium and phosphate, which are in turn needed for the normal mineralization of bone, muscle contraction, nerve conduction, and general cellular function in all cells of the body. Vitamin D achieves this after its conversion to the active form 1,25-dihydroxyvitamin D [1,25-$(OH)_2$D], or calcitriol. This active form regulates the transcription of a number of vitamin D-dependent genes which code for calcium-transporting proteins and bone matrix proteins.

Vitamin D also modulates the transcription of cell cycle proteins, which decrease cell proliferation and increase cell differentiation of a number of specialized cells of the body (e.g. osteoclastic precursors, enterocytes, keratinocytes). This property may explain the actions of vitamin D in bone resorption, intestinal calcium transport, and skin. Vitamin D also possesses immunomodulatory properties that may alter responses to infections in vivo. These cell differentiating and immunomodulatory properties underlie the reason why vitamin D derivatives are now used successfully in the treatment of psoriasis and other skin disorders.

3.1.1 Overview of vitamin D metabolism

Vitamin D, a seco-steroid, can either be made in the skin from a cholesterol-like precursor (7-dehydrocholesterol) by exposure to sunlight or can be provided pre-formed in the diet (1). The version made in the skin is referred to as vitamin D_3 whereas the dietary form can be vitamin D_3 or a closely-related molecule of plant origin known as vitamin D_2. Because vitamin D can be made in the skin, it should not strictly be called a vitamin, and some nutritional texts refer to the substance as a prohormone and to the two forms as colecalciferol (D_3) and ergocalciferol (D_2).

From a nutritional perspective, the two forms are metabolized similarly in humans, are equal in potency, and can be considered equivalent. It is now firmly established that vitamin D_3 is metabolized first in the liver to 25-hydroxyvitamin D (calcidiol) (2) and subsequently in the kidneys to

1,25-(OH)$_2$D (calcitriol) (3) to produce a biologically active hormone. The 1,25-(OH)$_2$D compound, like all vitamin D metabolites, is present in the blood complexed to the vitamin D-binding protein, a specific α-globulin. Calcitriol is believed to act on target cells in a similar way to a steroid hormone. Free hormone crosses the plasma membrane and interacts with a specific nuclear receptor known as the vitamin D receptor, a DNA-binding, zinc-finger protein with a relative molecular mass of 55 000 (4). This ligand-receptor complex binds to a specific vitamin D-responsive element and, with associated transcription factors (e.g. retinoid X receptor), enhances transcription of mRNAs which code for calcium-transporting proteins, bone matrix proteins, or cell cycle-regulating proteins (5). As a result of these processes, 1,25-(OH)$_2$D stimulates intestinal absorption of calcium and phosphate and mobilizes calcium and phosphate by stimulating bone resorption (6). These functions serve the common purpose of restoring blood levels of calcium and phosphate to normal when concentrations of the two ions are low.

Lately, interest has focused on other cellular actions of calcitriol. With the discovery of 1,25-(OH)$_2$D receptors in many classically non-target tissues such as brain, various bone marrow-derived cells, skin, and thymus (7), the view has been expressed that 1,25-(OH)$_2$D induces fusion and differentiation of macrophages (8, 9). This effect has been widely interpreted to mean that the natural role of 1,25-(OH)$_2$D is to induce osteoclastogenesis from colony forming units (i.e. granulatory monocytes in the bone marrow). Calcitriol also suppresses interleukin-2 production in activated T-lymphocytes (10, 11), an effect which suggests the hormone might play a role in immuno-modulation in vivo. Other tissues (e.g. skin) are directly affected by exogenous administration of vitamin D, though the physiologic significance of these effects is poorly understood. The pharmacologic effects of 1,25-(OH)$_2$D are profound and have resulted in the development of vitamin D analogues, which are approved for use in hyperproliferative conditions such as psoriasis (12).

Clinical assays measure 1,25-(OH)$_2$D$_2$ and 1,25-(OH)$_2$D$_3$, collectively called 1,25-(OH)$_2$D. Similarly, calcidiol is measured as 25-OH-D but it is a mixture of 25-OH-D$_2$ and 25-OH-D$_3$. For the purposes of this document, 1,25-(OH)$_2$D and 25-OH-D will be used to refer to calcitriol and calcidiol, respectively.

3.1.2 Calcium homeostasis

In calcium homeostasis, 1,25-(OH)$_2$D works in conjunction with parathyroid hormone (PTH) to produce its beneficial effects on the plasma levels of ionized calcium and phosphate (5, 13). The physiologic loop (Figure 3.1) starts with the calcium receptor of the parathyroid gland (14). When the level of

FIGURE 3.1
Calcium homeostasis

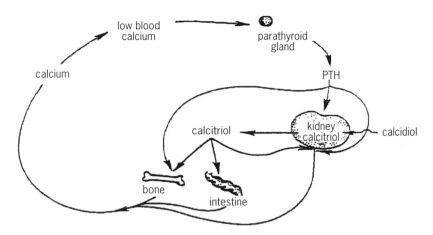

Source: adapted, with permission from the authors and publisher, from reference (13).

ionized calcium in plasma falls, PTH is secreted by the parathyroid gland and
stimulates the tightly regulated renal enzyme 25-OH-D-1-α-hydroxylase to
make more 1,25-$(OH)_2$D from the large circulating pool of 25-OH-D. The
resulting increase in 1,25-$(OH)_2$D (with the rise in PTH) causes an increase
in calcium transport within the intestine, bone, and kidney. All these events
raise plasma calcium levels back to normal, which in turn is sensed by the
calcium receptor of the parathyroid gland. The further secretion of PTH is
turned off not only by the feedback action of calcium, but also by a short
feedback loop involving 1,25-$(OH)_2$D directly suppressing PTH synthesis in
the parathyroid gland (not shown in Figure 3.1).

Although this model oversimplifies the events involved in calcium homeostasis, it clearly demonstrates that sufficient 25-OH-D must be available
to provide adequate 1,25-$(OH)_2$D synthesis and hence an adequate level
of plasma calcium; and similarly that vitamin D deficiency will result in
inadequate 25-OH-D and 1,25-$(OH)_2$D synthesis, inadequate calcium
homeostasis, and a constantly elevated PTH level (i.e. secondary
hyperparathyroidism).

It becomes evident from this method of presentation of the role of vitamin
D that the nutritionist can focus on the plasma levels of 25-OH-D and PTH
to gain an insight into vitamin D status. Not shown but also important is
the end-point of the physiologic action of vitamin D, namely, adequate
plasma calcium and phosphate ions that provide the raw materials for bone
mineralization.

3.2 Populations at risk for vitamin D deficiency

3.2.1 Infants

Infants constitute a population at risk for vitamin D deficiency because of relatively large vitamin D needs brought about by their high rate of skeletal growth. At birth, infants have acquired in utero the vitamin D stores that must carry them through the first months of life. A recent survey of French neonates revealed that 64% had 25-OH-D values below 30 nmol/l, the lower limit of the normal range (15). Breast-fed infants are particularly at risk because of the low concentrations of vitamin D in human milk (16). This problem is further compounded in some infants fed human milk by a restriction in exposure to ultraviolet (UV) light for seasonal, latitudinal, cultural, or social reasons. Infants born in the autumn months at extreme latitudes are particularly at risk because they spend the first 6 months of their life indoors and therefore have little opportunity to synthesize vitamin D in their skin during this period. Consequently, although vitamin D deficiency is rare in developed countries, sporadic cases of rickets are still being reported in many northern cities but almost always in infants fed human milk (17–20).

Infant formulas are supplemented with vitamin D at levels ranging from 40 international units (IU) or 1 mg/418.4 kJ to 100 IU or 2.5 mg/418.4 kJ, that provide approximately between 6 mg and 15 mg of vitamin D, respectively. These amounts of dietary vitamin D are sufficient to prevent rickets.

3.2.2 Adolescents

Another period of rapid growth of the skeleton occurs at puberty and increases the need not for the vitamin D itself, but for the active form 1,25-$(OH)_2D$. This need results from the increased conversion of 25-OH-D to 1,25-$(OH)_2D$ in adolescents (21). Unlike infants, however, adolescents usually spend more time outdoors and therefore usually are exposed to levels of UV light sufficient for synthesizing vitamin D for their needs. Excess production of vitamin D in the summer and early autumn months is stored mainly in the adipose tissue (22) and is available to sustain high growth rates in the winter months that follow. Insufficient vitamin D stores during this period of increased growth can lead to vitamin D insufficiency (23).

3.2.3 Elderly

Over the past 20 years, clinical research studies of the basic biochemical machinery for handling vitamin D have suggested an age-related decline in many key steps of vitamin D action (24), including the rate of skin synthesis, the rate of hydroxylation (leading to the activation to the hormonal form), and the response of target tissues (e.g. bone) (25). Not surprisingly, a number of independent studies from around the world have shown that there appears to be vitamin D deficiency in a subset of the elderly population, characterized by low blood levels of 25-OH-D coupled with elevations in plasma PTH and alkaline phosphatase (26). There is evidence that this vitamin D deficiency contributes to declining bone mass and increases the incidence of hip fractures (27). Although some of these studies may exaggerate the extent of the problem by focusing on institutionalized individuals or inpatients with decreased sun exposures, in general they have forced health professionals to re-address the vitamin D intake of this segment of society and look at potential solutions to correct the problem. Table 3.1 presents the findings of several studies that found that modest increases in vitamin D intakes (between 10 and 20 µg/day) reduce the rate of bone loss and the incidence of hip fractures.

These findings have led several agencies and researchers to suggest an increase in recommended vitamin D intakes for the elderly from 2.5–5 µg/day to a value that is able to maintain normal 25-OH-D levels in the elderly, such as 10–15 µg/day. This vitamin D intake results in lower rates of bone loss and is proposed for the middle-aged (50–70 years) and old-aged (>70 years) populations (33). The increased requirements are justified mainly on the grounds of the reduction in skin synthesis of vitamin D, a linear reduction occurring in both men and women that begins with the thinning of the skin at age 20 years (24).

3.2.4 Pregnant and lactating women

Elucidation of the changes in calciotropic hormones occurring during pregnancy and lactation has revealed a role for vitamin D in the former but not definitively in the latter. Even in pregnancy, the changes in vitamin D metabolism which occur, namely an increase in the maternal plasma levels of 1,25-$(OH)_2D$ (34) due to a putative placental synthesis of the hormone (35), do not seem to impinge greatly on the maternal vitamin D requirements. The concern that modest vitamin D supplementation might be deleterious to the fetus is not justified. Furthermore, because transfer of vitamin D from mother to fetus is important for establishing the neonate's growth rate, the goal of ensuring adequate vitamin D status with conventional prenatal vitamin D supplements probably should not be discouraged.

In lactating women there appears to be no direct role for vitamin D because increased calcium needs are regulated by the PTH-related peptide (36, 37), and recent studies have failed to show any change in vitamin D metabolites during lactation (38, 39). As stated above, the vitamin D content of human

TABLE 3.1

Randomized, controlled trials with dietary vitamin D supplements

Reference	Study group	n^a	Age (years) Mean	SD	Regimen	Duration (years)	Results
Dawson-Hughes et al., 1991 (28)	Healthy, postmenopausal women living independently	249	62	0.5	10 μg vitamin D + 400 mg calcium	1.0	Reduced late wintertime bone loss from vertebrae; Net spine BMD↑; No change in whole-body BMD
Chapuy et al., 1992 (29)	Healthy, elderly women living in nursing homes or in apartments for the elderly	3270	84	6	20 μg vitamin D + 1200 mg calcium	1.5	Hip fractures 43% ↓; Non-vertebral fractures 32% ↓; In subset (n = 56), BMD of proximal femur 2.7% ↑ in vitamin D group and 4.6% ↓ in placebo group
Chapuy et al., 1994 (30)[b]						3.0	Hip fractures 29% ↓; Non-vertebral fractures 24% ↓
Dawson-Hughes et al., 1995 (31)	Healthy postmenopausal women living independently	261	64	5	2.5 μg or 17.5 μg vitamin D + 500 mg calcium	2.0	Loss of BMD from femoral neck lower in 17.5 μg group (−1.06%) than in 2.5 μg group (−2.54%); No difference in BMD at spine
Lips et al., 1996 (32)	Healthy, elderly individuals living independently, in nursing homes, or in apartments for the elderly	2578 (1916 women, 662 men)	80	6	10 μg vitamin D	2.0	No difference in fracture incidence; In subset (n = 248) of women from nursing homes, BMD 2.3% ↑ after 2 years

SD, standard deviation; BMD, bone mineral density; ↑, increase; ↓, decrease.
[a] Number of subjects enrolled in the study.
[b] Same study as Chapuy et al. (29) after a further 1.5 years of treatment.
Source: adapted, with permission, from reference (25).

milk is low (*16*). Consequently, there is no great drain on maternal vitamin D reserves either to regulate calcium homeostasis or to supply the need of human milk. Because human milk is a poor source of vitamin D, rare cases of nutritional rickets are still found, but these are almost always in breast-fed infants deprived of sunlight exposure (*17–20*). Furthermore, there is little evidence that increasing calcium or vitamin D supplementation to lactating mothers results in an increased transfer of calcium or vitamin D in milk (*38*). Thus, the current thinking, based on a clearer understanding of the role of vitamin D in lactation, is that there is little purpose in recommending additional vitamin D for lactating women. The goal for mothers who breastfeed their infants seems to be merely to ensure good nutrition and sunshine exposure in order to ensure normal vitamin D status during the perinatal period.

3.3 Evidence used for estimating recommended intakes

3.3.1 Lack of accuracy in estimating dietary intake and skin synthesis

The unique problem of estimating total intake of a substance that can be provided in the diet or made in the skin by exposure to sunlight makes it difficult to derive adequate total intakes of vitamin D for the general population. Moreover, accurate food composition data are not available for vitamin D, accentuating the difficulty in estimating dietary intakes. Whereas two recent United States national surveys have avoided even attempting this task, the second National Health and Nutrition Examination Survey (NHANES II) estimated vitamin D intakes to be 2.9 µg/day and 2.3 µg/day for younger and older women, respectively. A recent study of elderly women by Kinyamu et al. (*40*) concurred with this assessment, finding an intake of 3.53 µg/day.

Skin synthesis is equally difficult to estimate, being affected by such imponderables as age, season, latitude, time of day, skin exposure, and sunscreen use. In vitamin D-replete individuals, estimates of skin synthesis are put at around 10 µg/day (*24, 41*), with total intakes estimated at 15 µg/day (*24*).

3.3.2 Use of plasma 25-OH-D as a measure of vitamin D status

Numerous recent studies have used plasma 25-OH-D as a measure of vitamin D status, and there is a strong presumptive relationship of this variable with bone status. Thus, it is not surprising that several nutritional committees (e.g. the Food and Nutrition Board of the United States National Academy of Sciences' Institute of Medicine in conjunction with Health Canada) have chosen to use a biochemical basis for estimating required intakes and have used these estimates to derive recommended intakes (*33*). The method used involves the estimation of the mean group dietary intake of vitamin D required to maintain the plasma 25-OH-D levels above 27 nmol/l, which is the level necessary to ensure normal bone health. Previously, many studies had established 27 nmol/l as the lower limit of the normal range (e.g. NHANES III [42]). This dietary intake of vitamin D for each population group was rounded to the nearest 50 IU (1.25 µg) and then doubled to cover the needs of all individuals within that group irrespective of sunlight exposure. This amount was termed *adequate intake* (AI) and was used in place of the recommended dietary allowance (RDA), which had been used by United States agencies since 1941. The present Expert Consultation decided to use these figures as recommended nutrient intakes (RNIs) because it considered this to be an entirely logical approach to estimating the vitamin D needs for the global population.

Because many studies had recommended increases in vitamin D intakes for the elderly, it might have been expected that the proposed increases in suggested intakes from 5 µg/day (the RDA in the United States [43] and the RNI in Canada [44]) to between 10 and 15 µg/day (AI) would be welcomed. However, a recent editorial in a prominent medical journal attacked the recommendations as being too conservative (45). Furthermore, an article in the same journal (46) reported the level of hypovitaminosis D to be as high as 57% in a population of ageing (mean age, 62 years) medical inpatients in the Boston area.

Of course, such inpatients are by definition sick and should not be used to calculate intakes of healthy individuals. Indeed, the new NHANES III study (42) of 18 323 healthy individuals from all regions of the United States suggests that approximately 5% had values of 25-OH-D below 27 nmol/l (see Table 3.2). Although the data are skewed by sampling biases that favour sample collection in the southern states in winter months and northern states in the summer months, even subsets of data collected in northern states in September give the incidence of low 25-OH-D in the elderly in the 6–18% range (47), compared with 57% in the institutionalized inpatient population (46) mentioned above. Ideally, such measurements in a healthy population should be made at the end of the winter months before UV irradiation has reached a strength sufficient to allow skin synthesis of vitamin D. Thus, the NHANES III study may still underestimate the incidence of hypovitaminosis D in a northern elderly population in winter. Nevertheless, in lieu of additional studies of selected human populations, it would seem that the recommendations of the Food and Nutrition Board are reasonable guidelines for vitamin D intakes, at least for the near future. This considered approach allows for a period of time to monitor the potential shortfalls of

TABLE 3.2
Frequency distribution of serum or plasma 25-OH-D: preliminary unweighted results from the third National Health and Nutrition Examination Survey, 1988–1994[a]

Percentile	25-OH-D[b] (ng/ml)[c]
1st	7.6
5th	10.9
10th	13.2
50th	24.4
90th	40.1
95th	45.9
99th	59.0

[a] Total number of samples used in data analysis: 18 323; mean: 25.89 ng/ml (±11.08). Values are for all ages, ethnicity groups, and both sexes.
[b] High values: four values between 90–98 ng/ml, one value of 160.3 ng/ml. Values <5 ng/ml (lowest standard) entered arbitrarily in the database as "3".
[c] Units: for 25-OH-D, 1 ng/ml = 2.5 nmol/l, 10 ng/ml = 25 nmol/l, 11 ng/ml = 28.5 nmol/l (low limit),
30 ng/ml = 75 nmol/l (normal), 60 ng/ml = 150 nmol/l (upper limit).
Source: reference (42).

the new recommendations as well as to assess whether the suggested guidelines can be achieved, a point that was repeatedly raised about the vitamin D RDA.

3.4 Recommended intakes for vitamin D

In recommending intakes for vitamin D, it must be recognized that in most locations in the world in a broad band around the equator (between latitudes 42°N and 42°S), the most physiologically relevant and efficient way of acquiring vitamin D is to synthesize it endogenously in the skin from 7-dehydrocholesterol by sun (UV) light exposure. In most situations, approximately 30 minutes of skin exposure (without sunscreen) of the arms and face to sunlight can provide all the daily vitamin D needs of the body (24). However, skin synthesis of vitamin D is negatively influenced by factors which may reduce the ability of the skin to provide the total needs of the individual (24):

- latitude and season—both influence the amount of UV light reaching the skin;
- the ageing process—thinning of the skin reduces the efficiency of this synthetic process;

- skin pigmentation—the presence of darker pigments in the skin interferes with the synthetic process because UV light cannot reach the appropriate layer of the skin;
- clothing—virtually complete covering of the skin for medical, social, cultural, or religious reasons leaves insufficient skin exposed to sunlight;
- sunscreen use—widespread and liberal use of sunscreen, though reducing skin damage by the sun, deleteriously affects synthesis of vitamin D.

Because not all of these problems can be solved in all geographic locations, particularly during winter at latitudes higher than 42° where synthesis is virtually zero, it is recommended that individuals not synthesizing vitamin D should correct their vitamin D status by consuming the amounts of vitamin D appropriate for their age group (Table 3.3).

TABLE 3.3
Recommended nutrient intakes (RNIs) for vitamin D, by group

Group	RNI (µg/day)[a]
Infants and children	
0–6 months	5
7–12 months	5
1–3 years	5
4–6 years	5
7–9 years	5
Adolescents	
10–18 years	5
Adults	
19–50 years	5
51–65 years	10
65+ years	15
Pregnant women	5
Lactating women	5

[a] Units: for vitamin D, 1 IU = 25 ng, 40 IU = 1 µg, 200 IU = 5 µg, 400 IU = 10 µg, 600 IU = 15 µg, 800 IU = 20 µg.

3.5 Toxicity

The adverse effects of high vitamin D intakes—hypercalciuria and hypercalcaemia—do not occur at the recommended intake levels discussed above. In fact, it is worth noting that the recommended intakes for all age groups are still well below the lowest observed adverse effect level of 50 µg/day and do not reach the "no observed adverse effect level" of 20 µg/day (*33, 48*). Outbreaks of idiopathic infantile hypercalcaemia in the United Kingdom in the post-World War II era led to the withdrawal of vitamin D fortification from all foods in that country because of concerns that they were due to hypervitaminosis D. There are some suggestions in the literature that these outbreaks of idiopathic infantile hypercalcaemia may have involved genetic and dietary components and were not due strictly to technical problems with over-fortification as was assumed (*49, 50*). In retrospect, the termination of the vitamin D fortification may have been counterproductive as it exposed segments of the United Kingdom community to vitamin D deficiency and may have discouraged other nations from starting vitamin D fortification programmes (*50*). This is all the more cause for concern because hypovitaminosis D is still a problem worldwide, particularly in developing countries, at high latitudes and in countries where skin exposure to sunlight is discouraged (*51*).

3.6 Recommendations for future research

Further research is needed to determine the following:

- whether vitamin D supplements during pregnancy have any positive effects later in life;
- whether vitamin D has a role in lactation;
- the long-term effects of high vitamin D intakes;
- whether dietary vitamin D supplements are as good as exposure to UV light;
- whether vitamin D is only needed for regulation of calcium and phosphate.

References

1. Feldman D, Glorieux FH, Pike JW. *Vitamin D*. New York, NY, Academic Press, 1997.
2. Blunt JW, DeLuca HF, Schnoes HK. 25-hydroxycholecalciferol. A biologically active metabolite of vitamin D3. *Biochemistry*, 1968, 7:3317–3322.
3. Fraser DR, Kodicek E. Unique biosynthesis by kidney of a biologically active vitamin D metabolite. *Nature*, 1970, 228:764–766.
4. Haussler MR. Vitamin D receptors: nature and function. *Annual Review of Nutrition*, 1986, 6:527–562.
5. Jones G, Strugnell S, DeLuca HF. Current understanding of the molecular actions of vitamin D. *Physiology Reviews*, 1998, 78:1193–1231.
6. DeLuca HF. The vitamin D story: a collaborative effort of basic science and clinical medicine. *FASEB Journal*, 1988, 2:224–236.
7. Pike JW. Vitamin D3 receptors: structure and function in transcription. *Annual Review of Nutrition*, 1991, 11:189–216.
8. Abe E et al. 1,25-dihydroxyvitamin D3 promotes fusion of mouse alveolar macrophages both by a direct mechanism and by a spleen cell-mediated indirect mechanism. *Proceedings of the National Academy of Sciences*, 1983, 80:5583–5587.
9. Bar-Shavit Z et al. Induction of monocytic differentiation and bone resorption by 1,25-dihydroxyvitamin D3. *Proceedings of the National Academy of Sciences*, 1983, 80:5907–5911.
10. Bhalla AK et al. Specific high affinity receptors for 1,25-dihydroxyvitamin D3

in human peripheral blood mononuclear cells: presence in monocytes and induction in T lymphocytes following activation. *Journal of Clinical Endocrinology and Metabolism*, 1983, 57:1308–1310.

11. Tsoukas CD, Provvedini DM, Manolagas SC. 1,25-dihydroxyvitamin D3: a novel immunoregulatory hormone. *Science*, 1984, 224:1438–1440.

12. Kragballe K. Vitamin D analogs in the treatment of psoriasis. *Journal of Cellular Biochemistry*, 1992, 49:46–52.

13. Jones G, DeLuca HF. HPLC of vitamin D and its metabolites. In: Makin HLJ, Newton R, eds. *High performance liquid chromatography and its application to endocrinology*. Berlin, Springer-Verlag, 1988:95–139 (Monographs on Endocrinology, volume 30).

14. Brown EM, Pollak M, Hebert SC. The extracellular calcium-sensing receptor: its role in health and disease. *Annual Review of Medicine*, 1998, 49:15–29.

15. Zeghund F et al. Subclinical vitamin D deficiency in neonates: definition and response to vitamin D supplements. *American Journal of Clinical Nutrition*, 1997, 65:771–778.

16. Specker BL, Tsang RC, Hollis BW. Effect of race and diet on human milk vitamin D and 25-hydroxyvitamin D. *American Journal of Diseases in Children*, 1985, 139:1134–1137.

17. Pettifor JM, Daniels ED. Vitamin D deficiency and nutritional rickets in children. In: Feldman D, Glorieux FH, Pike JW. *Vitamin D*. New York, NY, Academic Press, 1997:663–678.

18. Binet A, Kooh SW. Persistence of vitamin D deficiency rickets in Toronto in the 1990s. *Canadian Journal of Public Health*, 1996, 87:227–230.

19. Brunvand L, Nordshus T. Nutritional rickets—an old disease with new relevance. *Nordisk Medicin*, 1996, 111:219–221.

20. Gessner BD et al. Nutritional rickets among breast-fed black and Alaska native children. *Alaska Medicine*, 1997, 39:72–74.

21. Aksnes L, Aarskog D. Plasma concentrations of vitamin D metabolites at puberty: effect of sexual maturation and implications for growth. *Journal of Clinical Endocrinology and Metabolism*, 1982, 55:94–101.

22. Mawer EB et al. The distribution and storage of vitamin D and its metabolites in human tissues. *Clinical Science*, 1972, 43:413–431.

23. Gultekin A et al. Serum 25-hydroxycholecalciferol levels in children and adolescents. *Turkish Journal of Pediatrics*, 1987, 29:155–162.

24. Holick MF. Vitamin D—new horizons for the 21st century. McCollum Award Lecture. *American Journal of Clinical Nutrition*, 1994, 60:619–630.

25. Shearer MJ. The roles of vitamins D and K in bone health and osteoporosis prevention. *Proceedings of the Nutrition Society*, 1997, 56:915–937.

26. Chapuy M-C, Meunier PJ. Vitamin D insufficiency in adults and the elderly. In: Feldman D, Glorieux FH, Pike JW. *Vitamin D*. New York, NY, Academic Press, 1997:679–693.

27. Dawson-Hughes B et al. Effect of calcium and vitamin D supplementation on bone density in men and women 65 years of age or older. *New England Journal of Medicine*, 1997, 337:670–676.

28. Dawson-Hughes B et al. Effect of vitamin D supplementation on wintertime and overall bone loss in healthy postmenopausal women. *Annals of Internal Medicine*, 1991, 115:505–512.

29. Chapuy M-C et al. Vitamin D3 and calcium prevent hip fractures in elderly women. *New England Journal of Medicine*, 1992, 327:1637–1642.

30. Chapuy M-C et al. Effects of calcium and cholecalciferol treatment for three years on hip fractures in elderly women. *British Medical Journal*, 1994, 308:1081–1082.

31. Dawson-Hughes B et al. Rates of bone loss in postmenopausal women randomly assigned to one of two dosages of vitamin D. *American Journal of Clinical Nutrition*, 1995, 61:1140–1145.

32. Lips P et al. Vitamin D supplementation and fracture incidence in elderly persons: a randomized, placebo-controlled clinical trial. *Annals of Internal Medicine*, 1996, 124:400–406.

33. Food and Nutrition Board. *Dietary reference intakes for calcium, phosphorus, magnesium, vitamin D, and fluoride*. Washington, DC, National Academy Press, 1997.

34. Bouillon R et al. Influence of the vitamin D-binding protein on the serum concentration of 1,25-dihydroxyvitamin D3. Significance of the free 1,25-dihydroxyvitamin D3 concentration. *Journal of Clinical Investigation*, 1981, 67:589–596.

35. Delvin EE et al. In vitro metabolism of 25-hydroxycholecalciferol by isolated cells from human decidua. *Journal of Clinical Endocrinology and Metabolism*, 1985, 60:880–885.

36. Sowers MF et al. Elevated parathyroid hormone-related peptide associated with lactation and bone density loss. *Journal of the American Medical Association*, 1996, 276:549–554.

37. Prentice A. Calcium requirements of breast-feeding mothers. *Nutrition Reviews*, 1998, 56:124–127.

38. Sowers M et al. Role of calciotrophic hormones in calcium mobilization of lactation. *American Journal of Clinical Nutrition*, 1998, 67:284–291.

39. Kovacs CS, Kronenberg HM. Maternal-fetal calcium and bone metabolism during pregnancy, puerperium, and lactation. *Endocrine Reviews*, 1997, 18:832–872.

40. Kinyamu HK et al. Dietary calcium and vitamin D intake in elderly women: effect on serum parathyroid hormone and vitamin D metabolites. *American Journal of Clinical Nutrition*, 1998, 67:342–348.

41. Fraser DR. The physiological economy of vitamin D. *Lancet*, 1983, 1:969–972.

42. *National Health and Nutrition Examination Survey III, 1988–1994* [CD-ROM]. Hyatsville, MD, Centers for Disease Control and Prevention, 1998 (CD-ROM Series 11, No. 2A).

43. Subcommittee on the Tenth Edition of the Recommended Dietary Allowances, Food and Nutrition Board. *Recommended Dietary Allowances, 10th ed.* Washington, DC, National Academy Press, 1989.

44. *Nutrition recommendations (1990).* Ottawa, Health and Welfare Canada, 1990.

45. Utiger RD. The need for more vitamin D. *New England Journal of Medicine*, 1998, 338:828–829.

46. Thomas MK et al. Hypovitaminosis D in medical inpatients. *New England Journal of Medicine*, 1998, 338:777–783.

47. Looker AC, Gunter EW. Hypovitaminosis D in medical inpatients. *New England Journal of Medicine*, 1998, 339:344–345.

48. Lachance PA. International perspective: basis, need and application of recommended dietary allowances. *Nutrition Reviews*, 1998, 56:S2–S4.

49. Jones KL. Williams syndrome: an historical perspective of its evolution, natural history, and etiology. *American Journal of Medical Genetics*, 1990, 6(Suppl.):S89–S96.

50. Fraser D. The relation between infantile hypercalcemia and vitamin D—public health implications in North America. *Pediatrics*, 1967, 40:1050–1061.
51. Mawer EB, Davies M. Vitamin D deficiency, rickets and osteomalacia, a returning problem worldwide. In: Norman AW, Bouillon R, Thomasset M, eds. *Vitamin D. Chemistry, biology and clinical applications of the steroid hormone*. Riverside, CA, University of California, 1997:899–906.

4. Calcium

4.1 Introduction

It has been nearly 30 years since the last FAO/WHO recommendations on calcium intake were published in 1974 (*1*) and nearly 40 years since the experts' meeting in Rome (*2*), on whose findings these recommendations were based. During this time, a paradigm shift has occurred with respect to the involvement of calcium in the etiology of osteoporosis. The previous reports were written against the background of the Albright paradigm (*3*), according to which osteomalacia and rickets were due to calcium deficiency, vitamin D deficiency, or both, and osteoporosis was attributed to the failure of new bone formation secondary to negative nitrogen balance, osteoblast insufficiency, or both. The rediscovery of earlier information that calcium deficiency led to the development of osteoporosis (not rickets and osteomalacia) in experimental animals (*4*) resulted in a re-examination of osteoporosis in humans, notably in postmenopausal women. This re-examination yielded evidence in the late 1960s that menopausal bone loss was not due to a decrease in bone formation but rather to an increase in bone resorption (*5–8*); this has had a profound effect on our understanding of other forms of osteoporosis and has led to a new paradigm that is still evolving.

Although reduced bone formation may aggravate the bone loss process in elderly people (*9*) and probably plays a major role in corticosteroid osteo-porosis (*10*)—and possibly in osteoporosis in men (*11*)—bone resorption is increasingly held responsible for osteoporosis in women and for the bone deficit associated with hip fractures in elderly people of both sexes (*12*). Because bone resorption is also the mechanism whereby calcium deficiency destroys bone, it is hardly surprising that the role of calcium in the patho-genesis of osteoporosis has received increasing attention and that recom-mended calcium intakes have risen steadily in the past 35 years from the nadir which followed the publication of the report from the Rome meeting in 1962 (*13*). The process has been accelerated by the growing realization that insen-sible losses of calcium (e.g. via skin, hair, nails) need to be taken into account in the calculation of calcium requirements.

As the calcium allowances recommended for developed countries have been rising—and may still not have reached their peak—the gap between recommended and actual calcium intakes in developing countries has widened. The concept that calcium requirement may itself vary from culture to culture for dietary, genetic, lifestyle, and geographical reasons, is emerging. This report therefore seeks to make it clear that its main recommendations—like the latest recommendations from the European Union (*14*), Australia (*15*), Canada/United States (*16*), and the United Kingdom (*17*)—are largely based on data derived from the developed world and are not necessarily applicable to countries with different dietary cultures, different lifestyles, and different environments for which different calculations may be indicated.

4.2 Chemistry and distribution of calcium

Calcium is a divalent cation with an atomic weight of 40. In the elementary composition of the human body, it ranks fifth after oxygen, carbon, hydrogen, and nitrogen, and it makes up 1.9% of the body by weight (*18*). Carcass analyses show that calcium constitutes 0.1–0.2% of early fetal fat-free weight, rising to about 2% of adult fat-free weight. In absolute terms, this represents a rise from about 24 g (600 mmol) at birth to 1300 g (32.5 mol) at maturity, requiring an average daily positive calcium balance of 180 mg (4.5 mmol) during the first 20 years of growth (Figure 4.1).

FIGURE 4.1
Whole-body bone mineral (WB Min) (left axis) and whole-body calcium (WB Ca) (right axis) as a function of age as determined by total-body dual-energy X-ray absorptiometry

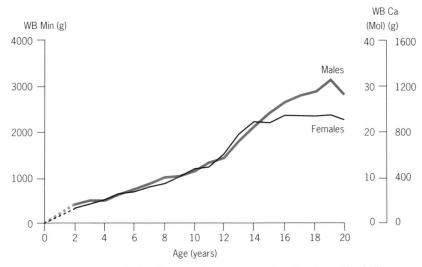

Source: based on data supplied by Dr Zanchetta, Instituto de Investigaciones Metabolicas, Buenos Aires, Argentina.

Nearly all (99%) of total body calcium is located in the skeleton. The remaining 1% is equally distributed between the teeth and soft tissues, with only 0.1% in the extracellular fluid (ECF). In the skeleton it constitutes 25% of the dry weight and 40% of the ash weight. The ECF contains ionized calcium at concentrations of about 4.8 mg/100 ml (1.20 mmol/l) maintained by the parathyroid–vitamin D system as well as complexed calcium at concentrations of about 1.6 mg/100 ml (0.4 mmol/l). In the plasma there is also a protein-bound calcium fraction, which is present at a concentration of 3.2 mg/100 ml (0.8 mmol/l). In the cellular compartment, the total calcium concentration is comparable with that in the ECF, but the free calcium concentration is lower by several orders of magnitude (*19*).

4.3 Biological role of calcium

Calcium salts provide rigidity to the skeleton and calcium ions play a role in many, if not most, metabolic processes. In the primitive exoskeleton and in shells, rigidity is generally provided by calcium carbonate, but in the vertebrate skeleton, it is provided by a form of calcium phosphate which approximates hydroxyapatite $[Ca_{10}(OH)_2(PO_4)_6]$ and is embedded in collagen fibrils.

Bone mineral serves as the ultimate reservoir for the calcium circulating in the ECF. Calcium enters the ECF from the gastrointestinal tract by absorption and from bone by resorption. Calcium leaves the ECF via the gastrointestinal tract, kidneys, and skin and enters into bone via bone formation (Figure 4.2). In addition, calcium fluxes occur across all cell membranes. Many neuromuscular and other cellular functions depend on the maintenance of the

FIGURE 4.2
Major calcium movements in the body

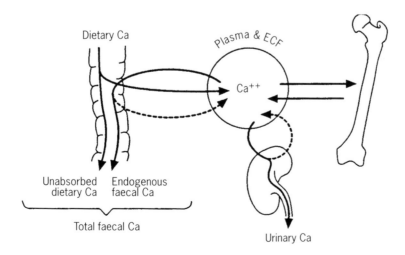

Dietary Ca

Plasma & ECF

Ca++

Unabsorbed dietary Ca Endogenous faecal Ca

Total faecal Ca

Urinary Ca

ionized calcium concentration in the ECF. Calcium fluxes are also important mediators of hormonal effects on target organs through several intracellular signalling pathways, such as the phosphoinositide and cyclic adenosine monophosphate systems. The cytoplasmic calcium concentration is regulated by a series of calcium pumps, which either concentrate calcium ions within the intracellular storage sites or extrude them from the cells (where they flow in by diffusion). The physiology of calcium metabolism is primarily directed towards the maintenance of the concentration of ionized calcium in the ECF. This concentration is protected and maintained by a feedback loop through calcium receptors in the parathyroid glands (20), which control the secretion of parathyroid hormone (see Figure 3.1). This hormone increases the renal tubular reabsorption of calcium, promotes intestinal calcium absorption by stimulating the renal production of 1,25-dihydroxyvitamin D or calcitriol [1,25-$(OH)_2$D], and, if necessary, resorbs bone. However, the integrity of the system depends critically on vitamin D status; if there is a deficiency of vitamin D, the loss of its calcaemic action (21) leads to a decrease in the ionized calcium and secondary hyperparathyroidism and hypophosphataemia. This is why experimental vitamin D deficiency results in rickets and osteomalacia whereas calcium deficiency gives rise to osteoporosis (4, 22).

4.4 Determinants of calcium balance

4.4.1 Calcium intake

In a strictly operational sense, calcium balance is determined by the relationship between calcium intake and calcium absorption and excretion. A striking feature of the system is that relatively small changes in calcium absorption and excretion can neutralize a high intake or compensate for a low one. There is a wide variation in calcium intake between countries, generally following the animal protein intake and depending largely on dairy product consumption. The lowest calcium intakes occur in developing countries, particularly in Asia, and the highest in developed countries, particularly in North America and Europe (Table 4.1).

4.4.2 Calcium absorption

Ingested calcium mixes with digestive juice calcium in the proximal small intestine from where it is absorbed by a process which has an active saturable component and a diffusion component (24–27). When calcium intake is low, calcium is mainly absorbed by active (transcellular) transport, but at higher intakes, an increasing proportion of calcium is absorbed by simple (paracellular) diffusion. The unabsorbed component appears in the faeces together with the unabsorbed component of digestive juice calcium known as endoge-

TABLE 4.1
Daily protein and calcium intakes in different regions of the world, 1987–1989

Region	Protein (g)			Calcium (mg)		
	Total	Animal	Vegetable	Total	Animal	Vegetable
North America	108.7	72.2	36.5	1031	717	314
Europe	102.0	59.6	42.4	896	684	212
Oceania	98.3	66.5	31.8	836	603	233
Other developed	91.1	47.3	43.8	565	314	251
USSR	106.2	56.1	50.1	751	567	184
All developed	103.0	60.1	42.9	850	617	233
Africa	54.1	10.6	43.5	368	108	260
Latin America	66.8	28.6	38.2	477	305	171
Near East	78.7	18.0	60.7	484	223	261
Far East	58.2	11.0	47.2	305	109	196
Other developing	55.8	22.7	33.1	432	140	292
All developing	59.9	13.3	46.6	344	138	206

Source: reference (23).

nous faecal calcium. Thus, the faeces contain unabsorbed dietary calcium and digestive juice calcium that was not reabsorbed (Figure 4.2).

True absorbed calcium is the total amount of calcium absorbed from the calcium pool in the intestines and therefore contains both dietary and digestive juice components. Net absorbed calcium is the difference between dietary calcium and faecal calcium and is numerically the same as true absorbed calcium minus endogenous faecal calcium. At zero calcium intake, all the faecal calcium is endogenous and represents the digestive juice calcium which has not been reabsorbed; net absorbed calcium at this intake is therefore negative to the extent of about 200 mg (5 mmol) (28, 29). When the intake reaches about 200 mg (5 mmol), dietary and faecal calcium become equal and net absorbed calcium is zero. As calcium intake increases, net absorbed calcium also increases, steeply at first but then, as the active transport becomes saturated, more slowly until the slope of absorbed on ingested calcium approaches linearity with an ultimate gradient of about 5–10% (24, 25, 30, 31). The relationship between intestinal calcium absorption and calcium intake, derived from 210 balance experiments performed in 81 individuals collected from the literature (32–39), is shown in Figure 4.3.

True absorption is an inverse function of calcium intake, falling from some 70% at very low intakes to about 35% at high intakes (Figure 4.4). Percentage net absorption is negative at low intake, becomes positive as intake increases, reaches a peak of about 35% at an intake of about 400 mg, and then falls off as intake increases further. True and net absorption converge as intake

FIGURE 4.3

The relationship between calcium intake and calcium absorbed (or excreted) calculated from 210 balance experiments in 81 subjects

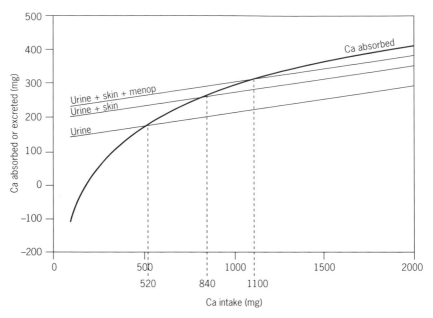

Equilibrium is reached at an intake of 520 mg, which rises to 840 mg when skin losses of 60 mg are added and to 1100 mg when menopausal loss is included. The curvilinear relationship between intestinal calcium absorption and calcium intake can be linearized by using the logarithm of calcium intake to yield the equation: $Ca_a = 174 \log_e Ca_i - 909 \pm 71$ (SD), where Ca_i represents ingested calcium and Ca_a net absorbed calcium in mg/day. The relationship between urinary calcium excretion and calcium intake is given by the equation: $Ca_u = 0.078 Ca_i + 137 \pm 11.2$ (SD), where Ca_u is urinary calcium and Ca_i calcium intake in mg/day.
Source: based on data from references (32–39).

rises because the endogenous faecal component that separates them becomes proportionately smaller.

Many factors influence the availability of calcium for absorption and the absorptive mechanism itself. In the case of the former, factors include the presence of substances which form insoluble complexes with calcium, such as the phosphate ion. The relatively high calcium–phosphate ratio of 2.2 in human milk compared with 0.77 in cow milk (18) may be a factor in the higher absorption of calcium from human milk than cow milk (see below).

Intestinal calcium absorption is mainly controlled by the serum concentration of 1,25-(OH)₂D (see Chapter 3). The activity of the 1-α-hydroxylase, which catalyses 1,25-(OH)₂D production from 25-hydroxyvitamin D (25-OH-D) in the kidneys, is negatively related to plasma calcium and phosphate concentrations and positively related to plasma parathyroid hormone concentrations (21). Thus the inverse relationship between calcium intake and

FIGURE 4.4
True and net calcium absorption as percentages of calcium intake

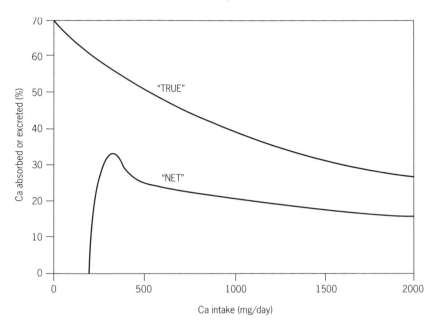

Note the great differences between these functions at low calcium intakes and their progressive convergence as calcium intake increases.

fractional absorption described above is enhanced by the inverse relationship between dietary calcium and serum 1,25-(OH)$_2$D (*21, 40, 41*).

Phytates, present in the husks of many cereals as well as in nuts, seeds, and legumes, can form insoluble calcium phytate salts in the gastrointestinal tract. Excess oxalates can precipitate calcium in the bowel but are not an important factor in most diets.

4.4.3 Urinary calcium

Urinary calcium is the fraction of the filtered plasma water calcium which is not reabsorbed in the renal tubules. At a normal glomerular filtration rate of 120 ml/min and an ultrafiltrable calcium concentration of 6.4 mg/100 ml (1.60 mmol/l), the filtered load of calcium is about 8 mg/min (0.20 mmol/min) or 11.6 g/day (290 mmol/day). Because the average 24-hour calcium excretion in subjects from developed countries is about 160–200 mg (4–5 mmol), it follows that 98–99% of the filtered calcium is usually reabsorbed in the renal tubules. However, calcium excretion is extremely sensitive to changes in filtered load. A decrease in plasma water calcium of only 0.17 mg/100 ml (0.043 mmol/l), which is barely detectable, was sufficient to account for a

65

decrease in urinary calcium of 63 mg (1.51 mmol) when 27 subjects changed from a normal- to a low-calcium diet (42). This very sensitive renal response to calcium deprivation combines with the inverse relationship between calcium intake and absorption to stabilize the plasma ionized calcium concentration and to preserve the equilibrium between calcium entering and leaving the ECF over a wide range of calcium intakes. However, there is always a significant obligatory loss of calcium in the urine (as there is in the faeces), even on a low calcium intake, simply because maintenance of the plasma ionized calcium and, therefore, of the filtered load, prevents total elimination of calcium from the urine. The lower limit for urinary calcium in developed countries is about 140 mg (3.5 mmol) but depends on protein and salt intakes. From this obligatory minimum, urinary calcium increases on intake with a slope of about 5–10% (30, 31, 43). In Figure 4.3, the relationship between urinary calcium excretion and calcium intake is represented by the line which intersects the absorbed calcium line at an intake of 520 mg.

4.4.4 Insensible losses

Urinary and endogenous faecal calcium are not the only forms of excreted calcium; losses through skin, hair, and nails also need to be taken into account. These are not easily measured, but a combined balance and isotope procedure has yielded estimates of daily insensible calcium losses in the range of 40–80 mg (1–2 mmol), which are unrelated to calcium intake (44, 45). Thus, the additional loss of a mean of 60 mg (1.5 mmol) as a constant to urinary calcium loss raises the level of dietary calcium at which absorbed and excreted calcium reach equilibrium from 520 to 840 mg (13 to 21 mmol) (Figure 4.3).

4.5 Criteria for assessing calcium requirements and recommended nutrient intakes

4.5.1 Methodology

Although it is well established that calcium deficiency causes osteoporosis in experimental animals, the contribution that calcium deficiency makes to osteoporosis in humans is much more controversial, in part due to the great variation in calcium intakes across the world (Table 4.1), which does not appear to be associated with any corresponding variation in the prevalence of osteoporosis. This issue is dealt with at greater length in the section on nutritional factors (see section 4.10); in this section we will simply define what is meant by calcium requirement and how it may be calculated.

The calcium requirement of an adult is generally recognized to be the intake required to maintain calcium balance and therefore skeletal integrity. The mean calcium requirement of adults is therefore the mean intake at which intake and output are equal; at present this can only be determined by balance studies conducted with sufficient care, and over a sufficiently long period of time to ensure reasonable accuracy and then corrected for insensible losses. The reputation of the balance technique has been harmed by a few studies with inadequate equilibration times and short collection periods, but this should not be allowed to detract from the value of the meticulous work of those who have collected faecal and urinary samples for weeks or months from subjects on well-defined diets. This meticulous work has produced valuable balance data, which are clearly valid; the mean duration of the 210 experiments from eight publications used in this report to derive the recommended intakes was 90 days with a range of 6–480 days. (The four 6-day balance studies in the series used a non-absorbable marker and are therefore acceptable.)

The usual way of determining mean calcium requirement from balance studies is by linear regression of calcium output (or calcium balance) on intake and calculation of the mean intake at which intake and output are equal (or balance is zero). This was probably first done in 1939 by Mitchell and Curzon (*46*), who arrived at a mean requirement of 9.8 mg/kg/day or about 640 mg/day (16 mmol) for a mean body weight of 65 kg. The same type of calculation was subsequently used by many others who arrived at requirements ranging from 200 mg/day (5 mmol/day) in male Peruvian prisoners (*47*) to 990 mg/day (24.75 mmol) in premenopausal women (*48*), but most values were about 600 mg/day (15 mmol) (*31*) without allowing for insensible losses. However, this type of simple linear regression yields a higher mean calcium requirement (640 mg in the 210 balance experiments used here) (Figure 4.5a) than the intercept of absorbed and excreted calcium (520 mg) (Figure 4.3) because it tends to underestimate the negative calcium balance at low intake and overestimate the positive balance at high intake. A better reflection of biological reality is obtained by deriving calcium output from the functions given previously (see section 4.4.2) and then regressing that output on calcium intake. This yields the result shown in Figure 4.5b where balance is more negative (i.e. the regression line is above the line of equality) at low intakes and less positive (i.e. the regression line is below the line of equality) at high intakes than in the linear model, and yields a zero balance at 520 mg, which is the same as that arrived at in Figure 4.3 when excreted and absorbed calcium were equal.

An alternative way of calculating calcium requirement is to determine the intake at which the mean maximum positive balance occurs. This has been done with a two-component, split, linear regression model in which calcium balance is regressed on intake to determine the threshold intake above which no further increase in calcium retention occurs (*49*). This may well be an appropriate way of calculating the calcium requirement of children and

FIGURE 4.5
Calcium output as a (a) linear and (b) non-linear function of calcium intake calculated from the same balances as Figure 4.3

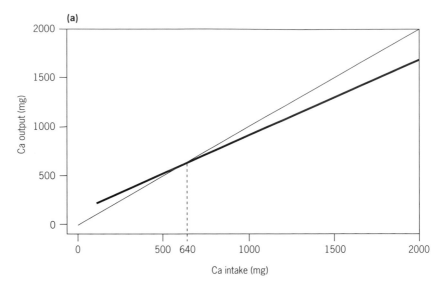

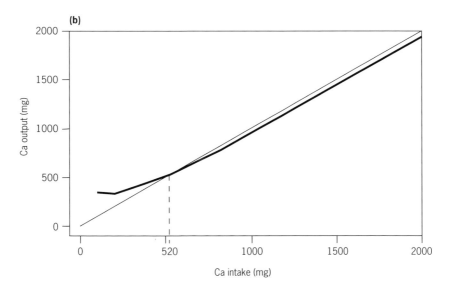

(a) The regression line crosses the line of equality at an intake of 640 mg. The equation is: $Ca_o = 0.779 Ca_i + 142$ where Ca_o is calcium output and Ca_i is calcium intake in mg/day. (b) The regression line crosses the line of equality at an intake of 520 mg. The equation is: $Ca_o = Ca_i - 174 \log_e Ca_i - 909 + 0.078 Ca_u + 137$ where Ca_o is calcium output, Ca_i is calcium intake, Ca_i is the insensible losses and Ca_u is urinary calcium in mg/day..
Source: based on data from references (32–39).

adolescents (and perhaps pregnant and lactating women) who need to be in positive calcium balance and in whom the difference between calcium intake and output is therefore relatively large and measurable by the balance technique. However, in normal adults the difference between calcium intake and output at high calcium intakes represents a very small difference between two large numbers, and this calculation, therefore, carries too great an error to calculate their requirement.

The Expert Consultation concurred that the most satisfactory way of calculating calcium requirement from current data is by using the intake level at which excreted calcium equals net absorbed calcium, which has the advantage of permitting separate analysis of the effects of changes in calcium absorption and excretion. This intercept has been shown in Figure 4.3 to occur at an intake of about 520 mg, but when insensible losses of calcium of 60 mg (1.5 mmol) (44, 45) are taken into account, the intercept rises to 840 mg, which was considered to be as close as it is possible to get at present to the calcium requirement of adults on Western-style diets. The intercept rises to about 1100 mg due to an increase in obligatory urinary calcium losses of 30 mg (0.75 mmol) at menopause (50). A value of 1100 mg was thus proposed as the mean calcium requirement of postmenopausal women (see below). However, this type of calculation cannot be easily applied to other high-risk populations (such as children) because there are not sufficient published data from these groups to permit a similar analysis of the relationship between calcium intake, absorption, and excretion. An alternative is to estimate how much calcium each population group needs to absorb to meet obligatory calcium losses and desirable calcium retention, and then to calculate the intake required to provide this rate of calcium absorption. This is what has been done in section 4.6.

4.5.2 Populations at risk for calcium deficiency

It is clear from Figure 4.1 that a positive calcium balance (i.e. net calcium retention) is required throughout growth, particularly during the first 2 years of life and during puberty and adolescence. These age groups therefore constitute populations at risk for calcium deficiency, as do pregnant women (especially in the last trimester), lactating women, postmenopausal women, and, possibly, elderly men.

4.6 Recommendations for calcium requirements

4.6.1 Infants

In the first 2 years of life, the daily calcium increment in the skeleton is about 100 mg (2.5 mmol) (51). The urinary calcium of infants is about 10 mg/day (0.25 mmol/day) and is virtually independent of intake (52–56);

insensible losses are likely to be similar in magnitude. Therefore, infants need to absorb some 120 mg (3 mmol) of calcium daily to allow for normal growth. What this represents in dietary terms can be calculated from calcium absorption studies in newborn infants (52–56). These studies suggest that the absorption of calcium from cow milk by infants is about 0.5 SD above the normal adult slope and from human milk is more than 1 SD above the normal adult slope. If this information is correct, different recommendations need to be made for infants depending on milk source. With human milk, an absorption of 120 mg (3 mmol) of calcium requires a mean intake of 240 mg (6 mmol) (Figure 4.6) and a recommended intake of say 300 mg (7.5 mmol), which is close to the amount provided in the average daily milk production of 750 ml. With cow milk, calcium intake needs to be about 300 mg (7.5 mmol) to meet the requirement (Figure 4.6) and the recommended intake 400 mg (10 mmol) (Table 4.2).

4.6.2 Children

The accumulation of whole-body calcium with skeletal growth is illustrated in Figure 4.1. It rises from about 120 g (3 mol) at age 2 years to 400 g (10 mol)

FIGURE 4.6
Calcium intakes required to provide the absorbed calcium necessary to meet calcium requirements at different stages in the lifecycle

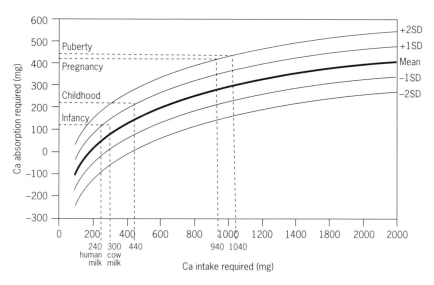

The solid lines represent the mean and range of calcium absorption as a function of calcium intake derived from the equation in Figure 4.3. The interrupted lines represent the estimated calcium absorption requirements and the corresponding intake requirements based on North American and western European data.
Source: based on data from references (32–39).

TABLE 4.2
Recommended calcium allowances based on North American and western European data

Group	Recommended intake (mg/day)
Infants and children	
0–6 months	
Human milk	300
Cow milk	400
7–12 months	400
1–3 years	500
4–6 years	600
7–9 years	700
Adolescents	
10–18 years	1300[a]
Adults	
Females	
19 years to menopause	1000
Postmenopause	1300
Males	
19–65 years	1000
65+ years	1300
Pregnant women (last trimester)	1200
Lactating women	1000

[a] Particularly during the growth spurt.

at age 9 years. These values can be converted into a daily rate of calcium accumulation from ages 2 to 9 years of about 120 mg (3 mmol), which is very similar to the amount calculated by Leitch and Aitken (*57*) from growth analyses. Although urinary calcium must rise with the growth-related rise in glomerular filtration rate, a reasonable estimate of the mean value from ages 2 to 9 years might be 60 mg (1.5 mmol) (*58*). When this is added to a daily skeletal increment of 120 mg (3 mmol) and a dermal loss of perhaps 40 mg (1.0 mmol), the average daily net absorbed calcium needs to be 220 mg (5.5 mmol) during this period. If the net absorption of calcium by children is 1 SD above that of adults, the average daily requirement during this period is about 440 mg (11 mmol) (Figure 4.6) and the average recommended intake is 600 mg (15 mmol)—somewhat lower in the earlier years and somewhat higher in the later years (Table 4.2).

4.6.3 Adolescents

As can be seen in Figure 4.1, a striking increase in the rate of skeletal calcium accretion occurs at puberty—from about ages 10 to 17 years. The peak rate of calcium retention in this period is 300–400 mg (7.5–10 mmol) daily (*57*); it occurs earlier in girls but continues longer in boys. To maintain a value of

300 mg (7.5 mmol) for the skeleton—taking into account 100 mg (2.5 mmol) for urinary calcium (58), and 40 mg (1.0 mmol) for insensible losses—the net absorbed calcium during at least part of this period needs to be 440 mg (11 mmol) daily. Even with the assumption of high calcium absorption (+2 SD), this requires an intake of 1040 mg (26.0 mmol) daily (Figure 4.6) and a recommended intake of 1300 mg (32.5 mmol) during the peak growth phase (Table 4.2). It is difficult to justify any difference between the allowances for boys and girls because, as mentioned above, although the growth spurt starts earlier in girls, it continues longer in boys. This recommended intake (which is close to that derived differently by Matkovic and Heaney [49, 58]) is not achieved by many adolescents even in developed countries (59–61), but the effects of this shortfall on their growth and bone status are unknown.

4.6.4 Adults

As indicated earlier and for the reasons given, the Consultation concluded that the mean apparent calcium requirement of adults in developed countries is about 520 mg (13 mmol) but that this is increased by insensible losses to some 840 mg (21 mmol) (Figure 4.3). This reasoning forms the basis of the recommended intake for adults of 1000 mg (Table 4.2).

4.6.5 Menopausal women

The most important single cause of osteoporosis—at least in developed countries—is probably menopause, which is accompanied by an unequivocal and sustained rise in obligatory urinary calcium of about 30 mg (0.75 mmol) daily (50, 62, 63). Because calcium absorption certainly does not increase at this time, and probably decreases (64, 65), this extra urinary calcium represents a negative calcium balance which is compatible with the average bone loss of about 0.5–1.0% per year after menopause. There is a consensus that these events are associated with an increase in bone resorption but controversy continues about whether this is the primary event, the response to an increased calcium demand, or both. The results of calcium trials are clearly relevant. Before 1997, there had been 20 prospective trials of calcium supplementation in 857 postmenopausal women and 625 control subjects; these trials collectively showed a highly significant suppression of bone loss through calcium supplementation (65). Another meta-analysis covering similar numbers showed that calcium supplementation significantly enhanced the effect of estrogen on bone (66). It is therefore logical to recommend sufficient additional calcium after menopause to cover at least the extra obligatory loss of calcium in the urine. The additional dietary calcium needed to meet an increased urinary loss of 30 mg (0.75 mmol) is 260 mg/day (6.5 mmol/day)

(Figure 4.3), which raises the daily requirement from 840 mg (21 mmol) to 1100 mg (27.5 mmol) and the recommended intake from 1000 to 1300 mg/day (25 to 32.5 mmol/day) (Table 4.2), which is a little higher than that recommended by Canada and the United States (*16*) (see section 4.8).

4.6.6 Ageing adults

Not enough is known about bone and calcium metabolism during ageing to enable calculation of the calcium requirements of older men and women with any confidence. Calcium absorption tends to decrease with age in both sexes (*67–69*) but whereas there is strong evidence that calcium requirement rises during menopause, corresponding evidence about ageing men is less convincing (*32, 36*). Nonetheless, as a precaution an extra allowance of 300 mg/day (7.5 mmol/day) for men over 65 years to raise their requirement to that of postmenopausal women was proposed (Table 4.2).

4.6.7 Pregnant women

The calcium content of the newborn infant is about 24 g (600 mmol). Most of this calcium is laid down in the last trimester of pregnancy, during which the fetus retains about 240 mg (6 mmol) of calcium daily (*51*). There is some evidence that pregnancy is associated with an increase in calcium absorption (associated with a rise in the plasma 1,25-$(OH)_2$ D level) (*70–72*). For a maternal urinary calcium of 120 mg (3 mmol) and a maternal skin loss of 60 mg (1.5 mmol), the absorbed calcium should be 420 mg (10.5 mmol) daily. To achieve this optimal calcium absorption, the corresponding calcium intake would need to be at least 940 mg (23.5 mmol) (Figure 4.6). The recommended nutrient intake was thus set at 1200 mg (30 mmol) (Table 4.2), which is similar to that proposed by Canada and the United States (*16*) (see section 4.8).

4.6.8 Lactating women

The calcium content of human milk is about 36 mg/100 ml (9 mmol/l) (*18*). A lactating woman produces about 750 ml of milk daily, which represents about 280 mg (7.0 mmol) of calcium. For a maternal urinary calcium of 100 mg/day (2.5 mmol/day) and a maternal skin loss of 60 mg/day (1.5 mmol/day), the required absorption is 440 mg/day (11 mmol/day)—the same as at puberty. If calcium absorption efficiency is maximal (i.e. 2 SD above the normal adult mean)—possibly because of the effect of prolactin on the production of 1,25-$(OH)_2$D (*72*)—the requirement would be about 1040 mg (26.0 mmol) and the recommended intake would be about 1300 mg (32.5 mmol). However, although it is known that bone is lost during lactation and restored after weaning (73, 74), early reports that this bone loss could be prevented by calcium supplementation (75) have not been confirmed in controlled studies (76–78).

The prevailing view now is that calcium absorption does not increase, and may even decrease, during lactation. It is increasingly thought that lactational bone loss is not a nutritional problem but may be due to the parathyroid hormone-related peptide secreted by the breast (79) and is therefore beyond the control of dietary calcium. In view of this uncertainty, the present recommendations do not include any extra calcium allowance during lactation (Table 4.2); any risk to adolescent mothers is covered by the general recommendation of 1300 mg for adolescents.

4.7 Upper limits

Because of the inverse relationship between fractional calcium absorption and calcium intake (Figure 4.4), a calcium supplement of 1000 mg (25 mmol) in conjunction with a Western-style diet only increases urinary calcium by about 60 mg (1.5 mmol). Urinary calcium also rises very slowly with intake (slope of 5–10%) and the risk of kidney stones from dietary hypercalciuria must therefore be negligible. In fact, it has been suggested that dietary calcium may protect against renal calculi because it binds dietary oxalate and reduces oxalate excretion (80, 81). Toxic effects of a high calcium intake have only been described when the calcium is given as the carbonate form in very high doses; this toxicity is caused as much by the alkali as by the calcium and is due to precipitation of calcium salts in renal tissue (milk-alkali syndrome) (82). However, in practice an upper limit on calcium intake of 3 g (75 mmol) is recommended.

4.8 Comparisons with other recommendations

The current recommendations of the European Union, Australia, Canada/ United States United States, and the United Kingdom are given in Table 4.3. The present Expert Consultation's recommendations for adults are very close to those of Canada and the United States but higher than those of Australia and the United Kingdom, which do not take into account insensible losses, and higher than those of the European Union, which assume 30% absorption of dietary calcium. The British and European values make no allowance for ageing or menopause. Recommendations for other high-risk groups are very similar in all five sets of recommendations except for the rather low allowance for infants by Canada and the United States. Nonetheless, despite this broad measure of agreement among developed countries, the Consultation had some

TABLE 4.3
Current calcium intake recommendations (mg/day)

Group	Australia 1991[a]	United Kingdom 1991[b]	European Union 1993[c]	Canada and United States 1997[d]
Pregnancy (last trimester)	1100	700	700	1000–1300
Lactation	1200	1250	1200	1000–1300
Infancy	300 (human milk)	525	400	210–270
	500 (cow milk)			
Childhood	530–800	350–550	400–550	500–800
Puberty and adolescence				
Boys	1000–1200	1000	1000	1300
Girls	800–1000	800	800	1300
Maturity				
Males	800	700	700	1000
Females	800	700	700	1000
Later life				
Males >65 years	800	700	700	1200
Postmenopausal women	1000	700	700	1200

[a] Recommended dietary intake (15).
[b] Reference nutrient intake (17).
[c] Population reference intake (14).
[d] Adequate intake (16).

misgivings about the application of these recommendations—all of which rely ultimately on data from white populations in developed countries—to developing countries where the requirements may be different for ethnic, dietary or geographical reasons.

4.9 Ethnic and environmental variations in the prevalence of osteoporosis

Variations in the worldwide prevalence of osteoporosis can be considered at several levels. The first level is genetic: is there a genetic (ethnic) difference in the prevalence of osteoporosis between racial groups within a given society? The second level is geographic: is there a difference in the prevalence of osteoporosis between countries at different latitudes? The third level might be termed cultural and involves lifestyle in general, and diet in particular. At each of these levels, the prevalence of osteoporosis can in theory be determined in at least two ways: from the distribution of bone density within the population and from the prevalence of fractures, notably hip fractures. In practice, hip fracture data (or mortality from falls in elderly people which has been used as a surrogate [83]) are more readily available than bone densitometry data, which are only slowly emerging from the developing world.

4.9.1 Ethnicity

Comparisons between racial groups within countries suggest substantial racial differences in the prevalence of osteoporosis. This was probably first noted by Trotter (*84*) when she showed that bone density (weight/volume) was significantly higher in skeletons from black than from Caucasian subjects in the United States. It was later shown that hip fracture rates were lower in blacks than Caucasians in South Africa (*85*) and the United States (*86*). These observations have been repeatedly confirmed (*87, 88*) without being fully explained but appear to be genetic in origin because the better bone status of Afro-Americans compared with Caucasians in the United States is already apparent in childhood (*89*) and cannot be accounted for by differences in body size (*90*). Nor can the difference in fracture rates between these two groups be explained by differences in hip axis length (*90*); it seems to be largely or wholly due to differences in bone density. Similarly, comparisons between Caucasians and Samoans in New Zealand (*91*) have shown the latter to have the higher bone densities. Asians have lower bone densities than Caucasians in New Zealand but these differences are largely accounted for by differences in body size (*91*). In the United States, fracture rates are lower among Asians than among Caucasians but this may be accounted for by their shorter hip axis length (*92*) and their lower incidence of falls (*93*). Bone density is generally lower in Asians than Caucasians within the United States (*94*) but again, this is largely accounted for by differences in body size (*95*). There are also lower hip fracture rates for Hispanics, Chinese, Japanese and Koreans than Caucasians living in the United States (*96, 97*). The conclusion must be that there are probably genetic factors influencing the prevalence of osteoporosis and fractures, but it is impossible to exclude the role of differences in diet and lifestyle between ethnic communities within a country.

4.9.2 Geography

There are wide geographical variations in hip fracture incidence which cannot be accounted for by ethnicity. In the United States, the age-adjusted incidence of hip fracture in Caucasian women aged 65 years and over varied with geography but was high everywhere—ranging from 700 to 1000 per 100 000 per year (*98*). Within Europe, the age-adjusted hip fracture rates ranged from 280 to 730 per 100 000 women in one study (*99*) and from 419 to 545 per 100 000 in another (*96*) in which the comparable rates were 52.9 in Chile, 94.0 in Venezuela, and 247 in Hong Kong per 100 000 per year. In another study (*100*), age-adjusted hip fracture rates in women in 12 European countries ranged from 46 per 100 000 per year in Poland to 504 per 100 000 in Sweden, with a marked positive gradient from south to north and from poor to rich. In Chinese populations, the hip fracture rate is much lower in Beijing (87–97 per 100 000) than in Hong Kong (181–353 per 100 000) (*101*) where the standard of living is higher. Thus, there are marked geographic variations in hip fracture rates within the same ethnic groups; this may be due to differences in diet but may also be due to variations in the supply of vitamin D from sunlight, both of which are discussed below.

4.9.3 Culture and diet

It can be concluded from the discussion above that there are probably ethnic and geographic differences in hip fracture rates. Intakes of calcium have been known for many years to vary greatly from one country to another, as is clearly shown in FAO food balance sheets (Table 4.1). Until fairly recently, it was widely assumed that low calcium intakes had no injurious consequences. This view of the global situation underpinned the very conservative adequate calcium intakes recommended by FAO/WHO in 1962 (*2*). At that time, osteoporosis was still regarded as a bone matrix disorder and the possibility that it could be caused by calcium deficiency was barely considered.

As previously stated, the paradigm has since changed. Calcium deficiency is taken more seriously now and the apparent discrepancy between calcium intake and bone status worldwide has attracted considerable attention. However, with the exception of calcium deficiency rickets reported from Nigeria (*102*), no satisfactory explanation has been found for the apparently low prevalence of osteoporosis in developing countries on low calcium intakes; on international comparisons on a larger scale, it is very difficult to separate genetic from environmental factors. Nonetheless, certain patterns have emerged which are likely to have biological significance, the most striking of which is the positive correlation between hip fracture rates and standard of living first noted by Hegsted when he observed that osteoporosis was largely a disease of affluent industrialized cultures (*103*). He based this conclusion on a previously published review of hip fracture rates in 10 countries (*104*) that strongly suggested a correlation between hip fracture rate and affluence. Another review of 19 regions and racial groups (*105*) confirmed this by showing a gradient of age- and sex-adjusted hip fracture rates from 31 per 100 000 in South African Bantu to 968 per 100 000 in Norway. In the analysis of hip fracture rates in Beijing and Hong Kong referred to above (*101*), it was noted that the rates in both cities were much lower than in the United States.

Many other publications point to the same conclusion—that hip fracture prevalence (and by implication osteoporosis) is related to affluence and, consequently, to animal protein intake, as Hegsted pointed out, but also, para-doxically, to calcium intake because of the strong correlation between calcium and protein intakes within and between societies. This could be explained if protein actually increased calcium requirement (see section 4.10).

4.9.4 The calcium paradox

The paradox that hip fracture rates are higher in developed countries where calcium intake is high than in developing countries where calcium intake is low probably has more than one explanation. Hegsted (*103*) was probably the first to note the close relationship between calcium and protein intakes across the world (which is also true within countries [*63*]) and to hint at, but dismiss, the possibility that the adverse effect of high protein intakes might outweigh the positive effect of high calcium intakes on calcium balance. He may have erred in dismissing this possibility since fracture risk has recently been shown to be a function of protein intake in North American women (*106*). There is also suggestive evidence that hip fracture rates (as judged by mortality from falls in elderly people across the world) are a func-tion of protein intake, national income, and latitude (*107*). The latter associ-ation is particularly interesting in view of the strong evidence of vitamin D deficiency in hip fracture patients in the developed world (*108–114*) and the successful prevention of such fractures with small doses of vitamin D and calcium (*115, 116*) (see Chapter 3). It is therefore possible that hip fracture rates may be related to protein intake, vitamin D status, or both, and that either of these factors could explain the calcium paradox.

4.10 Nutritional factors affecting calcium requirement

The calcium requirements proposed in Table 4.2 are based on data from devel-oped countries (notably Norway and the United States) and can only be applied with any confidence to countries and populations with similar dietary cultures. Other dietary cultures may entail different calcium requirements and call for different recommendations. In particular, the removal or addition of any nutrient that affects calcium absorption or excretion must have an effect on calcium requirement. Two such nutrients are sodium and animal protein, both of which increase urinary calcium and therefore must be presumed to increase calcium requirement. A third candidate is vitamin D because of its role in calcium homeostasis and calcium absorption.

4.10.1 Sodium

It has been known at least since 1961 that urinary calcium is related to urinary sodium (*117*) and that sodium administration raises calcium excretion, presumably because sodium competes with calcium for reabsorption in the renal tubules. Regarding the quantitative relationships between the renal handling of sodium and calcium, the filtered load of sodium is about 100 times that of calcium (in molar terms) but the clearance of these two elements is similar at about 1 ml/min, which yields about 99% reabsorption and 1% excretion for both (118). However, these are approximations which conceal the close dependence of urinary sodium on sodium intake and the weaker dependence of urinary calcium on calcium intake. It is an empirical fact that urinary sodium and calcium are significantly related in normal and hypercalciuric subjects on freely chosen diets (119–122). The slope of urinary calcium on sodium varies in published work from about 0.6% to 1.2% (in molar terms); a representative figure is about 1%, that is, 100 mmol of sodium (2.3 g) takes out about 1 mmol (40 mg) of calcium (63, 120). The biological significance of this relationship is supported by the accelerated osteoporosis induced by feeding salt to rats on low-calcium diets (123) and the effects of salt administration and salt restriction on markers of bone resorption in postmenopausal women (124, 125). Because salt restriction lowers urinary calcium, it is likely also to lower calcium requirement and, conversely, salt feeding is likely to increase calcium requirement. This is illustrated in Figure 4.7, which shows that lowering sodium intake by 100 mmol (2.3 g) from, for example, 150 to 50 mmol (3.45 to 1.15 g), reduces the theoretical calcium requirement from 840 mg (21 mmol) to 600 mg (15 mmol). However, the implications of this for global calcium requirements cannot be computed because information on sodium intake is available from only a very few countries (126).

4.10.2 Protein

The positive effect of dietary protein—particularly animal protein—on urinary calcium has also been known since at least the 1960s (127–129). One study found that 0.85 mg of calcium was lost for each gram of protein in the diet (130). A meta-analysis of 16 studies in 154 adult humans on protein intakes of up to 200 g found that 1.2 mg of calcium was lost in the urine for every 1-g rise in dietary protein (131). A small but more focused study showed a rise of 40 mg in urinary calcium when dietary animal protein was raised from 40 to 80 g (i.e. within the physiological range) (132). This ratio of urinary calcium to dietary protein (1 mg to 1 g) was adopted by the Expert Consultation as a representative value. This means that a 40-g reduction in animal protein intake from 60 to 20 g (roughly the difference between the developed and developing regions shown in Table 4.1) would reduce calcium requirement by the same amount as a 2.3-g reduction in dietary sodium (i.e. from 840 to 600 mg) (Figure 4.7).

FIGURE 4.7
The effect of varying protein or sodium intake on theoretical calcium requirement

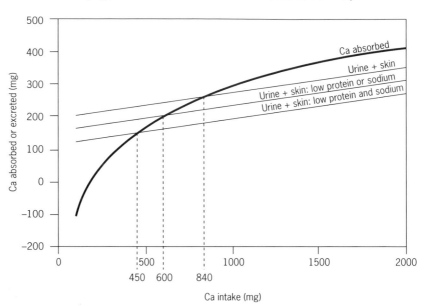

With a Western-style diet, absorbed calcium matches urinary and skin calcium at an intake of 840 mg (see Figure 4.3). Reducing animal protein intakes by 40 g reduces the intercept value and thus the requirement to 600 mg. Reducing both sodium and protein reduces the intercept value to 450 mg.
Source: based on data from references (*32–39*).

How animal protein exerts its effect on calcium excretion is not fully understood. A rise in glomerular filtration rate in response to protein has been suggested as one factor (*128*) but this is unlikely to be important in the steady state. The major mechanisms are thought to be the effect of the acid load contained in animal proteins and the complexing of calcium in the renal tubules by sulphate and phosphate ions released by protein metabolism (*133*, *134*). Urinary calcium is significantly related to urinary phosphate (as well as to urinary sodium), particularly in subjects on restricted calcium intakes or in the fasting state, and most of the phosphorus in the urine of people on Western-style diets comes from animal protein in the diet (*63*). Thus, the empirical observation that an intake of 1 g of protein results in 1 mg of calcium in the urine agrees very well with the phosphorus content of animal protein (about 1% by weight) and the observed relationship between calcium and phosphate in the urine (*63*). Similar considerations apply to urinary sulphate but it is probably less important than the phosphate ion because the association constant for calcium sulphate is lower than that for calcium phosphate (*135*).

4.10.3 Vitamin D

One of the first observations made on vitamin D after it had been identified in 1918 (*136*) was that it promoted calcium absorption (*137*). It is now well established that vitamin D (synthesized in the skin under the influence of sunlight) is converted to 25-OH-D in the liver and then to 1,25-$(OH)_2$D in the kidneys and that the latter metabolite controls calcium absorption (*21*) (see Chapter 3). However, plasma 25-OH-D closely reflects vitamin D nutritional status and because it is the substrate for the renal enzyme which produces 1,25-$(OH)_2$D, it could have an indirect effect on calcium absorption. The plasma level of 1,25-$(OH)_2$D is principally regulated by gene expression of 1-α-hydroxylase (CYP1α) and not by the plasma concentration of 25-OH-D. This has been seen consistently in animal studies, and the high calcium absorption (*138*) and high plasma concentrations of 1,25-$(OH)_2$D (*139*) observed in Gambian mothers are consistent with this type of adaptation. However, vitamin D synthesis may be compromised at high latitudes, to the degree that 25-OH-D levels may not be sufficient to sustain adequate 1,25-$(OH)_2$D levels and efficient intestinal calcium absorption—although this theory remains unproved.

Regardless of the mechanism of compromised vitamin D homeostasis, the differences in calcium absorption efficiency have a major effect on theoretical calcium requirement, as illustrated in Figure 4.8, which shows that an increase in calcium absorption of as little as 10% reduces the intercept of excreted and absorbed calcium (and therefore calcium requirement) from 840 to 680 mg. The figure also shows the great increase in calcium intake that is required as a result of any impairment of calcium absorption.

4.10.4 Implications

In light of the major reduction in theoretical calcium requirement which follows animal protein restriction, an attempt has been made to show (in Table 4.4) how the calcium allowances recommended in Table 4.2 could be modified to apply to countries where the animal protein intake per capita is around 20–40 g rather than around the 60–80 g typical of developed countries. These hypothetical allowances take into account the need to protect children, in whom skeletal needs are much more important determinants of calcium requirement than are urinary losses and in whom calcium supplementation is likely to have a beneficial effect, for example, as has been reported in the

FIGURE 4.8
The effect of varying calcium absorptive efficiency on theoretical calcium requirement

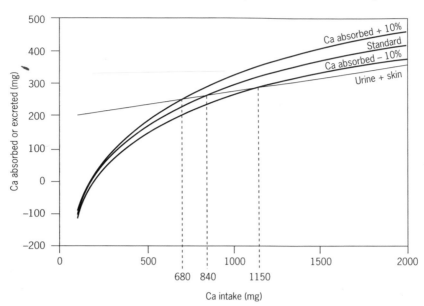

At normal calcium absorption, the intercept of urinary plus skin calcium meets absorbed calcium at an intake of 840 mg (see Figure 4.3). A 10% reduction in calcium absorption raises the intercept value and requirement to 1150 mg and a 10% increase in calcium absorption reduces it to 680 mg.
Source: based on data from references (*32–39*).

Gambia (*140*). However, adjustment for animal protein intake has a major effect on the recommended calcium allowances for adults as Table 4.4 shows. It also brings the allowances nearer to what the actual calcium intakes are in many parts of the world.

If sodium intakes were also lower in developing than in developed countries or urinary sodium were reduced for other reasons, such as increased sweat losses, the calcium requirement might be even lower, for example, 450 mg (Figure 4.7). This would be reduced still further by any increase in calcium absorption as illustrated in Figure 4.8, whether resulting from better vitamin D status because of increased sunlight exposure or for other reasons. Because the increase in calcium absorption in Gambian compared with British women is much more than 10% (*138*), this is likely to have a major—although not at present calculable—effect on calcium requirement there. However, the adjusted bone mineral density in Gambian women is reported to be some 20% lower in the spine (but not in the forearm) than in British women (*141*), a finding which emphasizes the need for more data from developing countries.

TABLE 4.4
**Theoretical calcium allowances based on an animal
protein intake of 20–40 g**

Group	Recommended intake (mg/day)
Infants and children	
0–6 months	
Human milk	300
Cow milk	400
7–12 months	450
1–3 years	500
4–6 years	550
7–9 years	700
Adolescents	
10–18 years	1000[a]
Adults	
Females	
19 years to menopause	750
Postmenopause	800
Males	
19–65 years	750
65+ years	800
Pregnant women (last trimester)	800
Lactating women	750

[a] Particularly during the growth spurt.

4.11 Conclusions

Calcium is an essential nutrient that plays a vital role in neuromuscular function, many enzyme-mediated processes and blood clotting, as well as providing rigidity to the skeleton by virtue of its phosphate salts. Its non-structural roles require the strict maintenance of ionized calcium concentration in tissue fluids at the expense of the skeleton if necessary and it is therefore the skeleton which is at risk if the supply of calcium falls short of the requirement.

Calcium requirements are determined essentially by the relationship between absorptive efficiency and excretory rate—excretion being through the bowel, kidneys, skin, hair, and nails. In adults, the rate of calcium absorption from the gastrointestinal tract needs to match the rate of all losses from the body if the skeleton is to be preserved; in children and adolescents, an extra input is needed to cover the requirements of skeletal growth.

Compared with that of other minerals, calcium economy is relatively inefficient. On most intakes, only about 25–30% of dietary calcium is effectively absorbed and obligatory calcium losses are relatively large. Dietary intake of calcium has to be large enough to ensure that the rate of absorption matches obligatory losses if skeletal damage is to be avoided. The system is subject to considerable interindividual variation in both calcium absorption and excretion for reasons that are not fully understood but which include vitamin D status, sodium and protein intake, age, and menopausal status in women. Although it needs to be emphasized that calcium deficiency and negative calcium balance must sooner or later lead to osteoporosis, this does not mean that all osteoporosis can be attributed to calcium deficiency. On the contrary, there may be more osteoporosis in the world from other causes. Nonetheless, it would probably be agreed that any form of osteoporosis must inevitably be aggravated by negative external calcium balance. Such negative balance—even for short periods—is prejudicial because it takes so much longer to rebuild bone than to destroy it. Bone that is lost, even during short periods of calcium deficiency, is only slowly replaced when adequate amounts of calcium become available.

In seeking to define advisable calcium intakes on the basis of physiological studies and clinical observations, nutrition authorities have to rely largely on data from developed countries living at relatively high latitudes. Although it is now possible to formulate recommendations that are appropriate to different stages in the lifecycle of the populations of these countries, extrapolation from these figures to other cultures and nutritional environments can only be tentative and must rely on what is known of nutritional and environmental effects on calcium absorption and excretion. Nonetheless, an attempt in this direction has been made, in full knowledge that the speculative calculations may be incorrect because of other variables not yet identified.

No reference has been made in this discussion to the possible beneficial effects of calcium in the prevention or treatment of pre-eclampsia (*142*), colon cancer (*143*), or hypertension (*144*) and no attempt has been made to use these conditions as end-points on which to base calcium intakes. In each of the above conditions, epidemiological data suggest an association with calcium intake, and experimentation with increased calcium intakes has now been tried. In each case the results have been disappointing, inconclusive, or negative (*145–147*) and have stirred controversy (*148–150*). Because there is no clear consensus about optimal calcium intake for prevention or treatment of these conditions and also no clear mechanistic ideas on how dietary calcium intakes affect them, it is not possible to allow for the effect of health outcomes in these areas on the present calcium recommendations. However, although the anecdotal information and positive effects of calcium observed in these three conditions cannot influence current recommendations, they do suggest that generous calcium allowances may confer other benefits besides protecting the skeleton. Similarly, no reference has been made to the effects of physical activity, alcohol, smoking, or other known risk factors on bone status because the effects of these variables on calcium requirement are beyond the realm of simple calculation.

4.12 Recommendations for future research

Future research should include the following:

- to recognize that there is an overwhelming need for more studies of calcium metabolism in developing countries;
- to investigate further the cultural, geographical, and genetic bases for differences in calcium intakes in different groups in developing countries;
- to establish the validity of different recommended calcium intakes based on animal protein and sodium intakes;
- to clarify the role of dietary calcium in pre-eclampsia, colon cancer, and hypertension;
- to study the relationship between latitude, sun exposure, and synthesis of vitamin D and intestinal calcium absorption in different geographical locations.

References

1. *Handbook on human nutritional requirements.* Rome, Food and Agriculture Organization of the United Nations, 1974.
2. FAO/WHO Expert Group. *Calcium requirements. Report of an FAO/WHO Expert Group.* Rome, Food and Agriculture Organization of the United Nations, 1962 (FAO Nutrition Meetings Report Series, No. 30).
3. Albright F, Reifenstein EC. *The parathyroid glands and metabolic bone disease.* Baltimore, MA, Williams & Wilkins, 1948.
4. Nordin BEC. Osteomalacia, osteoporosis and calcium deficiency. *Clinical Orthopaedics and Related Research*, 1960, 17:235–258.
5. Young MM, Nordin BEC. Effects of natural and artificial menopause on plasma and urinary calcium and phosphorus. *Lancet*, 1967, 2:118–120.
6. Stepan JJ et al. Bone loss and biochemical indices of bone remodeling in surgically induced postmenopausal women. *Bone*, 1987, 8:279–284.
7. Kelly PJ et al. Age and menopause-related changes in indices of bone turnover. *Journal of Clinical Endocrinology and Metabolism*, 1989, 69:1160–1165.
8. Christiansen C et al. Pathophysiological mechanisms of estrogen effect on bone metabolism. Dose–response relationships in early postmenopausal women. *Journal of Clinical Endocrinology and Metabolism*, 1982, 55: 1124–1130.
9. Parfitt AM. Osteomalacia and related disorders. In: Avioli LV, Krane SM, eds. *Metabolic bone disease and clinically related disorders*, 2nd ed. Philadelphia, PA, WB Saunders, 1990:329–396.
10. Need AG. Corticosteroid hormones. In: Nordin BEC, Need AG, Morris HA, eds. *Metabolic bone and stone disease*, 3rd ed. Edinburgh, Churchill Livingstone, 1993:43–62.
11. Horowitz M. Osteoporosis in men. In: Nordin BEC, Need AG, Morris HA, eds. *Metabolic bone and stone disease*, 3rd ed. Edinburgh, Churchill Livingstone, 1993:70–78.
12. Lips P et al. Histomorphometric profile and vitamin D status in patients with

femoral neck fracture. *Metabolic Bone Disease and Related Research*, 1982, 4:85–93.

13. Truswell S. Recommended dietary intakes around the world. Report by Committee 1/5 of the International Union of Nutritional Sciences. *Nutrition Abstracts and Reviews*, 1983, 53:939–1119.

14. Scientific Committee for Food. *Nutrient and energy intakes for the European Community*. Luxembourg, Office for Official Publications of the European Communities, 1993 (Reports of the Scientific Committee for Food, Thirty-first Series).

15. *Recommended dietary intakes for use in Australia*. Canberra, National Health and Medical Research Council, 1991.

16. Food and Nutrition Board. *Dietary reference intakes for calcium, phosphorus, magnesium, vitamin D, and fluoride*. Washington, DC, National Academy Press, 1997.

17. Department of Health. *Dietary reference values for food energy and nutrients for the United Kingdom. Report of the Panel on Dietary Reference Values of the Committee on Medical Aspects of Food Policy*. London, Her Majesty's Stationery Office, 1991.

18. Nordin BEC. Nutritional considerations. In: Nordin BEC, ed. *Calcium, phosphate and magnesium metabolism*. Edinburgh, Churchill Livingstone, 1976:1–35.

19. Robertson WG, Marshall RW. Ionized calcium in body fluids. *Critical Reviews in Clinical Laboratory Sciences*, 1981, 15:85–125.

20. Brown EM, Hebert SC. Calcium-receptor-regulated parathyroid and renal function. *Bone*, 1997, 20:303–309.

21. Jones G, Strugnell SA, DeLuca HF. Current understanding of the molecular actions of vitamin D. *Physiological Reviews*, 1998, 78:1193–1231.

22. Wu DD et al. Regional patterns of bone loss and altered bone remodeling in response to calcium deprivation in laboratory rabbits. *Calcified Tissue International*, 1990, 47:18–23.

23. *Production yearbook, Vol. 44, 1990*. Rome, Food and Agriculture Organization of the United Nations, 1991.

24. Ireland P, Fordtran JS. Effect of dietary calcium and age on jejunal calcium absorption in humans studied by intestinal perfusion. *Journal of Clinical Investigation*, 1973, 52:2672–2681.

25. Heaney RP, Saville PD, Recker RR. Calcium absorption as a function of calcium intake. *Journal of Laboratory and Clinical Medicine*, 1975, 85: 881–890.

26. Wilkinson R. Absorption of calcium, phosphorus and magnesium. In: Nordin BEC, ed. *Calcium, phosphate and magnesium metabolism*. Edinburgh, Churchill Livingstone, 1976:36–112.

27. Marshall DH. Calcium and phosphate kinetics. In: Nordin BEC, ed. *Calcium, phosphate and magnesium metabolism*. Edinburgh, Churchill Livingstone, 1976:257–297.

28. Heaney RP, Skillman TG. Secretion and excretion of calcium by the human gastrointestinal tract. *Journal of Laboratory and Clinical Medicine*, 1964, 64:29–41.

29. Nordin BEC, Horsman A, Aaron J. Diagnostic procedures. In: Nordin BEC, ed. *Calcium, phosphate and magnesium metabolism*. Edinburgh, Churchill Livingstone, 1976:469–524.

30. Marshall DH, Nordin BEC, Speed R. Calcium, phosphorus and magnesium requirement. *Proceedings of the Nutrition Society*, 1976, 35:163–173.
31. Nordin BEC, Marshall DH. Dietary requirements for calcium. In: Nordin BEC, ed. *Calcium in human biology.* Berlin, Springer-Verlag, 1988, 447–471.
32. Bogdonoff MD, Shock NW, Nichols MP. Calcium, phosphorus, nitrogen, and potassium balance studies in the aged male. *Journal of Gerontology*, 1953, 8:272–288.
33. Clarkson EM et al. The effect of a high intake of calcium and phosphate in normal subjects and patients with chronic renal failure. *Clinical Science*, 1970, 39:693–704.
34. Johnston FA, McMillan TJ, Derby-Falconer G. Calcium retained by young women before and after adding spinach to the diet. *Journal of the American Dietetic Association*, 1952, 28:933–938.
35. Malm OJ. Calcium requirement and adaptation in adult men. *Scandinavian Journal of Clinical Laboratory Investigation*, 1958, 10(Suppl. 36):S1–S289.
36. Owen EC, Irving JT, Lyall A. The calcium requirements of older male subjects with special reference to the genesis of senile osteoporosis. *Acta Medica Scandinavica*, 1940, 103:235–250.
37. Steggerda FR, Mitchell HH. The calcium requirement of adult man and the utilization of the calcium in milk and in calcium gluconate. *Journal of Nutrition*, 1939, 17:253–262.
38. Steggerda FR, Mitchell HH. Further experiments on the calcium requirement of adult man and the utilization of the calcium in milk. *Journal of Nutrition*, 1941, 21:577–588.
39. Steggerda FR, Mitchell HH. Variability in the calcium metabolism and calcium requirements of adult human subjects. *Journal of Nutrition*, 1946, 31:407–422.
40. Gallagher JC et al. Intestinal calcium absorption and serum vitamin D metabolites in normal subjects and osteoporotic patients. *Journal of Clinical Investigation*, 1979, 64:729–736.
41. Wishart JM et al. Relations between calcium intake, calcitriol, polymorphisms of the vitamin D receptor gene, and calcium absorption in premenopausal women. *American Journal of Clinical Nutrition*, 1997, 65:798–802.
42. MacFadyen IJ et al. Effect of variation in dietary calcium on plasma concentration and urinary excretion of calcium. *British Medical Journal*, 1965, 1:161–164.
43. Heaney RP, Recker RR, Ryan RA. Urinary calcium in perimenopausal women: normative values. *Osteoporosis International*, 1999, 9:13–18.
44. Charles P et al. Calcium metabolism evaluated by ^{47}Ca kinetics: estimation of dermal calcium loss. *Clinical Science*, 1983, 65:415–422.
45. Hasling C et al. Calcium metabolism in postmenopausal osteoporosis: the influence of dietary calcium and net absorbed calcium. *Journal of Bone and Mineral Research*, 1990, 5:939–946.
46. Mitchell HH, Curzon EG. The dietary requirement of calcium and its significance. *Actualités scientifiques et industrielles, volume 771 (nutrition)*. Paris, Hermann & Cie, 1939.
47. Hegsted DM, Moscoso I, Collazos CHC. Study of minimum calcium requirements by adult men. *Journal of Nutrition*, 1952, 46:181–201.
48. Heaney RP, Recker RR, Saville PD. Menopausal changes in calcium balance performance. *Journal of Laboratory and Clinical Medicine*, 1978, 92:953–963.

49. Matkovic V, Heaney RP. Calcium balance during human growth: evidence for threshold behavior. *American Journal of Clinical Nutrition*, 1992, 55:992–996.

50. Nordin BEC et al. Biochemical variables in pre- and postmenopausal women: reconciling the calcium and estrogen hypotheses. *Osteoporosis International*, 1999, 9:351–357.

51. American Academy of Pediatrics Committee on Nutrition. Calcium requirements in infancy and childhood. *Pediatrics*, 1978, 62:826–832.

52. Williams ML et al. Calcium and fat absorption in neonatal period. *American Journal of Clinical Nutrition*, 1970, 23:1322–1330.

53. Hanna FM, Navarrete DA, Hsu FA. Calcium-fatty acid absorption in term infants fed human milk and prepared formulas simulating human milk. *Pediatrics*, 1970, 45:216–224.

54. Widdowson EM. Absorption and excretion of fat, nitrogen, and minerals from "filled" milks by babies one week old. *Lancet*, 1965, 2: 1099–1105.

55. Shaw JCL. Evidence for defective skeletal mineralization in low birthweight infants: the absorption of calcium and fat. *Pediatrics*, 1976, 57:16–25.

56. Widdowson EM et al. Effect of giving phosphate supplements to breast-fed babies on absorption and excretion of calcium, strontium, magnesium and phosphorus. *The Lancet*, 1963, 2:1250–1251.

57. Leitch I, Aitken FC. The estimation of calcium requirements: a re-examination. *Nutrition Abstracts and Reviews*, 1959, 29:393–411.

58. Matkovic V. Calcium metabolism and calcium requirements during skeletal modeling and consolidation of bone mass. *American Journal of Clinical Nutrition*, 1991, 54(Suppl. 1):S245–S260.

59. Abrams SA, Stuff JE. Calcium metabolism in girls: current dietary intakes lead to low rates of calcium absorption and retention during puberty. *American Journal of Clinical Nutrition*, 1994, 60:739–743.

60. Truswell AS, Darnton-Hill I. Food habits of adolescents. *Nutrition Reviews*, 1981, 39:73–88.

61. Marino DD, King JC. Nutritional concerns during adolescence. *Pediatric Clinics of North America*, 1980, 27:125–139.

62. Prince RL et al. The effects of menopause and age in calcitropic hormones: a cross-sectional study of 655 healthy women aged 35 to 90. *Journal of Bone and Mineral Research*, 1995, 10:835–842.

63. Nordin BEC, Polley KJ. Metabolic consequences of the menopause. A cross-sectional, longitudinal, and intervention study on 557 normal post-menopausal women. *Calcified Tissue International*, 1987, 41(Suppl. 1):S1–S59.

64. Heaney RP et al. Calcium absorption in women: relationships to calcium intake, estrogen status, and age. *Journal of Bone and Mineral Research*, 1989, 4:469–475.

65. Nordin BEC. Calcium and osteoporosis. *Nutrition*, 1997, 13:664–686.

66. Nieves JW et al. Calcium potentiates the effect of estrogen and calcitonin on bone mass: review and analysis. *American Journal of Clinical Nutrition*, 1998, 67:18–24.

67. Morris HA et al. Calcium absorption in normal and osteoporotic post-menopausal women. *Calcified Tissue International*, 1991, 49:240–243.

68. Ebeling PR et al. Influence of age on effects of endogenous 1,25-dihydroxy-vitamin D on calcium absorption in normal women. *Calcified Tissue International*, 1994, 55:330–334.

69. Need AG et al. Intestinal calcium absorption in men with spinal osteoporosis. *Clinical Endocrinology*, 1998, 48:163–168.
70. Heaney RP, Skillman TG. Calcium metabolism in normal human pregnancy. *Journal of Clinical Endocrinology and Metabolism*, 1971, 33:661–670.
71. Kent GN et al. The efficiency of intestinal calcium absorption is increased in late pregnancy but not in established lactation. *Calcified Tissue International*, 1991, 48:293–295.
72. Kumar R et al. Elevated 1,25-dihydroxyvitamin D plasma levels in normal human pregnancy and lactation. *Journal of Clinical Investigation*, 1979, 63:342–344.
73. Kent GN et al. Human lactation: forearm trabecular bone loss, increased bone turnover, and renal conservation of calcium and inorganic phosphate with recovery of bone mass following weaning. *Journal of Bone and Mineral Research*, 1990, 5:361–369.
74. López JM et al. Bone turnover and density in healthy women during breastfeeding and after weaning. *Osteoporosis International*, 1996, 6: 153–159.
75. Chan GM et al. Effects of increased dietary calcium intake upon the calcium and bone mineral status of lactating adolescent and adult women. *American Journal of Clinical Nutrition*, 1987, 46:319–323.
76. Prentice A et al. Calcium requirements of lactating Gambian mothers: effects of a calcium supplement on breast-milk calcium concentration, maternal bone mineral content and urinary calcium excretion. *American Journal of Clinical Nutrition*, 1995, 62:58–67.
77. Kalkwarf HJ et al. The effect of calcium supplementation on bone density during lactation and after weaning. *New England Journal of Medicine*, 1997, 337:523–528.
78. Allen LH. Women's dietary calcium requirements are not increased by pregnancy or lactation. *American Journal of Clinical Nutrition*, 1998, 67:591–592.
79. Sowers MF et al. Elevated parathyroid hormone-related peptide associated with lactation and bone density loss. *Journal of the American Medical Association*, 1996, 276:549–554.
80. Curhan GC et al. Comparison of dietary calcium with supplemental calcium and other nutrients as factors affecting the risk for kidney stones in women. *Annals of Internal Medicine*, 1997, 126:497–504.
81. Curhan GC et al. A prospective study of dietary calcium and other nutrients and the risk of symptomatic kidney stones. *New England Journal of Medicine*, 1993, 328:833–838.
82. Burnett CH et al. Hypercalcaemia without hypercalciuria or hypophosphatemia, calcinosis and renal insufficiency. A syndrome following prolonged intake of milk and alkali. *New England Journal of Medicine*, 1949, 240:787–794.
83. Eddy TP. Deaths from domestic falls and fractures. *British Journal of Preventive and Social Medicine*, 1972, 26:173–179.
84. Trotter M, Broman GE, Peterson RR. Densities of bones of white and Negro skeletons. *Journal of Bone and Joint Surgery*, 1960, 42(A):50–58.
85. Solomon L. Osteoporosis and fracture of the femoral neck in the South African Bantu. *Journal of Bone and Joint Surgery*, 1968, 50(B2):2–13.
86. Bollet AJ, Engh G, Parson W. Sex and race incidence of hip fractures. *Archives of Internal Medicine*, 1965, 116:191–194.

87. Cohn SH et al. Comparative skeletal mass and radial bone mineral content in black and white women. *Metabolism*, 1977, 26:171–178.

88. DeSimone DP et al. Influence of body habitus and race on bone mineral density of the midradius, hip, and spine in aging women. *Journal of Bone and Mineral Research*, 1989, 5:827–830.

89. Bell NH et al. Demonstration that bone mass is greater in black than in white children. *Journal of Bone and Mineral Research*, 1991, 6:719–723.

90. Nelson DA et al. Ethnic differences in regional bone density, hip axis length, and lifestyle variables among healthy black and white men. *Journal of Bone and Mineral Research*, 1995, 10:782–787.

91. Cundy T et al. Sources of interracial variation in bone mineral density. *Journal of Bone and Mineral Research*, 1995, 10:368–373.

92. Cummings SR et al. Racial differences in hip axis lengths might explain racial differences in rates of hip fracture. *Osteoporosis International*, 1994, 4: 226–229.

93. Davis JW et al. Incidence rates of falls among Japanese men and women living in Hawaii. *Journal of Clinical Epidemiology*, 1997, 50:589–594.

94. Yano K et al. Bone mineral measurements among middle-aged and elderly Japanese residents in Hawaii. *American Journal of Epidemiology*, 1984, 119:751–764.

95. Ross PD et al. Body size accounts for most differences in bone density between Asian and Caucasian women. *Calcified Tissue International*, 1996, 59:339–343.

96. Silverman SL, Madison RE. Decreased incidence of hip fracture in Hispanics, Asians, and blacks: California hospital discharge data. *American Journal of Public Health*, 1988, 78:1482–1483.

97. Lauderdale D et al. Hip fracture incidence among elderly Asian-American populations. *American Journal of Epidemiology*, 1997, 146:502–509.

98. Villa ML, Nelson L. Race, ethnicity and osteoporosis. In: Marcus R, Feldman D, Kelsey J, eds. *Osteoporosis.* San Diego, CA, Academic Press, 1996:435–447.

99. Bacon WE et al. International comparison of hip fracture rates in 1988–89. *Osteoporosis International*, 1996, 6:69–75.

100. Johnell A et al. The apparent incidence of hip fracture in Europe: a study of national register sources. *Osteoporosis International*, 1992, 2:298–302.

101. Xu L et al. Very low rates of hip fracture in Beijing, People's Republic of China: the Beijing Osteoporosis Project. *American Journal of Epidemiology*, 1996, 144:901–907.

102. Thacher TD et al. A comparison of calcium, vitamin D, or both for nutritional rickets in Nigerian children. *New England Journal of Medicine*, 1999, 341:563–568.

103. Hegsted DM. Calcium and osteoporosis. *Journal of Nutrition*, 1986, 116: 2316–2319.

104. Gallagher JC et al. Epidemiology of fractures of the proximal femur in Rochester, Minnesota. *Clinical Orthopaedics and Related Research*, 1980, 150:163–171.

105. Maggi S et al. Incidence of hip fractures in the elderly. A cross-national analysis. *Osteoporosis International*, 1991, 1:232–241.

106. Feskanich D et al. Protein consumption and bone fractures in women. *American Journal of Epidemiology*, 1996, 143:472–479.

107. Nordin BEC. Calcium in health and disease. *Food, Nutrition and Agriculture*, 1997, 20:13–24.
108. Aaron JE et al. Frequency of osteomalacia and osteoporosis in fractures of the proximal femur. *Lancet*, 1974, 2:229–233.
109. Aaron JE, Gallagher JC, Nordin BEC. Seasonal variation of histological osteomalacia in femoral neck fractures. *Lancet*, 1974, 2:84–85.
110. Baker MR et al. Plasma 25-hydroxy vitamin D concentrations in patients with fractures of the femoral neck. *British Medical Journal*, 1979, 1:589.
111. Morris HA et al. Vitamin D and femoral neck fractures in elderly South Australian women. *Medical Journal of Australia*, 1984, 140:519–521.
112. von Knorring J et al. Serum levels of 25-hydroxyvitamin D, 24,25-dihydroxyvitamin D and parathyroid hormone in patients with femoral neck fracture in southern Finland. *Clinical Endocrinology*, 1982, 17:189–194.
113. Pun KK et al. Vitamin D status among patients with fractured neck of femur in Hong Kong. *Bone*, 1990, 11:365–368.
114. Lund B, Sorenson OH, Christensen AB. 25-hydroxycholecalciferol and fractures of the proximal femur. *Lancet*, 1975, 2:300–302.
115. Chapuy MC et al. Vitamin D₃ and calcium to prevent hip fractures in elderly women. *New England Journal of Medicine*, 1992, 327:1637–1642.
116. Boland R. Role of vitamin D in skeletal muscle function. *Endocrine Reviews*, 1986, 7:434–448.
117. Walser M. Calcium clearance as a function of sodium clearance in the dog. *American Journal of Physiology*, 1961, 200:769–773.
118. Nordin BEC, Need AG. The effect of sodium on calcium requirement. In: Draper HH, ed. *Advances in nutritional research. Volume 9. Nutrition and osteoporosis.* New York, NY, Plenum Press, 1994:209–230.
119. Goulding A, Lim PE. Effects of varying dietary salt intake on the fasting excretion of sodium, calcium and hydroxyproline in young women. *New Zealand Medical Journal*, 1983, 96:853–854.
120. Sabto J et al. Influence of urinary sodium on calcium excretion in normal individuals. *Medical Journal of Australia*, 1984, 140:354–356.
121. Kleeman CR et al. Effect of variations in sodium intake on calcium excretion in normal humans. *Proceedings of the Society for Experimental Biology*, 1964, 115:29–32.
122. Epstein FH. Calcium and the kidney. *American Journal of Medicine*, 1968, 45:700–714.
123. Goulding A, Campbell D. Dietary NaCl loads promote calciuria and bone loss in adult oophorectomized rats consuming a low calcium diet. *Journal of Nutrition*, 1983, 113:1409–1414.
124. McParland BE, Goulding A, Campbell AJ. Dietary salt affects biochemical markers of resorption and formation of bone in elderly women. *British Medical Journal*, 1989, 299:834–835.
125. Need AG et al. Effect of salt restriction on urine hydroxyproline excretion in postmenopausal women. *Archives of Internal Medicine*, 1991, 151:757–759.
126. Elliott P et al. Intersalt revisited: further analyses of 24-hour sodium excretion and blood pressure within and across populations. *British Medical Journal*, 1996, 312:1249–1253.
127. Hegsted DM, Linkswiler HM. Long-term effects of level of protein intake on calcium metabolism in young adult women. *Journal of Nutrition*, 1981, 111:244–251.

128. Margen S et al. Studies in calcium metabolism. I. The calciuretic effect of dietary protein. *American Journal of Clinical Nutrition*, 1974, 27:584–589.
129. Linkswiler HM et al. Protein-induced hypercalciuria. *Federation Proceedings*, 1981, 40:2429–2433.
130. Heaney RP. Protein intake and the calcium economy. *Journal of the American Dietetic Association*, 1993, 93:1259–1260.
131. Kerstetter JE, Allen LH. Dietary protein increases urinary calcium. *Journal of Nutrition*, 1989, 120:134–136.
132. Nordin BEC et al. Dietary calcium and osteoporosis. In: Pietinen P, Nishida C, Khaltaev N, eds. *Proceedings of the Second WHO Symposium on Health Issues for the 21st Century: Nutrition and Quality of Life, Kobe, Japan, 24–26 November 1993*. Geneva, World Health Organization, 1996:181–198 (WHO/NUT/95.7).
133. Schuette SA, Zemel MB, Linkswiler HM. Studies on the mechanism of protein-induced hypercalciuria in older men and women. *Journal of Nutrition*, 1980, 110:305–315.
134. Schuette SA et al. Renal acid, urinary cyclic AMP, and hydroxyproline excretion as affected by level of protein, sulfur amino acid, and phosphorus intake. *Journal of Nutrition*, 1981, 111:2106–2116.
135. Need AG, Horowitz M, Nordin BEC. Is the effect of dietary protein on urine calcium due to its phosphate content? *Bone*, 1998, 23(Suppl.):SA344.
136. Mellanby E. The part played by an "accessory factor" in the production of experimental rickets. A further demonstration of the part played by accessory food factors in the aetiology of rickets. *Journal of Physiology*, 1918, 52:11–53.
137. Telfer SV. Studies in calcium and phosphorus metabolism. *Quarterly Journal of Medicine*, 1926, 20:1–6.
138. Fairweather-Tait S et al. Effect of calcium supplements and stage of lactation on the calcium absorption efficiency of lactating women accustomed to low calcium intakes. *American Journal of Clinical Nutrition*, 1995, 62:1188–1192.
139. Prentice A et al. Biochemical markers of calcium and bone metabolism during 18 months of lactation in Gambian women accustomed to a low calcium intake and in those consuming a calcium supplement. *Journal of Clinical Endocrinology and Metabolism*, 1998, 83:1059–1066.
140. Dibba B et al. Effect of calcium supplementation on bone mineral accretion in Gambian children accustomed to a low calcium diet. *American Journal of Clinical Nutrition*, 2000, 71:544–549.
141. Aspray TJ et al. Low bone mineral content is common but osteoporotic fractures are rare in elderly rural Gambian women. *Journal of Bone and Mineral Research*, 1996, 11:1019–1025.
142. Bucher HC et al. Effect of calcium supplementation on pregnancy-induced hypertension and pre-eclampsia. *Journal of the American Medical Association*, 1996, 275:1113–1117.
143. Garland CF, Garland FC, Gorham ED. Can colon cancer incidence and death rates be reduced with calcium and vitamin D? *American Journal of Clinical Nutrition*, 1991, 54(Suppl.):S193–S201.
144. McCarron DA. Role of adequate dietary calcium intake in the prevention and management of salt-sensitive hypertension. *American Journal of Clinical Nutrition*, 1997, 65(Suppl.):S712–S716.
145. Joffe GM et al. The relationship between abnormal glucose tolerance

and hypertensive disorders of pregnancy in healthy nulliparous women. *American Journal* of *Obstetrics and Gynecology*, 1998, 179:1032–1037.

146. Martinez ME, Willett WC. Calcium, vitamin D, and colorectal cancer: a review of the epidemiologic evidence. *Cancer Epidemiology, Biomarkers and Prevention*, 1998, 7:163–168.

147. Resnick LM. The role of dietary calcium in hypertension: a hierarchical overview. *American Journal of Hypertension*, 1999, 12:99–112.

148. DerSimonian R, Levine RJ. Resolving discrepancies between a meta-analysis and a subsequent large controlled trial. *Journal of the American Medical Association*, 1999, 282:664–670.

149. Mobarhan S. Calcium and the colon: recent findings. *Nutrition Reviews*, 1999, 57:124–126.

150. McCarron DA, Reusser ME. Finding consensus in the dietary calcium-blood pressure debate. *Journal of the American College of Nutrition*, 1999, 18(Suppl.):S398–S405.

5. Vitamin E

5.1 Role of vitamin E in human metabolic processes

A large body of scientific evidence indicates that reactive free radicals are involved in many diseases, including heart disease and cancers (*1*). Cells contain many potentially oxidizable substrates such as polyunsaturated fatty acids (PUFAs), proteins, and DNA. Therefore, a complex antioxidant defence system normally protects cells from the injurious effects of endogenously produced free radicals as well as from species of exogenous origin such as cigarette smoke and pollutants. Should our exposure to free radicals exceed the protective capacity of the antioxidant defence system, a phenomenon often referred to as oxidative stress (*2*), then damage to biological molecules may occur. There is considerable evidence that disease causes an increase in oxidative stress; therefore, consumption of foods rich in antioxidants, which are potentially able to quench or neutralize excess radicals, may play an important role in modifying the development of disease.

Vitamin E is the major lipid-soluble antioxidant in the cell antioxidant defence system and is exclusively obtained from the diet. The term "vitamin E" refers to a family of eight naturally-occurring homologues that are synthesized by plants from homogentisic acid. All are derivatives of 6-chromanol and differ in the number and position of methyl groups on the ring structure. The four tocopherol homologues (*d*-α-, *d*-β-, *d*-γ-, and *d*-δ-) have a saturated 16-carbon phytyl side chain, whereas the four tocotrienols (*d*-α-, *d*-β-, *d*-γ-, and *d*-δ-) have three double bonds on the side chain. There is also a widely available synthetic form, *dl*-α-tocopherol, prepared by coupling trimethylhydroquinone with isophytol. This consists of a mixture of eight stereoisomers in approximately equal amounts; these isomers are differentiated by rotations of the phytyl chain in various directions that do not occur naturally.

For dietary purposes, vitamin E activity is expressed as α-tocopherol equivalents (α-TEs). One α-TE is the activity of 1 mg *RRR*-α-tocopherol (*d*-α-tocopherol). To estimate the α-TE of a mixed diet containing natural forms of vitamin E, the number of milligrams of β-tocopherol should be multiplied by 0.5, γ-tocopherol by 0.1, and α-tocotrienol by 0.3. Any of the synthetic all-*rac-*

α-tocopherols (*dl*-α-tocopherol) should be multiplied by 0.74. One milligram of the latter compound in the acetate form is equivalent to 1 IU of vitamin E.

Vitamin E is an example of a phenolic antioxidant. Such molecules readily donate the hydrogen from the hydroxyl (-OH) group on the ring structure to free radicals, making them unreactive. On donating the hydrogen, the phenolic compound itself becomes a relatively unreactive free radical because the unpaired electron on the oxygen atom is usually delocalized into the aromatic ring structure thereby increasing its stability (*3*).

The major biological role of vitamin E is to protect PUFAs and other components of cell membranes and low-density lipoprotein (LDL) from oxidation by free radicals. Vitamin E is located primarily within the phospholipid bilayer of cell membranes. It is particularly effective in preventing lipid peroxidation—a series of chemical reactions involving the oxidative deterioration of PUFAs (see Chapter 8 on antioxidants). Elevated levels of lipid peroxidation products are associated with numerous diseases and clinical conditions (*4*). Although vitamin E is primarily located in cell and organelle membranes where it can exert its maximum protective effect, its concentration may only be one molecule for every 2000 phospholipid molecules. This suggests that after its reaction with free radicals it is rapidly regenerated, possibly by other antioxidants (*5*).

Absorption of vitamin E from the intestine depends on adequate pancreatic function, biliary secretion, and micelle formation. Conditions for absorption are like those for dietary lipid, that is, efficient emulsification, solubilization within mixed bile salt micelles, uptake by enterocytes, and secretion into the circulation via the lymphatic system (*6*). Emulsification takes place initially in the stomach and then in the small intestine in the presence of pancreatic and biliary secretions. The resulting mixed micelle aggregates the vitamin E molecules, solubilizes the vitamin E, and then transports it to the brush border membrane of the enterocyte, probably by passive diffusion. Within the enterocyte, tocopherol is incorporated into chylomicrons and secreted into the intracellular space and lymphatic system and subsequently into the blood stream. Tocopherol esters, present in processed foods and vitamin supplements, must be hydrolysed in the small intestine before absorption.

Vitamin E is transported in the blood by the plasma lipoproteins and erythrocytes. Chylomicrons carry tocopherol from the enterocyte to the liver, where they are incorporated into parenchymal cells as chylomicron remnants. The catabolism of chylomicrons takes place in the systemic circulation through the action of cellular lipoprotein, lipase. During this process tocopherol can be transferred to high-density lipoproteins (HDLs). The tocopherol in HDLs can transfer to other circulating lipoproteins, such as LDLs and very low-density lipoproteins (VLDLs) (7). During the conversion of VLDL to LDL in the circulation, some α-tocopherol remains within the core lipids and is thus incorporated in LDL. Most α-tocopherol then enters the cells of peripheral tissues within the intact lipoprotein through the LDL receptor pathway, although some may be taken up by membrane binding sites recognizing apolipoprotein A-I and A-II present on HDL (8).

Although the process of absorption of all the tocopherol homologues in the diet is similar, the α form predominates in blood and tissue. This is due to the action of binding proteins that preferentially select the α form over other forms. In the first instance, a 30-kDa binding protein unique to the liver cytoplasm preferentially incorporates α-tocopherol in the nascent VLDL (9). This form also accumulates in non-hepatic tissues, particularly at sites where free radical production is greatest, such as in the membranes of mitochondria and endoplasmic reticulum in the heart and lungs (10).

Hepatic intracellular transport may be expedited by a 14.2-kDa binding protein that binds α-tocopherol in preference to the other homologues (11). Other proteinaceous sites with apparent tocopherol-binding abilities have been found on erythrocytes, adrenal membranes, and smooth muscle cells (12). These may serve as vitamin E receptors which orient the molecule within the membrane for optimum antioxidant function.

These selective mechanisms explain why vitamin E homologues have markedly differing antioxidant abilities in biological systems and they illustrate the important distinction between the in vitro antioxidant effectiveness of a substance in the stabilization of, for example, a food product and its in vivo potency as an antioxidant. From a nutritional perspective, the most important form of vitamin E is α-tocopherol; this is corroborated in animal model tests of biopotency which assess the ability of the various homologues to prevent fetal absorption and muscular dystrophies (Table 5.1).

Plasma vitamin E concentrations vary little over a wide range of dietary intakes. Even daily supplements of the order of 1600 IU/day for 3 weeks only increased plasma levels by 2–3 times and on cessation of treatment, plasma levels returned to pretreatment levels in 5 days (13). Similarly, tissue concentrations only increased by 2–3 times when patients undergoing heart surgery were given 300 mg/day of the natural stereoisomer for 2 weeks preoperatively (14). Kinetic studies with deuterated tocopherol (15) suggest that there is rapid equilibration of new tocopherol in erythrocytes, liver, and spleen but that turnover in other tissues such as heart, muscle, and adipose tissue is much slower. The brain is markedly resistant to depletion of, and repletion with, vitamin E (16). This presumably reflects an adaptive mechanism to avoid detrimental oxidative reactions in this key organ.

TABLE 5.1
Approximate biological activity of naturally-occurring tocopherols and tocotrienols compared with d-α-tocopherol

Common name	Biological activity compared with d-α-tocopherol (%)
d-α-tocopherol	100
d-β-tocopherol	50
d-γ-tocopherol	10
d-δ-tocopherol	3
d-α-tocotrienol	30
d-β-tocotrienol	5
d-γ-tocotrienol	Unknown
d-δ-tocotrienol	Unknown

The primary oxidation product of α-tocopherol is α-tocopheryl quinone that can be conjugated to yield the glucuronate after prior reduction to the hydroquinone. This glucuronide is excreted in the bile as such or further degraded in the kidneys to α-tocopheronic acid glucuronide and hence excreted in the bile. Those vitamin E homologues not preferentially selected by the hepatic binding proteins are eliminated during the process of nascent VLDL secretion in the liver and probably excreted via the bile (*17*). Some vitamin E may also be excreted via skin sebaceous glands (*18*).

5.2 Populations at risk for vitamin E deficiency

There are many signs of vitamin E deficiency in animals, most of which are related to damage to cell membranes and leakage of cell contents to external fluids. Disorders provoked by traces of peroxidized PUFAs in the diets of animals with low vitamin E status include cardiac or skeletal myopathies, neuropathies, and liver necrosis (*19*) (Table 5.2). Muscle and neurological problems are also a consequence of human vitamin E deficiency (*20*). Early diagnostic signs of deficiency include leakage of muscle enzymes such as creatine kinase and pyruvate kinase into plasma, increased levels of lipid peroxidation products in plasma, and increased erythrocyte haemolysis.

The assessment of the vitamin E requirement for humans is confounded by the very rare occurrence of clinical signs of deficiency because these usually only develop in infants and adults with fat-malabsorption syndromes or liver disease, in individuals with genetic anomalies in transport or binding proteins, and possibly in premature infants (*19, 21*). This suggests that diets contain sufficient vitamin E to satisfy nutritional needs.

Work with several animal models (*22*) suggests that increasing intakes of vitamin E inhibits the progression of vascular disease by preventing the oxi-

TABLE 5.2
Diseases and syndromes in animals associated with vitamin E deficiency and excess intakes of polyunsaturated fatty acids

Syndrome	Affected organ or tissue	Species
Encephalomalacia	Cerebellum	Chick
Exudative diathesis	Vascular	Turkey
Microcytic anaemia	Blood, bone marrow	Chick
Macrocytic anaemia	Blood, bone marrow	Monkey
Pancreatic fibrosis	Pancreas	Chick, mouse
Liver necrosis	Liver	Pig, rat
Muscular degeneration	Skeletal muscle	Pig, rat, mouse
Microangiopathy	Heart muscle	Pig, lamb, calf
Kidney degeneration	Kidney tubules	Monkey, rat
Steatitis	Adipose tissue	Pig, chick
Testicular degeneration	Testes	Pig, calf, chick
Malignant hyperthermia	Skeletal muscle	Pig

Source: provided by GG Duthie, Rowett Research Institute, Aberdeen, United Kingdom.

dation of LDL. It is thought that oxidized lipoprotein is a key event in the development of the atheromatous plaque, which may ultimately occlude the blood vessel (*23*).

Human studies, however, have been less consistent in providing evidence for a role of vitamin E in preventing heart disease. Vitamin E supplements reduce ex vivo oxidizability of plasma LDLs but there is no correlation between ex vivo lipoprotein oxidizability and endogenous vitamin E levels in an unsupplemented population (*24*). Similarly, the few randomized double blind placebo-controlled intervention trials conducted to date with human volunteers, which focused on the relationship between vitamin E and cardio-vascular disease, have yielded inconsistent results. There was a marked reduction in non-fatal myocardial infarction in patients with coronary artery disease (as defined by angiogram) who were randomly assigned to take pharmacologic doses of vitamin E (400 and 800 mg/day) or a placebo in the Cambridge Heart Antioxidant Study involving 2000 men and women (*25*). However, the incidence of major coronary events in male smokers who received 20 mg/day of vitamin E for approximately 6 years was not reduced in a study using α-tocopherol and β-carotene supplementation (*26*). Furthermore, in the Medical Research Council/British Heart Foundation trial involving 20 536 patients with heart disease who received vitamin E (600 mg), vitamin C (250 mg) and β-carotene (20 mg) or a placebo daily for 5 years, there were no significant reductions in all-cause mortality, or in deaths due to vascular or non-vascular causes (*27*). It was concluded that these antioxidant supplements provided no measurable health benefits for these patients.

Epidemiological studies suggest that dietary vitamin E influences the risk of cardiovascular disease. Gey et al. (28) reported that lipid-standardized plasma vitamin E concentrations in middle-aged men across 16 European countries predicted 62% of the variance in the mortality from ischaemic heart disease. In the United States both the Nurses Health Study (29), which involved 87000 females in an 8-year follow-up, and the Health Professionals Follow-up Study of 40000 men (30) concluded that persons taking supplements of 100 mg/day or more of vitamin E for at least 2 years had approximately a 40% lower incidence of myocardial infarction and cardiovascular mortality than those who did not. However, there was no influence of dietary vitamin E alone on incidence of cardiovascular disease when those taking supplements were removed from the analyses. A possible explanation for the significant relationship between dietary vitamin E and cardiovascular disease in European countries but not in the United States may be found in the fact that across Europe populations consume foods with widely differing amounts of vitamin E. Sunflower seed oil, which is rich in α-tocopherol, tends to be consumed more widely in the southern European countries where a lower incidence of cardiovascular disease is reported, than in northern European countries where soybean oil, which contains more of the γ form, is preferred (31) (Table 5.3). A study carried out which compared plasma α-tocopherol and γ-tocopherol concentrations in middle-aged men and women in Toulouse (southern France) with Belfast (Northern Ireland) found that the concentrations of γ-tocopherol in Belfast were twice as high as those in Toulouse; α-tocopherol concentrations were identical in men in both countries but higher in women in Belfast than in Toulouse ($P < 0.001$) (32).

It has also been suggested that vitamin E supplementation (200–400 mg/day) may be appropriate therapeutically to moderate some aspects of degenerative diseases such as Parkinson disease, reduce the severity of neurologic disorders such as tardive dyskinesia, prevent periventricular haemorrhage in pre-term babies, reduce tissue injury arising from ischaemia and reperfusion during surgery, delay cataract development, and improve mobility in arthritis sufferers (33). However, very high doses may also induce adverse pro-oxidant effects (34), and the long-term advantages of such treatments have not been proven. In fact, a double blind study to determine the influence of vitamin E (200 mg/day) for 15 months on respiratory tract infections in non-institutionalized persons over 60 years found no difference in incidence between groups, but that the number of symptoms and duration of fever and restricted activity were greater in those receiving the vitamin (35).

TABLE 5.3
Cross-country correlations between coronary heart disease mortality in men and the supply of vitamin E homologues across 24 European countries

Homologue	Correlation coefficient, r
Total vitamin E	−0.386
d-α-tocopherol	−0.753[a]
d-β-tocopherol	−0.345
d-γ-tocopherol	−0.001
d-δ-tocopherol	0.098
d-α-tocotrienol	−0.072
d-β-tocotrienol	−0.329
d-γ-tocotrienol	−0.210

[a] The correlation with d-α-tocopherol is highly significant ($P < 0.001$) whereas all other correlations do not achieve statistical significance.
Source: based on reference (*31*).

5.3 Dietary sources and possible limitations to vitamin E supply

Because vitamin E is naturally present in plant-based diets and animal products and is often added by manufacturers to vegetable oils and processed foods, intakes are probably adequate to avoid overt deficiency in most situations. Exceptions may be during ecologic disasters and cultural conflicts resulting in food deprivation and famine.

Analysis of the FAO country food balance sheets indicates that about half the α-tocopherol in a typical northern European diet, such as in the United Kingdom, is derived from vegetable oils (*31*). Animal fats, vegetables, and meats each contribute about 10% to the total per capita supply and fruit, nuts, cereals, and dairy products each contribute about 4%. Eggs, fish, and pulses contribute less than 2% each.

There are marked differences in per capita α-tocopherol supply among different countries ranging from approximately 8–10 mg/person/day (e.g. Finland, Iceland, Japan, and New Zealand) to 20–25 mg/person/day (e.g. France, Greece, and Spain) (*31*). This variation can be ascribed mainly to the type and quantity of dietary oils used in different countries and the proportion of the different homologues in the oils (Table 5.4). For example, sunflower seed oil contains approximately 55 mg α-tocopherol/100 g in contrast to soybean oil that contains only 8 mg/100 ml (*36*).

TABLE 5.4
Vitamin E content of vegetable oils (mg tocopherol/100 g)

Oil	α-tocopherol	γ-tocopherol	δ-tocopherol	α-tocotrienol
Coconut	0.5	0	0.6	0.5
Maize (corn)	11.2	60.2	1.8	0
Palm	25.6	31.6	7.0	14.3
Olive	5.1	Trace	0	0
Peanut	13.0	21.4	2.1	0
Soybean	10.1	59.3	26.4	0
Wheatgerm	133.0	26.0	27.1	2.6
Sunflower	48.7	5.1	0.8	0

Source: reference (36).

5.4 Evidence used for estimating recommended intakes

In the case of the antioxidants (see Chapter 8), it was decided that there was insufficient evidence to enable a recommended nutrient intake (RNI) to be based on the additional health benefits obtainable from nutrient intakes above those usually found in the diet. Despite its important biological antioxidant properties, there is no consistent evidence that supplementing the diet with vitamin E protects against chronic disease. The main function of vitamin E, which appears to be that of preventing oxidation of PUFAs, has nevertheless been used by the present Consultation as the basis for proposing RNIs for vitamin E because of the considerable evidence in different animal species that low levels of vitamin E combined with an excess of PUFAs give rise to a wide variety of clinical signs.

There is very little clinical evidence of deficiency disease in humans except in certain inherited conditions where the metabolism of vitamin E is disturbed. Even biochemical evidence of poor vitamin E status in both adults and children is minimal. Meta-analysis of data collected within European countries indicates that optimum intakes may be implied when plasma concentrations of vitamin E exceed 25–30 μmol/l of lipid-standardized α-tocopherol (37). However, this approach should be treated with caution, as plasma vitamin E concentrations do not necessarily reflect intakes or tissue reserves because only 1% of the body tocopherol may be in the blood (38) and the amount in the circulation is strongly influenced by circulating lipid (39); nevertheless, a lipid-standardized vitamin E concentration (e.g. a tocopherol–cholesterol ratio) greater than 2.25 (calculated as μmol/mmol) is believed to represent satisfactory vitamin E status (38, 39). The erythrocytes of subjects with values below this concentration of vitamin E may show evidence of an increasing tendency to haemolyse when exposed to oxidizing agents and thus, such values should be taken as an indication of biochemical deficiency (40). However, the development of clinical evidence of vitamin E deficiency (e.g. muscle damage or neurologic lesions) can take several years of exposure to extremely low vitamin E levels (41).

Dietary intakes of PUFAs have been used to assess the adequacy of vitamin E intakes by United States and United Kingdom advisory bodies. PUFAs are very susceptible to oxidation and their increased intake, without a concomitant increase in vitamin E, can lead to a reduction in plasma vitamin E concentrations (42) and to elevations in some indexes of oxidative damage in human volunteers (43). However, diets high in PUFAs tend also to be high in vitamin E, and to set a dietary recommendation based on extremes of PUFA intake would deviate considerably from median intakes of vitamin E in most populations of industrialized countries. Hence 'safe' allowances for the United Kingdom (men 10 and women 7 mg/day) (44) and 'arbitrary' allowances for the United States (men 10 and women 8 mg/day) (45) for vitamin E intakes approximate the median intake in those countries. It is worth noting that only 11 (0.7%) out of 1629 adults in the 1986–1987 British Nutrition Survey had α-tocopherol–cholesterol ratios <2.25. Furthermore, although the high intake of soybean oil, with its high content of γ-tocopherol, substitutes for the intake of α-tocopherol in the British diet, a comparison of α-tocopherol–cholesterol ratios found almost identical results in two groups of randomly-selected, middle-aged adults in Belfast (Northern Ireland) and Toulouse (France), two countries with very different intakes of α-tocopherol (36) and cardiovascular risk (32).

It has been suggested that when the main PUFA in the diet is linoleic acid, a d-α-tocopherol–PUFA ratio of 0.4 (expressed as mg tocopherol per g PUFA) is adequate for adult humans (46, 47). This ratio has been recommended in the United Kingdom for infant formulas (48). Use of this ratio to calculate the vitamin E requirements of men and women with energy intakes of 2550 and 1940 kcal/day, respectively, and containing PUFAs at 6% of the energy intake (approximately 17 g and 13 g, respectively), (44) produced values of 7 and 5 mg/day of α-TEs, respectively. In both the United States and the United Kingdom, median intakes of α-TE are in excess of these amounts and the α-tocopherol–PUFA ratio is approximately 0.6 (49), which is well above the value of 0.4 that would be considered adequate for this ratio. The Nutrition Working Group of the International Life Sciences Institute Europe (50) has suggested an intake of 12 mg α-tocopherol for a daily intake of 14 g PUFAs to compensate for the high consumption of soybean oil in certain countries, where over 50% of vitamin E intake is accounted for by the less biologically active γ form. As indicated above, however, plasma concentrations of α-tocopherol in subjects from Toulouse and Belfast suggest that an increased amount of dietary vitamin E is not necessary to maintain satisfactory plasma concentrations (*32*).

At present, data are not sufficient to formulate recommendations for vitamin E intake for different age groups except for infancy. There is some indication that newborn infants, particularly if born prematurely, are vulnerable to oxidative stress because of low body stores of vitamin E, impaired absorption, and reduced transport capacity resulting from low concentrations of circulating low-density lipoproteins at birth (*51*). However, term infants nearly achieve adult plasma vitamin E concentrations in the first week (*52*) and although the concentration of vitamin E in early human milk can be variable, after 12 days it remains fairly constant at 0.32 mg α-TE/100 ml milk (*53*). Thus a human-milk-fed infant consuming 850 ml would have an intake of 2.7 mg α-TE. It seems reasonable that formula milk should not contain less than 0.3 mg α-TE/100 ml of reconstituted feed and not less than 0.4 mg α-TE/g PUFA.

No specific recommendations concerning the vitamin E requirements in pregnancy and lactation have been made by other advisory bodies (*44, 45*) mainly because there is no evidence of vitamin E requirements different from those of other adults and, presumably, also because the increased energy intake during these periods would compensate for the increased needs for infant growth and milk synthesis.

5.5 Toxicity

Vitamin E appears to have very low toxicity, and amounts of 100–200 mg of the synthetic all-*rac*-α-tocopherol are consumed widely as supplements (*29, 30*). Evidence of pro-oxidant damage has been associated with the feeding of supplements but usually only at very high doses (e.g. >1000 mg/day) (*34*). Nevertheless, the recent report from The Netherlands of increased severity of respiratory tract infections in persons over 60 years who received 200 mg vitamin E per day for 15 months, should be noted in case that is also an indication of a pro-oxidant effect (*35*).

5.6 Recommendations for future research

More investigation is required of the role of vitamin E in biological processes which do not necessarily involve its antioxidant function. These processes include:

- structural roles in the maintenance of cell membrane integrity;
- anti-inflammatory effects by direct and regulatory interaction with the prostaglandin synthetase complex of enzymes which participate in the metabolism of arachidonic acid;
- DNA synthesis;
- interaction with the immune response;
- regulation of intercellular signalling and cell proliferation through modulation of protein kinase C.

Additionally, more investigation is required of the growing evidence that inadequate vitamin E status may increase susceptibility to infection particularly by allowing the genomes of certain relatively benign viruses to convert to more virulent strains (54).

There is an important need to define optimum vitamin E intakes for younger groups of healthy persons since supplements for people who are already ill appear ineffective and can possibly be harmful in the elderly. Intervention trials with morbidity and mortality end-points will take years to complete, although the European Prospective Investigations on Cancer which has already been underway for more than 10 years (55) may provide some relevant information. One possible approach to circumvent this delay is to assess the effects of different intakes of vitamin E on biomarkers of oxidative damage to lipids, proteins, and DNA as their occurrence in vivo is implicated in many diseases, including vascular disease and certain cancers. However, clinical studies will always remain the gold standard.

References

1. Diplock AT. Antioxidants and disease prevention. *Molecular Aspects of Medicine*, 1994, 15:293–376.
2. Sies H. Oxidative stress: an introduction. In: Sies H, ed. *Oxidative stress: oxidants and antioxidants*. London, Academic Press, 1993:15–22.
3. Scott G. *Antioxidants in science, technology, medicine and nutrition*. Chichester, Albion Publishing, 1997.
4. Duthie GG. Lipid peroxidation. *European Journal of Clinical Nutrition*, 1993, 47:759–764.
5. Kagan VE. Recycling and redox cycling of phenolic antioxidants. *Annals of the New York Academy of Sciences*, 1998, 854:425–434.
6. Gallo-Torres HE. Obligatory role of bile for the intestinal absorption of vitamin E. *Lipids*, 1970, 5:379–384.
7. Traber MG et al. *RRR*- and *SRR*-α-tocopherols are secreted without discrimination in human chylomicrons, but *RRR*-α-tocopherol is preferentially secreted in very low density lipoproteins. *Journal of Lipid Research*, 1990, 31:675–685.
8. Traber MG. Regulation of human plasma vitamin E. In: Sies H, ed. *Antioxi-

dants in disease mechanisms and therapeutic strategies. San Diego, CA, Academic Press, 1996:49–63.

9. Traber MG, Kayden HJ. Preferential incorporation of α-tocopherol vs. γ-tocopherol in human lipoproteins. *American Journal of Clinical Nutrition*, 1989, 49:517–526.

10. Kornbrust DJ, Mavis RD. Relative susceptibility of microsomes from lung, heart, liver, kidney, brain and testes to lipid peroxidation: correlation with vitamin E content. *Lipids*, 1979, 15:315–322.

11. Dutta-Roy AK et al. Purification and partial characterisation of an α-tocopherol-binding protein from rabbit heart cytosol. *Molecular and Cellular Biochemistry*, 1993, 123:139–144.

12. Dutta-Roy AK et al. Vitamin E requirements, transport, and metabolism: role of α-tocopherol-binding proteins. *Journal of Nutritional Biochemistry*, 1994, 5:562–570.

13. Esterbauer H et al. The role of lipid peroxidation and antioxidants in oxidative modification of LDL. *Free Radicals in Biology and Medicine*, 1992, 13:341–390.

14. Mickle DAG et al. Effect of orally administered α-tocopherol acetate on human myocardial α-tocopherol levels. *Cardiovascular Drugs and Therapy*, 1991, 5:309–312.

15. Traber MG, Ramakrishnan R, Kayden HJ. Human plasma vitamin E kinetics demonstrate rapid recycling of plasma *RRR*-α-tocopherol. *Proceedings of the National Academy of Sciences*, 1994, 91:10005–10008.

16. Bourne J, Clement M. Kinetics of rat peripheral nerve, forebrain and cerebellum α-tocopherol depletion: comparison with different organs. *Journal of Nutrition*, 1991, 121:1204–1207.

17. Drevon CA. Absorption, transport and metabolism of vitamin E. *Free Radical Research Communications*, 1991, 14:229–246.

18. Shiratori T. Uptake, storage and excretion of chylomicra-bound 3H-alpha-tocopherol by the skin of the rat. *Life Sciences*, 1974, 14:929–935.

19. McLaren DS et al. Fat soluble vitamins. In: Garrow JS, James WPT, eds. *Human nutrition and dietetics*. Edinburgh, Churchill Livingstone, 1993: 208–238.

20. Sokol RJ. Vitamin E deficiency and neurologic disease. *Annual Review of Nutrition*, 1988, 8:351–373.

21. Traber MG et al. Impaired ability of patients with familial isolated vitamin E deficiency to incorporate α-tocopherol into lipoproteins secreted by the liver. *Journal of Clinical Investigation*, 1990, 85:397–407.

22. Williams RJ et al. Dietary vitamin E and the attenuation of early lesion development in modified Watanabe rabbits. *Atherosclerosis*, 1992, 94:153–159.

23. Steinberg D et al. Beyond cholesterol. Modifications of low-density lipoprotein that increase its atherogenicity. *New England Journal of Medicine*, 1989, 320:915–924.

24. Dieber-Rotheneder M et al. Effect of oral supplementation with *d*-α-tocopherol on the vitamin E content of human low density lipoprotein and resistance to oxidation. *Journal of Lipid Research*, 1991, 32:1325–1332.

25. Stephens NG et al. Randomised control trial of vitamin E in patients with coronary disease: Cambridge Heart Antioxidant Study (CHAOS). *Lancet*, 1996, 347:781–786.

26. Rapola J et al. Randomised trial of alpha-tocopherol and beta-carotene sup-

plements on incidence of major coronary events in men with previous myocardial infarction. *Lancet*, 1997, 349:1715–1720.

27. Heart Protection Study Group. MRC/BHF heart protection study of antioxidant vitamin supplementation in 20536 high-risk individuals: a randomised placebo-controlled trial. *Lancet*, 2002, 360:23–33.

28. Gey KF et al. Inverse correlation between plasma vitamin E and mortality from ischaemic heart disease in cross-cultural epidemiology. *American Journal of Clinical Nutrition*, 1991, 53(Suppl.):S326–S334.

29. Stampler MJ et al. Vitamin E consumption and risk of coronary heart disease in women. *New England Journal of Medicine*, 1993, 328:1444–1449.

30. Rimm EB et al. Vitamin E consumption and risk of coronary heart disease in men. *New England Journal of Medicine*, 1993, 328:1450–1456.

31. Bellizzi MC et al. Vitamin E and coronary heart disease: the European paradox. *European Journal of Clinical Nutrition*, 1994, 48:822–831.

32. Howard AN et al. Do hydroxy carotenoids prevent coronary heart disease? A comparison between Belfast and Toulouse. *International Journal of Vitamin and Nutrition Research*, 1996, 66:113–118.

33. Packer L. Vitamin E: biological activity and health benefits. Overview. In: Packer L, Fuchs J, eds. *Vitamin E in health and disease.* New York, NY, Marcel Dekker, 1993:977–982.

34. Brown KM, Morrice PC, Duthie GG. Erythrocyte vitamin E and plasma ascorbate concentrations in relation to erythrocyte peroxidation in smokers and non-smokers: dose–response of vitamin E supplementation. *American Journal of Clinical Nutrition*, 1997, 65:496–502.

35. Graat JM, Schouten EG, Kok FJ. Effect of daily vitamin E and multivitamin mineral supplementation on acute respiratory tract infections in elderly persons: a randomized controlled trial. *Journal of the American Medical Association*, 2002, 288:715–721.

36. Slover HT. Tocopherols in foods and fats. *Lipids*, 1971, 6:291–296.

37. Gey KF. Vitamin E and other essential antioxidants regarding coronary heart disease: risk assessment studies. In: Packer L, Fuchs J, eds. *Vitamin E in health and disease.* New York, NY, Marcel Dekker, 1993:589–634.

38. Horwitt MK et al. Relationship between tocopherol and serum lipid levels for the determination of nutritional adequacy. *Annals of the New York Academy of Sciences*, 1972, 203:223–236 .

39. Thurnham DI et al. The use of different lipids to express serum tocopherol: lipid ratios for the measurement of vitamin E status. *Annals of Clinical Biochemistry*, 1986, 23:514–520.

40. Leonard PJ, Losowsky MS. Effect of alpha-tocopherol administration on red cell survival in vitamin E deficient human subjects. *American Journal of Clinical Nutrition*, 1971, 24:388–393.

41. Horwitt MK. Interpretation of human requirements for vitamin E. In: Machlin L, ed. *Vitamin E, a comprehensive treatise.* New York, NY, Marcel Dekker, 1980:621–636.

42. Bunnell RH, De Ritter, Rubin SH. Effect of feeding polyunsaturated fatty acids with a low vitamin E diet on blood levels of tocopherol in men performing hard physical labor. *American Journal of Clinical Nutrition*, 1975, 28:706–711.

43. Jenkinson A et al. Dietary intakes of polyunsaturated fatty acids and indices of oxidative stress in human volunteers. *European Journal of Clinical Nutrition*, 1999, 53:523–528.

44. Department of Health. *Dietary reference values for food energy and nutrients for the United Kingdom.* London, Her Majesty's Stationery Office, 1991 (Report on Health and Social Subjects, No. 41).

45. Subcommittee on the Tenth Edition of the Recommended Dietary Allowances, Food and Nutrition Board. *Recommended dietary allowances,* 10th ed. Washington, DC, National Academy Press, 1989.

46. Bieri JG, Evarts RP. Tocopherols and fatty acids in American diets: the recommended allowance for vitamin E. *Journal of the American Dietetic Association,* 1973, 62:147–151.

47. Witting LA, Lee L. Dietary levels of vitamin E and polyunsaturated fatty acids and plasma vitamin E. *American Journal of Clinical Nutrition,* 1975, 28:571–576.

48. Department of Health and Social Security. *Artificial feeds for the young infant.* London, Her Majesty's Stationery Office, 1980 (Report on Health and Social Subjects, No. 18).

49. Gregory JR et al. *The Dietary and Nutritional Survey of British Adults.* London, Her Majesty's Stationery Office, 1990.

50. Nutrition Working Group of the International Life Science Institute Europe. Recommended daily amounts of vitamins and minerals in Europe. *Nutrition Abstracts and Reviews* (Series A), 1990, 60:827–842.

51. Lloyd JK. The importance of vitamin E in nutrition. *Acta Pediatrica Scandinavica,* 1990, 79:6–11.

52. Kelly FJ et al. Time course of vitamin E repletion in the premature infant. *British Journal of Nutrition,* 1990, 63:631–638.

53. Jansson L, Akesson B, Holmberg L. Vitamin E and fatty acid composition of human milk. *American Journal of Clinical Nutrition,* 1981, 34:8–13.

54. Beck MA. The influence of antioxidant nutrients on viral infection. *Nutrition Reviews,* 1998, 56:S140–S146.

55. Riboli E. Nutrition and cancer: background and rationale of the European Prospective Investigation into Cancer (EPIC). *Annals of Oncology,* 1992, 3:783–791.

6. Vitamin K

6.1 Introduction

Vitamin K is an essential fat-soluble micronutrient, which is needed for a unique post-translational chemical modification in a small group of proteins with calcium-binding properties, collectively known as vitamin K-dependent proteins or Gla proteins. Thus far, the only unequivocal role of vitamin K in health is in the maintenance of normal coagulation. The vitamin K-dependent coagulation proteins are synthesized in the liver and comprise factors II, VII, IX, and X, which have a haemostatic role (i.e. they are procoagulants that arrest and prevent bleeding), and proteins C and S, which have an anticoagulant role (i.e. they inhibit the clotting process). Despite this duality of function, the overriding effect of nutritional vitamin K deficiency is a bleeding tendency caused by the relative inactivity of the procoagulant proteins. Vitamin K-dependent proteins synthesized by other tissues include the bone protein osteocalcin and matrix Gla protein, though their functions remain to be clarified.

6.2 Biological role of vitamin K

Vitamin K is the family name for a series of fat-soluble compounds which have a common 2-methyl-1,4-naphthoquinone nucleus but differ in the structures of a side chain at the 3-position. They are synthesized by plants and bacteria. In plants the only important molecular form is phylloquinone (vitamin K_1), which has a phytyl side chain. Bacteria synthesize a family of compounds called menaquinones (vitamin K_2), which have side chains based on repeating unsaturated 5-carbon (prenyl) units. These are designated menaquinone-n (MK-n) according to the number (n) of prenyl units. Some bacteria also synthesize menaquinones in which one or more of the double bonds is saturated. The compound 2-methyl-1,4-naphthoquinone (common name menadione) may be regarded as a provitamin because vertebrates can convert it to MK-4 by adding a 4-prenyl side chain at the 3-position.

The biological role of vitamin K is to act as a cofactor for a specific carboxylation reaction that transforms selective glutamate (Glu) residues to γ-carboxyglutamate (Gla) residues (*1, 2*). The reaction is catalysed by a micro-somal enzyme, γ-glutamyl, or vitamin K-dependent carboxylase, which in turn is linked to a cyclic salvage pathway known as the vitamin K epoxide cycle (Figure 6.1).

The four vitamin K-dependent procoagulants (factor II or prothrombin, and factors VII, IX, and X) are serine proteases that are synthesized in the liver and then secreted into the circulation as inactive forms (zymogens). Their biological activity depends on their normal complement of Gla residues, which are efficient chelators of calcium ions. In the presence of Gla residues and calcium ions these proteins bind to the surface membrane phospholipids of platelets and endothelial cells where, together with other cofactors, they form membrane-bound enzyme complexes. When coagulation is initiated, the zymogens of the four vitamin K-dependent clotting factors are cleaved to

FIGURE 6.1
The vitamin K epoxide cycle

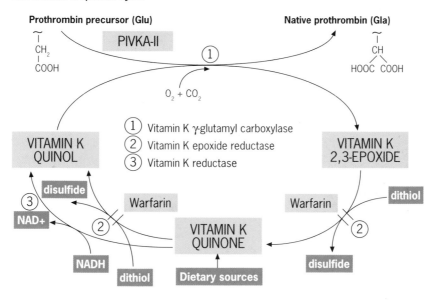

Scheme shows the cyclic metabolism of vitamin K in relation to the conversion of glutamate (Glu) to γ-carboxyglutamate (Gla) residues for the coagulation protein prothrombin. A general term for the glutamate precursors of vitamin K-dependent proteins is "proteins induced by vitamin K absence", abbreviated PIVKA. For prothrombin (factor II), the glutamate precursor is known as PIVKA-II. The active form of vitamin K needed for carboxylation is the reduced form, vitamin K quinol. Known enzyme reactions are numbered 1, 2, and 3. The carboxylation reaction is driven by a vitamin K-dependent carboxylase activity (reaction 1), which simultaneously converts vitamin K quinol to vitamin K 2,3-epoxide. Vitamin K 2,3-epoxide is reduced back to the quinone and then to the quinol by vitamin K epoxide reductase (reaction 2). The reductase activity denoted reaction 2 is dithiol dependent and is inhibited by coumarin anticoagulants such as warfarin. Dietary vitamin K may enter the cycle via an NADPH-dependent vitamin K reductase activity (reaction 3), which is not inhibited by warfarin.

yield the active protease clotting factors (1–3). Two other vitamin K-dependent proteins, protein C and protein S, play a regulatory role in the inhibition of coagulation. The function of protein C is to degrade phospholipid-bound activated factors V and VIII in the presence of calcium. Protein S acts as a synergistic cofactor to protein C by enhancing the binding of activated protein C to negatively charged phospholipids. There is evidence that protein S is synthesized by several tissues including the blood vessel wall and bone and may have other functions besides its well-established role as a coagulation inhibitor. Yet another vitamin K-dependent plasma protein (protein Z) is suspected to have a haemostatic role but its function is currently unknown.

Apart from the coagulation proteins, several other vitamin K-dependent proteins have been isolated from bone, cartilage, kidney, lungs, and other tissues (4, 5). Only two, osteocalcin and matrix Gla protein (MGP), have been well characterized. Both are found in bone but MGP also occurs in cartilage, blood vessel walls, and other soft tissues. It seems likely that one function of MGP is to inhibit mineralization (6). Thus far, no clear biological role for osteocalcin has been established despite its being the major non-collagenous bone protein synthesized by osteoblasts (7–9). This failure to establish a biological function for osteocalcin has hampered studies of the possible detrimental effects of vitamin K deficiency on bone health. Evidence of a possible association of a suboptimal vitamin K status with increased fracture risk remains to be confirmed (7–9).

6.3 Overview of vitamin K metabolism

6.3.1 Absorption and transport

Dietary vitamin K, mainly phylloquinone, is absorbed chemically unchanged from the proximal intestine after solubilization into mixed micelles composed of bile salts and the products of pancreatic lipolysis (10). In healthy adults the efficiency of absorption of phylloquinone in its free form is about 80% (10, 11). Within the intestinal mucosa the vitamin is incorporated into chylomicrons, is secreted into the lymph, and enters the blood via the lacteals (11, 12). Once in the circulation, phylloquinone is rapidly cleared (10) at a rate consistent with its continuing association with chylomicrons and the chylomicron remnants, which are produced by lipoprotein lipase hydrolysis at the surface of capillary endothelial cells (13). After an overnight fast, more than half of the circulating phylloquinone is still associated with triglyceride-rich lipoproteins, with the remainder being equally distributed between low-density and high-density lipoproteins (13). Although phylloquinone is the major circulating form of vitamin K, MK-7 is also present in plasma, at lower concentrations and with a lipoprotein distribution similar to phylloquinone (13). Although phylloquinone in blood must have been derived exclusively from the diet, it is not known whether circulating menaquinones such as MK-7 are derived from the diet, intestinal flora, or a combination of these sources.

6.3.2 Tissue stores and distribution

Until the 1970s, the liver was the only known site of synthesis of vitamin K-dependent proteins and hence was presumed to be the only significant storage site for the vitamin. However, the discovery of vitamin K-dependent processes and proteins in a number of extra-hepatic tissues suggests that this may not be the case (see section 6.2).

Human liver stores normally comprise about 90% menaquinones and 10% phylloquinone (14, 15). There is evidence that the phylloquinone liver stores are very labile; under conditions of severe dietary depletion, liver concentrations were reduced to about 25% of their initial levels after only 3 days (15). This high turnover of hepatic reserves of phylloquinone is in accord with the high losses of this vitamer through excretion (10).

Knowledge of hepatic stores of phylloquinone in different population groups is limited. Adult hepatic stores in a United Kingdom study were about 11 pmol/g (14) whereas in a study from Japan they were about two-fold higher (15). Such reserves are about 20 000–40 000-fold lower than those for retinol for relative daily intakes of phylloquinone that are only about 10-fold lower than those of vitamin A (16).

The relationship between hepatic and total-body stores of vitamin K is not known. Other sites of storage may be adipose tissue and bone; both are known to be sites where vitamin K-bearing chylomicrons and chylomicron remnants may be taken up. It has been reported that the predominant vitamer in human cortical and trabecular bone is phylloquinone; unlike the situation in liver, no menaquinones higher than MK-8 were detected (17).

In contrast to the hepatic preponderance of long-chain menaquinones, the major circulating form of vitamin K is invariably phylloquinone. The menaquinones MK-7, and possibly MK-8, are also present but the common hepatic forms, MKs 9–13, are not detectable in blood plasma (16, 18). This may be a consequence of a different route of absorption (e.g. the possibility of a portal route for long-chain MKs versus the established lymphatic route for phylloquinone), but might also suggest that once in the liver, the lipophilic long-chain menaquinones are not easily mobilized (16, 18, 19).

6.3.3 Bioactivity

Very little information exists on the relative effectiveness of the different hepatic forms of K vitamins with respect to the coagulation function of vitamin K in humans. This information is important because of the preponderance of long-chain menaquinones in human liver. Early bioassay data from rats suggested that long-chain menaquinones (MK-7, -9, and -10) were more efficient than phylloquinone in reversing vitamin K deficiency when single doses were given parenterally and that their sustained effect on vitamin K status may be due to their slower hepatic turnover (18, 19). Groenen-van Dooren et al. (20) also observed a longer duration of the biological response of MK-9 compared with phylloquinone in vitamin K-deficient rats. On the other hand, Will and Suttie (21) showed that when given orally, the dietary requirement for MK-9 for the maintenance of prothrombin synthesis in rats is higher than that for phylloquinone. They also reported that the initial hepatic turnover of MK-9 was two- to three-fold slower than that of phylloquinone.

Suttie (18) emphasized that the existence of a large pool of menaquinones in human liver does not necessarily mean that menaquinones make a proportionately greater contribution to the maintenance of vitamin K sufficiency. In humans, however, the development of subclinical signs of vitamin K deficiency detected in dietary phylloquinone restriction studies argues against this, especially when placed alongside the lack of change of hepatic menaquinone stores (15). One explanation is that many of the hepatic menaquinones are not biologically available to the microsomal γ-glutamyl carboxylase because of their different subcellular location; for instance, they may be located in the mitochondria and possibly other non-microsomal sites (18).

6.3.4 Excretion

Vitamin K is extensively metabolized in the liver and excreted in the urine and bile. In tracer experiments about 20% of an injected dose of phylloquinone was recovered in the urine whereas about 40–50% was excreted in the faeces via the bile (10); the proportion excreted was the same regardless of whether the injected dose was 1 mg or 45 µg. It seems likely, therefore, that about 60–70% of the amount of phylloquinone absorbed from each meal will ultimately be lost to the body by excretion. These results suggest that the body stores of phylloquinone are being constantly replenished.

The main urinary excretory products have been identified as carboxylic acids with 5- and 7-carbon side chains, which are excreted as glucuronide conjugates (10). The biliary metabolites have not been clearly identified but are initially excreted as water-soluble conjugates and become lipid soluble during their passage through the gastrointestinal tract, probably through deconjugation by the intestinal flora. There is no evidence for body stores of vitamin K being conserved by an enterohepatic circulation. Vitamin K itself is too lipophilic to be excreted in the bile and the side chain-shortened carboxylic acid metabolites are not biologically active.

6.4 Populations at risk for vitamin K deficiency
6.4.1 Vitamin K deficiency bleeding in infants

In infants up to around age 6 months, vitamin K deficiency, although rare, represents a significant public health problem throughout the world (*19, 22, 23*). The deficiency syndrome is traditionally known as haemorrhagic disease of the newborn. More recently, in order to give a better definition of the cause, it has been termed vitamin K deficiency bleeding (VKDB).

The time of onset of VKDB is now thought to be more unpredictable than previously supposed; currently three distinct syndromes are recognized: early, classic, and late VKDB (Table 6.1). Until the 1960s, VKDB was considered to be solely a problem of the first week of life. Then, in 1966, came the first reports from Thailand of a new vitamin K deficiency syndrome that typically presented between 1 and 2 months of life and which is now termed late VKDB. In 1977 Bhanchet and colleagues (*24*), who had first described this syndrome, summarized their studies of 93 affected Thai infants, estab-

TABLE 6.1
Classification of vitamin K deficiency bleeding of the newborn infant

Syndrome	Time of presentation	Common bleeding sites	Comments
Early VKDB	0–24 hours	Cephalohaematoma, intracranial, intrathoracic, intra-abdominal	Maternal drugs are a frequent cause (e.g. warfarin, anti-convulsants)
Classic VKDB	1–7 days	Gastrointestinal, skin, nasal, circumcision	Mainly idiopathic; maternal drugs are sometimes a cause
Late VKDB	1–12 weeks	Intracranial, skin, gastrointestinal	Mainly idiopathic, but may be a presenting feature of underlying disease (e.g. cystic fibrosis, α-1-antitrypsin deficiency, biliary atresia); some degree of cholestasis often present

VKDB, vitamin K deficiency bleeding.
Source: reference (*19*).

lishing the idiopathic history, preponderance of breast-fed infants (98%), and high incidence of intracranial bleeding (63%). More reports from south-east Asia and Australia followed, and in 1983 McNinch et al. (25) reported the return of VKDB in the United Kingdom. This increased incidence was ascribed to a decrease in the practice of vitamin K prophylaxis and to an increased trend towards exclusive human-milk feeding (25).

Without vitamin K prophylaxis, the incidence of late VKDB (per 100 000 births), based on acceptable surveillance data, has been estimated to be 4.4 in the United Kingdom, 7.2 in Germany, and as high as 72 in Thailand (26). Of real concern is that late VKDB, unlike the classic form, has a high incidence of death or severe and permanent brain damage resulting from intracranial haemorrhage (19, 22, 23).

Epidemiological studies worldwide have identified two major risk factors for both classic and late VKDB: exclusive human-milk feeding and the failure to give any vitamin K prophylaxis (19, 22, 23). The increased risk for infants fed human milk compared with formula milk is probably related to the relatively low concentrations of vitamin K (phylloquinone) in breast milk compared with formula milks (27–29). For classic VKDB, studies using the detection of under-carboxylated prothrombin or proteins induced by vitamin K absence (PIVKA-II) as a marker of subclinical vitamin K deficiency have suggested that it is the low cumulative intake of human milk in the first week of life rather than an abnormally low milk concentration per se that seems to be of greater relevance (30, 31). Thus, classic VKDB may be related, at least in part, to a failure to establish early breast-feeding practices.

For late VKDB other factors seem to be important because the deficiency syndrome occurs when breastfeeding is well established and mothers of affected infants seem to have normal concentrations of vitamin K in their milk (31). For instance, some (although not all) infants who develop late haemorrhagic disease of the newborn are later found to have abnormalities of liver function that may affect their bile acid production and result in a degree of malabsorption of vitamin K. The degree of cholestasis may be mild and its course may be transient and self-correcting, but affected infants will have an increased dietary requirement for vitamin K because of reduced absorption efficiency.

6.4.2 Vitamin K prophylaxis in infants

As bleeding can occur spontaneously and because no screening test is available, it is now common paediatric practice to protect all infants by giving vitamin K supplements in the immediate perinatal period. Vitamin K prophylaxis has had a chequered history but in recent years has become a high-profile issue of public health in many countries throughout the world. The reasons for this are two-fold. First, there is now a convincing body of evidence showing that without vitamin K prophylaxis, infants have a small but real risk of dying from, or being permanently brain damaged by, vitamin K deficiency in the first 6 months of life (*19, 22, 23*). The other, much less certain evidence stems from a reported epidemiological association between vitamin K given intramuscularly (but not orally) and the later development of childhood cancer (*32*). The debate, both scientific and public, which followed this and other publications has led to an increase in the use of multiple oral supplements instead of the traditional single intramuscular injection (usually of 1 mg phylloquinone) given at birth. Although most of the subsequent epidemiological studies have not confirmed any cancer link with vitamin K prophylaxis, the issue is still not resolved (*33, 34*).

6.4.3 Vitamin K deficiency in adults

In adults, primary vitamin K-deficient states that manifest as bleeding are almost unknown except when the absorption of the vitamin is impaired as a result of an underlying pathology (*1*).

6.5 Sources of vitamin K

6.5.1 Dietary sources

High-performance liquid chromatography can be used to accurately determine the major dietary form of vitamin K (phylloquinone) in foods, and food tables are being compiled for Western diets (*16, 35, 36*). Phylloquinone is distributed ubiquitously throughout the diet, and the range of concentrations in different food categories is very wide. In general, the relative values in vegetables confirm the known association of phylloquinone with photosynthetic tissues, with the highest values (normally in the range 400–700 μg/100 g) being found in green leafy vegetables. The next best sources are certain vegetable oils (e.g. soybean, rapeseed, and olive), which contain 50–200 μg/100 g; other vegetable oils, such as peanut, corn, sunflower, and safflower, however, contain much lower amounts of phylloquinone (1–10 μg/100 g). The great differences between vegetable oils with respect to vitamin K content obviously present problems for calculating the phylloquinone contents of oil-containing foods when the type of oil is not known.

Menaquinones seem to have a more restricted distribution in the diet than does phylloquinone. Menaquinone-rich foods are those with a bacterial fermentation stage. Yeasts, however, do not synthesize menaquinones. In the typical diet of developed countries, nutritionally significant amounts of long-chain menaquinones have been found in animal livers and fermented foods such as cheeses. The Japanese food *natto* (fermented soybeans) has a menaquinone content even higher than the phylloquinone content of green leafy vegetables.

The relative dietary importance of MK-4 is more difficult to evaluate because concentrations in foods may well depend on geographic differences in the use of menadione in animal husbandry. MK-4 may be synthesized in animal tissues from menadione supplied in animal feed. Another imponderable factor is the evidence that animal tissues and dairy produce may contain some MK-4 as a product of tissue synthesis from phylloquinone itself (*37*).

Knowledge of the vitamin K content of human milk has been the subject of methodologic controversies with a 10-fold variation in reported values of phylloquinone concentrations of mature human milk (*38*). Where milk sampling and analytical techniques have met certain criteria for their validity, the phylloquinone content of mature milk has generally ranged between 1 and 4 µg/l, with average concentrations near the lower end of this range (*28, 29, 38*). However, there is considerable intra- and intersubject variation, and levels are higher in colostral milk than in mature milk (*28*). Menaquinone concentrations in human milk have not been accurately determined but appear to be much lower than those of phylloquinone. Phylloquinone concentrations in infant formula milk range from 3 to 16 µg/l in unsupplemented formulas and up to 100 µg/l in fortified formulas (*26*). Currently most formulas are fortified; typical phylloquinone concentrations are about 50 µg/l.

6.5.2 Bioavailability of vitamin K from foods

Very little is known about the bioavailability of the K vitamins from different foods. It has been estimated that the efficiency of absorption of phylloquinone from boiled spinach (eaten with butter) is no greater than 10% (*39*) compared with an estimated 80% when phylloquinone is given in its free form (*10, 11*). This poor absorption of phylloquinone from green leafy vegetables may be explained by its location in chloroplasts and tight association with the thylakoid membrane, where naphthoquinone plays a role in photosynthesis. In comparison, the bioavailability of MK-4 from butter artificially enriched with this vitamer was more than two-fold higher than that of phylloquinone from spinach (*39*). The poor extraction of phylloquinone from leafy vegetables, which as a category represents the single greatest food source of phylloquinone, may place a different perspective on the relative importance of other foods with lower concentrations of phylloquinone (e.g. those containing soybean and rapeseed oils) but in which the vitamin is not tightly bound and its bioavailability likely to be greater. Even before bioavailability was taken into account, fats and oils that are contained in mixed dishes were found to make an important contribution to the phylloquinone content of the United States diet (*40*) and in a United Kingdom study, contributed 30% of the total dietary intake (*41*).

No data exist on the efficiency of intestinal absorption of dietary long-chain menaquinones. Because the lipophilic properties of menaquinones are greater than those of phylloquinone, it is likely that the efficiency of their absorption, in the free form, is low, as has been suggested by animal studies (*18, 21*).

6.5.3 Importance of intestinal bacterial synthesis as a source of vitamin K

Intestinal microflora synthesize large amounts of menaquinones, which are potentially available as a source of vitamin K (*42*). Quantitative measurements at different sites of the human intestine have demonstrated that most of these menaquinones are present in the distal colon (*42*). Major forms produced are MK-10 and MK-11 by *Bacteroides*, MK-8 by *Enterobacter*, MK-7 by *Veillonella*, and MK-6 by *Eubacterium lentum*. It is noteworthy that menaquinones with very long chains (MKs 10–13) are known to be synthesized by members of the anaerobic genus *Bacteroides*, and are found in large concentrations in the intestinal tract but have not been detected in significant amounts in foods. The widespread presence of MKs 10–13 in human livers at high concentrations (*14, 15*) therefore suggests that these forms, at least, originate from intestinal synthesis (*16*).

It is commonly held that animals and humans obtain a significant fraction of their vitamin K requirement from direct absorption of menaquinones produced by microfloral synthesis (*43*), but conclusive experimental evidence documenting the site and extent of absorption is singularly lacking (*18, 19, 23*). The most promising site of absorption is the terminal ileum, where there are some menaquinone-producing bacteria as well as bile salts. However, the balance of evidence suggests that the bioavailability of bacterial menaquinones is poor because they are for the most part tightly bound to the bacterial cytoplasmic membrane and also because the largest pool is present in the colon, which lacks bile salts for their solubilization (*19, 23*).

6.6 Information relevant to the derivation of recommended vitamin K intakes

6.6.1 Assessment of vitamin K status

Conventional coagulation assays are useful for detecting overt vitamin K-deficient states, which are associated with a risk of bleeding. However, they offer only a relatively insensitive insight into vitamin K nutritional status and the detection of subclinical vitamin K-deficient states. A more sensitive measure of vitamin K sufficiency can be obtained from tests that detect under-carboxylated species of vitamin K-dependent proteins. In states of vitamin K deficiency, under-carboxylated species of the vitamin K-dependent coagulation proteins are released from the liver into the blood; their levels increase with the degree of severity of vitamin K deficiency. These under-carboxylated forms (PIVKA) are unable to participate in the normal coagulation cascade because they are unable to bind calcium. The measurement of under-carboxylated prothrombin (PIVKA-II) is the most useful and sensitive homeostatic marker of subclinical vitamin K deficiency (see also section 6.4.1). Importantly, PIVKA-II is detectable in plasma before any changes occur in conventional coagulation tests. Several types of assay for PIVKA-II have been developed which vary in their sensitivity (44).

In the same way that vitamin K deficiency causes PIVKA-II to be released into the circulation from the liver, a deficit of vitamin K in bone will cause the osteoblasts to secrete under-carboxylated species of osteocalcin (ucOC) into the bloodstream. It has been proposed that the concentration of circulating ucOC reflects the sufficiency of vitamin K for the carboxylation of this Gla protein in bone tissue (7, 45). Most assays for ucOC are indirect in that they rely on the differential absorption of carboxylated and under-carboxylated forms to hydroxyapatite and are thus difficult to interpret (46).

Other criteria of vitamin K sufficiency that have been used are plasma measurements of phylloquinone and the measurement of urinary Gla. It is expected and found that the excretion of urinary Gla is decreased in individuals with vitamin K deficiency.

6.6.2 Dietary intakes in infants and their adequacy

The average intake of phylloquinone in infants fed human milk during the first 6 months of life has been reported to be less than 1 µg/day; this is approximately 100-fold lower than the intake in infants fed a typical supplemented formula (29). This large disparity between intakes is reflected in plasma levels (Table 6.2).

Using the detection of PIVKA-II as a marker of subclinical deficiency, a study from Germany concluded that a minimum daily intake of about 100 ml of colostral milk (that supplies about 0.2–0.3 µg of phylloquinone) is sufficient for normal haemostasis in a baby of about 3 kg during the first week of life (30, 47). Similar conclusions were reached in a Japanese study which showed a linear correlation between the prevalence of PIVKA-II and the volume of breast milk ingested over 3 days (48); 95% of infants with

TABLE 6.2
Dietary intakes and plasma levels of phylloquinone in human-milk-fed versus formula-fed infants aged 0–6 months

Age (weeks)	Phylloquinone intake (µg/day)		Plasma phylloquinone (µg/l)	
	Human-milk-fed[a]	Formula-fed[b]	Human-milk-fed	Formula-fed
6	0.55	45.4	0.13	6.0
12	0.74	55.5	0.20	5.6
26	0.56	52.2	0.24	4.4

[a] Breast-milk concentrations of phylloquinone averaged 0.86, 1.14, and 0.87 µg/l at 6, 12, and 26 weeks, respectively.
[b] All infants were fed a formula containing phylloquinone at 55 µg/l.
Source: reference (29).

detectable PIVKA-II had average daily intakes of less than about 120 ml, but the marker was not detectable when intakes reached 170 ml/day.

6.6.3 Factors of relevance to classical vitamin K deficiency bleeding

The liver stores of vitamin K in the neonate differ both qualitatively and quantitatively from those in adults. First, phylloquinone levels at birth are about one fifth those in adults and second, bacterial menaquinones are undetectable (14). It has been well established that placental transport of vitamin K to the human fetus is difficult (19, 22). The limited available data suggest that hepatic stores of menaquinones build up gradually after birth, becoming detectable at around the second week of life but only reaching adult concentrations after 1 month of age (14, 49). A gradual increase in liver stores of menaquinones may reflect the gradual colonization of the gut by enteric microflora.

A practical problem in assessing the functional status of vitamin K in the neonatal period is that there are both gestational and postnatal increases in the four vitamin K-dependent procoagulant factors which are unrelated to vitamin K status (50). This means that unless the deficiency state is quite severe, it is very difficult to interpret clotting factor activities as a measure of vitamin K sufficiency. Immunoassays are the best diagnostic tool for determining the adequacy of vitamin K stores in neonates, as they detect levels of PIVKA-II. The use of this marker has clearly shown that there is a temporary dip in the vitamin K status of infants exclusively fed human milk in the first few days after birth (30, 47, 48, 51, 52). The fact that the degree of this dip is associated with human-milk intakes (30, 47, 48) and is less evident or absent in infants given formula milk (30, 48, 52) or prophylactic vitamin K at birth (48, 51, 52) shows that the detection of PIVKA-II reflects a dietary lack of vitamin K (see also section 6.4.1).

6.6.4 Factors of relevance to late vitamin K deficiency bleeding

The natural tendency for human-milk-fed infants to develop a subclinical vitamin K deficiency in the first 2–3 days of life is self-limiting. Comparisons between untreated human-milk-fed infants and those who had received vitamin K or supplementary feeds clearly suggest that improvement in vitamin K-dependent clotting activity is due to an improved vitamin K status. After the first week, vitamin K-dependent clotting activity increases are more gradual, and it is not possible to differentiate—from clotting factor assays— between the natural postnatal increase in the synthesis of the core proteins and the increase achieved through an improved vitamin K status.

Use of the most sensitive assays for PIVKA-II show that there is still evidence of suboptimal vitamin K status in infants solely fed human milk between the ages of 1 and 2 months (52, 53). Deficiency signs are less common in infants who have received adequate vitamin K supplementation (52, 53) or who have been formula fed (52).

6.6.5 Dietary intakes in older infants, children, and adults and their adequacy

The only comprehensive national survey of phylloquinone intakes across all age groups (except infants aged 0–6 months) is that of the United States Food and Drug Administration Total Diet Study, which was based on the 1987–88 Nationwide Food Consumption Survey (40). For infants and children from the age of 6 months to 16 years, average phylloquinone intakes were above the current United States recommended dietary allowance (RDA) values for their respective age groups, more so for children up to 10 years than from 10 to 16 years (Table 6.3) (40). No studies have been conducted that assess functional markers of vitamin K sufficiency in children.

Intakes for adults in the Total Diet Study (Table 6.3) were also close to or slightly higher than the current United States RDA values of 80 μg for men and 65 μg for women, although intakes were slightly lower than the RDA in the 25–30-years age group (54). There is some evidence from an evaluation of all the United States studies that older adults have higher dietary intakes of phylloquinone than do younger adults (55).

The results from the United States are very similar to a detailed, seasonality study conducted in the United Kingdom in which mean intakes in men and women (aged 22–54 years) were 72 and 64 μg/day, respectively; no significant sex or seasonal variations were found (56). Another United Kingdom study suggested that intakes were lower in people who work as manual labourers and in smokers, reflecting the lower intakes of green vegetables and high-phylloquinone content vegetable oil in these groups (57).

120

TABLE 6.3

Mean dietary intakes of phylloquinone from the United States Food and Drug Administration Total Diet Study (TDS) based on the 1987–88 Nationwide Food Consumption Survey compared with the recommended dietary allowance (RDA), by group

Group	No.[a]	Phylloquinone intake (μg/day)	
		TDS[b]	RDA[c]
Infants			
6 months	141	77	10
Children			
2 years	152	24	15
6 years	154	46	20
10 years	119	45	30
Females, 14–16 years	188	52	45–55
Males, 14–16 years	174	64	45–65
Younger adults			
Females, 25–30 years	492	59	65
Males, 25–30 years	386	66	80
Females, 40–45 years	319	71	65
Males, 40–45 years	293	86	80
Older adults			
Females, 60–65 years	313	76	65
Males, 60–65 years	238	80	80
Females, 70+ years	402	82	65
Males, 70+ years	263	80	80

[a] The number of subjects as stratified by age and/or sex.
[b] Total Diet Study, 1990 (*40*).
[c] Recommended dietary allowance, 1989 (*54*).

Several dietary restriction and repletion studies have attempted to assess the adequacy of vitamin K intakes in adults (*55*, *58*). It is clear from these studies that volunteers consuming less than 10 μg/day of phylloquinone do not show any changes in conventional coagulation tests even after several weeks, unless other measures to reduce the efficiency of absorption are introduced. However, a diet containing only 2–5 μg/day of phylloquinone fed for 2 weeks did result in an increase of PIVKA-II and a 70% decrease in plasma phylloquinone (*59*). Similar evidence of a subclinical vitamin K deficiency coupled with an increased urinary excretion of Gla was found when dietary intakes of phylloquinone were reduced from about 80 to about 40 μg/day for 21 days (*60*). A repletion phase in this study was consistent with a human dietary vitamin K requirement (for its coagulation role) of about 1 μg/kg body weight/day.

The most detailed and controlled dietary restriction and repletion study conducted to date in healthy human subjects is that by Ferland et al. (*61*). In this study 32 healthy subjects in two age groups (20–40 and 60–80 years) were fed a mixed diet containing about 80 μg/day of phylloquinone, which is the RDA for adult males in the United States (54). After 4 days on this baseline diet there was a 13-day depletion period during which the subjects were fed a diet containing about 10 μg/day. After this depletion phase the subjects entered a 16-day repletion period during which, over 4-day intervals, they were sequentially repleted with 5, 15, 25, and 45 μg of phylloquinone. The depletion protocol had no effect on conventional coagulation and specific factor assays but did induce a significant increase in PIVKA-II in both age groups. The most dramatic change was in plasma levels of phylloquinone, which fell to about 15% of the values determined on day 1. The drop in plasma phylloquinone also suggested that the average dietary intake of these particular individuals before they entered the study had been greater than the baseline diet of 80 μg/day. The repletion protocol failed to bring the plasma phylloquinone levels of the young subjects back above the lower limit of the normal range (previously established in healthy adults) and the plasma levels in the elderly group rose only slightly above this lower limit in the last 4 days. Another indication of a reduced vitamin K status in the young group was the fall in urinary output of Gla (to 90% of baseline) that was not seen in the elderly group; this suggested that the younger subjects were more susceptible to the effects of an acute deficiency than were the older subjects.

One important dietary intervention study measured the carboxylation status of the bone vitamin K-dependent protein, osteocalcin, in response to altered dietary intakes of phylloquinone (62). This was a crossover study which evaluated the effect in young adults of increasing the dietary intake of phylloquinone to 420 μg/day for 5 days from a baseline intake of 100 μg/day. Although total concentrations of osteocalcin were not affected, ucOC fell dramatically in response to the 420 μg diet and by the end of the 5-day supplementation period was 41% lower than the baseline value. After the return to the mixed diet, the ucOC percentage rose significantly but after 5 days had not returned to pre-supplementation values. This study suggests that the carboxylation of osteocalcin in bone might require higher dietary intakes of vitamin K than those needed to sustain its haemostatic function.

6.7 Recommendations for vitamin K intakes
6.7.1 Infants 0–6 months
Consideration of the requirements of vitamin K for infants up to age 6 months is complicated by the need to prevent a rare but potentially devastating bleeding disorder which is caused by vitamin K deficiency. To protect the few affected infants, most developed and some developing countries have instituted a blanket prophylactic policy to protect infants at risk, a policy that is

endorsed by the present Consultation (Table 6.4). The numbers of infants at risk without such a programme has a geographic component, the risk being more prevalent in Asia, and a dietary component, with solely human-milk-fed babies having the highest risk (*22, 23, 27*). Of the etiologic factors, some of which may still be unrecognized, one factor in some infants is mild cholestasis. The problem of overcoming a variable and, in some infants, inefficient absorption is the likely reason that oral prophylactic regimens, even with two or three pharmacologic doses (1 mg phylloquinone), have occasionally failed to prevent VKDB (*63*). This makes it difficult to design an effective oral prophylaxis regimen that is comparable in efficacy with the previous "gold standard" of 1 mg phylloquinone given by intramuscular injection at birth. As previously stated, intramuscular prophylaxis fell out of favour in several countries after the epidemiological report and subsequent controversy that this administration route may be linked to childhood cancer (*32–34*).

TABLE 6.4
Recommended nutrient intakes (RNIs) for vitamin K, by group

Group	RNI[a] (µg/day)
Infants and children	
0–6 months	5[b]
7–12 months	10
1–3 years	15
4–6 years	20
7–9 years	25
Adolescents	
Females, 10–18 years	35–55
Males, 10–18 years	35–55
Adults	
Females	
19–65 years	55
65+ years	55
Males	
19–65 years	65
65+ years	65
Pregnant women	55
Lactating women	55

[a] The RNI for each group is based on a daily intake of approximately 1 µg/kg body weight of phylloquinone.
[b] This intake cannot be met by infants who are exclusively breastfed (see Table 6.2). To prevent bleeding due to vitamin K deficiency, it is recommended that all breast-fed infants should receive vitamin K supplementation at birth according to nationally approved guidelines. Vitamin K formulations and prophylactic regimes differ from country to country. Guidelines range from a single intramuscular injection (usually 1 mg of phylloquinone) given at birth to multiple oral doses given over the first few weeks of life.

Infants who have been entirely fed with supplemented formulas are well protected against VKDB and on intakes of around 50μg/day have plasma levels that are about 10-fold higher than the adult average of about 1.0 nmol/l (0.5 μg/l) (29) (Table 6.2). Clearly then, an optimal intake would lie below an intake of 50μg/day. Cornelissen et al. (64) evaluated the effectiveness of giving infants a daily supplement of 25 μg phylloquinone after they had received a single oral dose of 1 mg at birth. This regimen resulted in median plasma levels at ages 4, 8, and 12 weeks of around 2.2 nmol/l (1.0 μg/l) when sampled 20–28 hours after the most recent vitamin K dose; this level corresponds to the upper end of the adult fasting range. In 12-week-old infants supplemented with this regime, the median plasma level was about four-fold higher than that in a control group of unsupplemented infants (1.9 versus 0.5 nmol/l). Also none of the 50 supplemented infants had detectable PIVKA-II at 12 weeks compared with 15 of 131 infants (11.5%) in the control group. This regime has now been implemented in the Netherlands and surveillance data on late VKDB suggest that it may be as effective as parenteral vitamin K prophylaxis (63).

The fact that VKDB is epidemiologically associated with breastfeeding means that it is not prudent to base requirements solely on normal intakes of human milk and justifies the setting of a higher value that can only be met by some form of supplementation. The current United States RDA for infants is 5μg/day for the first 6 months (the greatest period of risk for VKDB) and 10μg/day during the second 6 months (54). These intakes are based on the adult RDA of 1μg/kg body weight/day. However, if the vitamin K content of human milk is assumed to be about 2μg/l, exclusively breast-fed infants aged 0–6 months may ingest only 20% of their presumed daily requirement of 5μg (54). Whether a figure of 5μg/day is itself safe is uncertain. In the United Kingdom the dietary reference value for infants is set at 10μg/day, which in relation to body weight (2μg/kg) is about double the estimate for adults (65). It was set with reference to the upper end of possible human milk concentrations plus a further qualitative addition to allow for the absence of hepatic menaquinones in early life and the presumed reliance on dietary vitamin K alone.

The association of VKDB with breastfeeding does not mean that most infants are at risk of developing VKDB, as this is a rare vitamin K deficiency syndrome. In contrast to measurements of PIVKA-II levels, comparisons of vitamin K-dependent clotting activities have shown no detectable differences between infants fed human milk and those fed artifical formula. The detection of PIVKA-II with normal functional levels of vitamin K-dependent coagulation factors does not imply immediate or even future haemorrhagic risk for a particular individual. The major value of PIVKA-II measurements in infants is to assess the prevalence of suboptimal vitamin K status in population studies. However, because of the potential consequences of VKDB, the paediatric profession of most countries agrees that some form of vitamin K supplementation is necessary even though there are widespread differences in actual practice.

6.7.2 Infants (7–12 months), children, and adults

In the past, the requirements for vitamin K have only considered its classical function in coagulation; an RDA has been given for vitamin K in the United States (54, 58) and a safe and adequate intake level given in the United Kingdom (65). In both countries the adult RDA or adequate intake have been set at a value of 1 μg/kg body weight/day. Thus, in the United States the RDA for a 79-kg man is listed as 80 μg/day and for a 63-kg woman as 65 μg/day (54).

At the time previous recommendations were set there were few data on dietary intakes of vitamin K (mainly phylloquinone) in different populations. The development of more accurate and wide-ranging food databases is now helping to redress this information gap. The results of several dietary intake studies carried out in the United States and the United Kingdom suggest that the average intakes for adults are very close to the respective recommendations of each country. In the United States, preliminary intake data also suggest that average intakes of phylloquinone in children and adolescents exceed the RDA; in 6-month-old infants the intakes exceeded the RDA of 10 μg by nearly eight-fold (40), reflecting the use of supplemented formula foods. Because there is no evidence of even subclinical deficiencies of haemostatic function, a daily intake of 1 μg/kg may still be used as the basis for the recommended nutrient intake (RNI). There is no basis as yet for making different recommendations for pregnant and lactating women (Table 6.4).

The question remains whether the RNI should be raised to take into account recent evidence that the requirements for the optimal carboxylation of vitamin K-dependent proteins in other tissues are greater than those for coagulation. There is certainly evidence that the γ-carboxylation of osteocalcin can be improved by intakes somewhere between 100 and 420 μg/day (62). If an RNI for vitamin K sufficiency is to be defined as that amount necessary for the optimal carboxylation of all vitamin K-dependent proteins, including osteocalcin, then it seems clear that this RNI would lie somewhere above the current intakes of many, if not most, of the population in the United States and the United Kingdom. However, because a clearly defined metabolic role and biochemical proof of the necessity for fully γ-carboxylated osteocalcin for bone health is currently lacking, it would be unwise to make such a recommendation at this time.

6.8 Toxicity

When taken orally, natural K vitamins seem free of toxic side effects. This apparent safety is bourne out by the common clinical administration of phylloquinone at doses of 10–20 mg or greater. Some patients with chronic fat malabsorption regularly ingest doses of this size without evidence of any harm. However, synthetic preparations of menadione or its salts are best avoided for nutritional purposes, especially for vitamin prophylaxis in neonates. Besides lacking intrinsic biological activity, the high reactivity of its unsubstituted 3-position has been associated with neonatal haemolysis and liver damage.

6.9 Recommendations for future research

The following are recommended areas for future research:

- prevalence, causes, and prevention of VKDB in infants in different population groups;
- bioavailability of dietary phylloquinone (and menaquinones) from foods and menaquinones from intestinal flora;
- significance of menaquinones to human requirements for vitamin K;
- the physiological roles of vitamin K-dependent proteins in functions other than coagulation;
- the significance of under-carboxylated vitamin K-dependent proteins and suboptimal vitamin K status to bone and cardiovascular health.

References

1. Suttie JW. Vitamin K. In: Diplock AD, ed. *Fat-soluble vitamins: their biochemistry and applications*. London, Heinemann, 1985:225–311.
2. Furie B, Furie BC. Molecular basis of vitamin K-dependent γ-carboxylation. *Blood*, 1990, 75:1753–1762.
3. Davie EW. Biochemical and molecular aspects of the coagulation cascade. *Thrombosis and Haemostasis*, 1995, 74:1–6.
4. Vermeer C. γ-Carboxyglutamate-containing proteins and the vitamin K-dependent carboxylase. *Biochemical Journal*, 1990, 266:625–636.
5. Ferland G. The vitamin K-dependent proteins: an update. *Nutrition Reviews*, 1998, 56:223–230.
6. Luo G et al. Spontaneous calcification of arteries and cartilage in mice lacking matrix Gla protein. *Nature*, 1997, 386:78–81.
7. Vermeer C, Jie K-S, Knapen MHJ. Role of vitamin K in bone metabolism. *Annual Review of Nutrition*, 1995, 15:1–22.
8. Binkley NC, Suttie JW. Vitamin K nutrition and osteoporosis. *Journal of Nutrition*, 1995, 125:1812–1821.

9. Shearer MJ. The roles of vitamins D and K in bone health and osteoporosis prevention. *Proceedings of the Nutrition Society*, 1997, 56:915–937.

10. Shearer MJ, McBurney A, Barkhan P. Studies on the absorption and metabolism of phylloquinone (vitamin K_1) in man. *Vitamins and Hormones*, 1974, 32:513–542.

11. Shearer MJ, Barkhan P, Webster GR. Absorption and excretion of an oral dose of tritiated vitamin K_1 in man. *British Journal of Haematology*, 1970, 18:297–308.

12. Blomstrand R, Forsgren L. Vitamin K_1-^{3}H in man: its intestinal absorption and transport in the thoracic duct lymph. *Internationale Zeitschrift für Vitaminsforschung*, 1968, 38:45–64.

13. Kohlmeier M et al. Transport of vitamin K to bone in humans. *Journal of Nutrition*, 1996, 126(Suppl.):S1192–S1196.

14. Shearer MJ et al. The assessment of human vitamin K status from tissue measurements. In: Suttie JW, ed. *Current advances in vitamin K research*. New York, NY, Elsevier, 1988:437–452.

15. Usui Y et al. Vitamin K concentrations in the plasma and liver of surgical patients. *American Journal of Clinical Nutrition*, 1990, 51:846–852.

16. Shearer MJ, Bach A, Kohlmeier M. Chemistry, nutritional sources, tissue distribution and metabolism of vitamin K with special reference to bone health. *Journal of Nutrition*, 1996, 126(Suppl.): S1181–S1186.

17. Hodges SJ et al. Detection and measurement of vitamins K_1 and K_2 in human cortical and trabecular bone. *Journal of Bone and Mineral Research*, 1993, 8:1005–1008.

18. Suttie JW. The importance of menaquinones in human nutrition. *Annual Review of Nutrition*, 1995, 15:399–417.

19. Shearer MJ. Vitamin K metabolism and nutriture. *Blood Reviews*, 1992, 6:92–104.

20. Groenen-van Dooren MMCL et al. Bioavailability of phylloquinone and menaquinones after oral and colorectal administration in vitamin K-deficient rats. *Biochemical Pharmacology*, 1995, 50:797–801.

21. Will BH, Suttie JW. Comparative metabolism of phylloquinone and menaquinone-9 in rat liver. *Journal of Nutrition*, 1992, 122:953–958.

22. Lane PA, Hathaway WE. Vitamin K in infancy. *Journal of Pediatrics*, 1985, 106:351–359.

23. Shearer MJ. Fat-soluble vitamins: vitamin K. *Lancet*, 1995, 345:229–234.

24. Bhanchet P et al. A bleeding syndrome in infants due to acquired prothrombin complex deficiency: a survey of 93 affected infants. *Clinical Pediatrics*, 1977, 16:992–998.

25. McNinch AW, Orme RL, Tripp JH. Haemorrhagic disease of the newborn returns. *Lancet*, 1983, 1:1089–1090.

26. von Kries R, Hanawa Y. Neonatal vitamin K prophylaxis. Report of the Scientific and Standardization Subcommittee on Perinatal Haemostasis. *Thrombosis and Haemostasis*, 1993, 69:293–295.

27. Haroon Y et al. The content of phylloquinone (vitamin K_1) in human milk, cows' milk and infant formula foods determined by high-performance liquid chromatography. *Journal of Nutrition*, 1982, 112:1105–1117.

28. von Kries R et al. Vitamin K_1 content of maternal milk: influence of the stage of lactation, lipid composition, and vitamin K_1 supplements given to the mother. *Pediatric Research*, 1987, 22:513–517.

29. Greer FR et al. Vitamin K status of lactating mothers, human milk and breast-feeding infants. *Pediatrics*, 1991, 88:751–756.

30. von Kries R, Becker A, Göbel U. Vitamin K in the newborn: influence of nutritional factors on acarboxy-prothrombin detectability and factor II and VII clotting activity. *European Journal of Pediatrics*, 1987, 146:123–127.

31. von Kries R, Shearer MJ, Göbel U. Vitamin K in infancy. *European Journal of Pediatrics*, 1988, 147:106–112.

32. Golding J et al. Childhood cancer, intramuscular vitamin K, and pethidine given during labour. *British Medical Journal*, 1992, 305:341–346.

33. Draper G, McNinch A. Vitamin K for neonates: the controversy. *British Medical Journal*, 1994, 308:867–868.

34. von Kries R. Neonatal vitamin K prophylaxis: the Gordian knot still awaits untying. *British Medical Journal*, 1998, 316:161–162.

35. Booth SL, Davidson KW, Sadowski JA. Evaluation of an HPLC method for the determination of phylloquinone (vitamin K_1) in various food matrices. *Journal of Agricultural and Food Chemistry*, 1994, 42:295–300.

36. Booth SL et al. Vitamin K_1 (phylloquinone) content of foods: a provisional table. *Journal of Food Composition and Analysis*, 1993, 6:109–120.

37. Thijssen HHW, Drittij-Reijnders MJ. Vitamin K distribution in rat tissues: dietary phylloquinone is a source of tissue menaquinone-4. *British Journal of Nutrition*, 1994, 72:415–425.

38. Canfield LM, Hopkinson JM. State of the art vitamin K in human milk. *Journal of Pediatric Gastroenterology and Nutrition*, 1989, 8:430–441.

39. Gijsbers BLMG, Jie K-SG, Vermeer C. Effect of food composition on vitamin K absorption in human volunteers. *British Journal of Nutrition*, 1996, 76:223–229.

40. Booth SL, Pennington JAT, Sadowski JA. Food sources and dietary intakes of vitamin K-1 (phylloquinone) in the American diet: data from the FDA Total Diet Study. *Journal of the American Dietetic Association*, 1996, 96:149–154.

41. Fenton ST et al. Nutrient sources of phylloquinone (vitamin K_1) in Scottish men and women [abstract]. *Proceedings of the Nutrition Society*, 1997, 56:301.

42. Conly JM, Stein K. Quantitative and qualitative measurements of K vitamins in human intestinal contents. *American Journal of Gastroenterology*, 1992, 87:311–316.

43. Davidson S, Passmore R, Eastwood MA. *Davidson and Passmore human nutrition and dietetics*, 8th ed. Edinburgh, Churchill Livingstone, 1986.

44. Widdershoven J et al. Four methods compared for measuring des-carboxy-prothrombin (PIVKA-II). *Clinical Chemistry*, 1987, 33:2074–2078.

45. Vermeer C, Hamulyák K. Pathophysiology of vitamin K-deficiency and oral anticoagulants. *Thrombosis and Haemostasis*, 1991, 66:153–159.

46. Gundberg CM et al. Vitamin K status and bone health: an analysis of methods for determination of undercarboxylated osteocalcin. *Journal of Clinical Endocrinology and Metabolism*, 1998, 83: 258–266.

47. von Kries R et al. Vitamin K deficiency and vitamin K intakes in infants. In: Suttie JW, ed. *Current advances in vitamin K research*. New York, NY, Elsevier, 1988:515–523.

48. Motohara K et al. Relationship of milk intake and vitamin K supplementation to vitamin K status in newborns. *Pediatrics*, 1989, 84:90–93.

49. Kayata S et al. Vitamin K_1 and K_2 in infant human liver. *Journal of Pediatric Gastroenterology and Nutrition*, 1989, 8:304–307.

50. McDonald MM, Hathaway WE. Neonatal hemorrhage and thrombosis. *Seminars in Perinatology*, 1983, 7:213–225.

51. Motohara K, Endo F, Matsuda I. Effect of vitamin K administration on carboxy-prothrombin (PIVKA-II) levels in newborns. *Lancet*, 1985, 2:242–244.

52. Widdershoven J et al. Plasma concentrations of vitamin K_1 and PIVKA-II in bottle-fed and breast-fed infants with and without vitamin K prophylaxis at birth. *European Journal of Pediatrics*, 1988, 148:139–142.

53. Motohara K, Endo F, Matsuda I. Vitamin K deficiency in breast-fed infants at one month of age. *Journal of Pediatric Gastroenterology and Nutrition*, 1986, 5:931–933.

54. Subcommittee on the Tenth Edition of the Recommended Dietary Allowances, Food and Nutrition Board. *Recommended dietary allowances*, 10th ed. Washington, DC, National Academy Press, 1989.

55. Booth SL, Suttie JW. Dietary intake and adequacy of vitamin K. *Journal of Nutrition*, 1998, 128:785–788.

56. Price R et al. Daily and seasonal variation in phylloquinone (vitamin K_1) intake in Scotland [abstract]. *Proceedings of the Nutrition Society*, 1996, 55:244.

57. Fenton S et al. Dietary vitamin K (phylloquinone) intake in Scottish men [abstract]. *Proceedings of the Nutrition Society*, 1994, 53:98.

58. Suttie JW. Vitamin K and human nutrition. *Journal of the American Dietetic Association*, 1992, 92:585–590.

59. Allison PM et al. Effects of a vitamin K-deficient diet and antibiotics in normal human volunteers. *Journal of Laboratory and Clinical Medicine*, 1987, 110:180–188.

60. Suttie JW et al. Vitamin K deficiency from dietary restriction in humans. *American Journal of Clinical Nutrition*, 1988, 47:475–480.

61. Ferland G, Sadowski JA, O'Brien ME. Dietary induced subclinical vitamin K deficiency in normal human subjects. *Journal of Clinical Investigation*, 1993, 91:1761–1768.

62. Sokoll LJ et al. Changes in serum osteocalcin, plasma phylloquinone, and urinary γ-carboxyglutamic acid in response to altered intakes of dietary phylloquinone in human subjects. *American Journal of Clinical Nutrition*, 1997, 65:779–784.

63. Cornelissen M et al. Prevention of vitamin K deficiency bleeding: efficacy of different multiple oral dose schedules of vitamin K. *European Journal of Pediatrics*, 1997, 156:126–130.

64. Cornelissen EAM et al. Evaluation of a daily dose of 25 μg vitamin K_1 to prevent vitamin K deficiency in breast-fed infants. *Journal of Pediatric Gastroenterology and Nutrition*, 1993, 16:301–305.

65. Department of Health. *Dietary reference values for food energy and nutrients for the United Kingdom.* London, Her Majesty's Stationery Office, 1991 (Report on Health and Social Subjects No. 41).

7. Vitamin C

7.1 Introduction

Vitamin C (chemical names: ascorbic acid and ascorbate) is a six-carbon lactone which is synthesized from glucose by many animals. Vitamin C is synthesized in the liver in some mammals and in the kidney in birds and reptiles. However, several species—including humans, non-human primates, guinea pigs, Indian fruit bats, and Nepalese red-vented bulbuls—are unable to synthesize vitamin C. When there is insufficient vitamin C in the diet, humans suffer from the potentially lethal deficiency disease scurvy (*1*). Humans and primates lack the terminal enzyme in the biosynthetic pathway of ascorbic acid, L-gulonolactone oxidase, because the gene encoding for the enzyme has undergone substantial mutation so that no protein is produced (*2*).

7.2 Role of vitamin C in human metabolic processes

7.2.1 Background biochemistry

Vitamin C is an electron donor (reducing agent or antioxidant), and probably all of its biochemical and molecular roles can be accounted for by this function. The potentially protective role of vitamin C as an antioxidant is discussed in the antioxidants chapter of this report (see Chapter 8).

7.2.2 Enzymatic functions

Vitamin C acts as an electron donor for 11 enzymes (*3, 4*). Three of those enzymes are found in fungi but not in humans or other mammals (*5, 6*) and are involved in reutilization pathways for pyrimidines and the deoxyribose moiety of deoxynucleosides. Of the eight remaining human enzymes, three participate in collagen hydroxylation (*7–9*) and two in carnitine biosynthesis (*10, 11*); of the three enzymes which participate in collagen hydroxylation, one is necessary for biosynthesis of the catecholamine norepinephrine (*12, 13*), one is necessary for amidation of peptide hormones (*14, 15*), and one is involved in tyrosine metabolism (*4, 16*).

Ascorbate interacts with enzymes having either monooxygenase or dioxygenase activity. The monooxygenases, dopamine β-monooxygenase and peptidyl-glycine α-monooxygenase, incorporate a single oxygen atom into a substrate, either a dopamine or a glycine-terminating peptide. The dioxygenases incorporate two oxygen atoms in two different ways: the enzyme 4-hydroxyphenylpyruvate dioxygenase incorporates two oxygen atoms into one product; the other dioxygenase incorporates one oxygen atom into succinate and one into the enzyme-specific substrate.

7.2.3 Miscellaneous functions

Concentrations of vitamin C appear to be high in gastric juice. Schorah et al. (17) found that the concentrations of vitamin C in gastric juice were several-fold higher (median, 249 μmol/l; range, 43–909 μmol/l) than those found in the plasma of the same normal subjects (median, 39 μmol/l; range, 14–101 μmol/l). Gastric juice vitamin C may prevent the formation of N-nitroso compounds, which are potentially mutagenic (18). High intakes of vitamin C correlate with reduced gastric cancer risk (19), but a cause-and-effect relationship has not been established. Vitamin C protects low-density lipoproteins ex vivo against oxidation and may function similarly in the blood (20) (see Chapter 8).

A common feature of vitamin C deficiency is anaemia. The antioxidant properties of vitamin C may stabilize folate in food and in plasma; increased excretion of oxidized folate derivatives in humans with scurvy has been reported (21). Vitamin C promotes absorption of soluble non-haem iron possibly by chelation or simply by maintaining the iron in the reduced (ferrous, Fe^{2+}) form (22, 23). The effect can be achieved with the amounts of vitamin C obtained in foods. However, the amount of dietary vitamin C required to increase iron absorption ranges from 25 mg upwards and depends largely on the amount of inhibitors, such as phytates and polyphenols, present in the meal (24). (See Chapter 13 for further discussion.)

7.3 Consequences of vitamin C deficiency

From the 15th century, scurvy was dreaded by seamen and explorers forced to subsist for months on diets of dried beef and biscuits. Scurvy was described by the Crusaders during the sieges of numerous European cities, and was also a result of the famine in 19th century Ireland. Three important manifestations of scurvy—gingival changes, pain in the extremities, and haemorrhagic manifestations—precede oedema, ulcerations, and ultimately death. Skeletal and vascular lesions related to scurvy probably arise from a failure of osteoid formation. In infantile scurvy the changes are mainly at the sites of most active bone growth; characteristic signs are a pseudoparalysis of the limbs caused by extreme pain on movement and caused by haemorrhages under the periosteum, as well as swelling and haemorrhages of the gums surrounding erupting teeth (25). In adults, one of the early principle adverse effects of the collagen-related pathology may be impaired wound healing (26).

Vitamin C deficiency can be detected from early signs of clinical deficiency, such as the follicular hyperkeratosis, petechial haemorrhages, swollen or bleeding gums, and joint pain, or from the very low concentrations of ascorbate in plasma, blood, or leukocytes. The Sheffield studies (26, 27) and the later studies in Iowa (28, 29) were the first major attempts to quantify vitamin C requirements. The studies indicated that the amount of vitamin C required to prevent or cure early signs of deficiency is between 6.5 and 10 mg/day. This range represents the lowest physiological requirement. The Iowa studies (28, 29) and Kallner et al. (30) established that at tissue saturation, whole-body vitamin C content is approximately 20 mg/kg, or 1500 mg, and that during depletion vitamin C is lost at a rate of 3% of whole-body content per day.

Clinical signs of scurvy appear in men at intakes lower than 10 mg/day (27) or when the whole-body content falls below 300 mg (28). Such intakes are associated with plasma ascorbate concentrations below 11 µmol/l or leukocyte levels less than $2 \, nmol/10^8$ cells. However, plasma concentrations fall to around 11 µmol/l even when dietary vitamin C is between 10 and 20 mg/day. At intakes greater than 25–35 mg/day, plasma concentrations start to rise steeply, indicating a greater availability of vitamin C for metabolic needs. In general, plasma ascorbate closely reflects the dietary intake and ranges between 20 and 80 µmol/l. During infection or physical trauma, the number of circulating leukocytes increases and these take up vitamin C from the plasma (31, 32). Therefore, both plasma and leukocyte levels may not be very precise indicators of body content or status at such times. However, leukocyte ascorbate remains a better indicator of vitamin C status than plasma ascorbate most of the time and only in the period immediately after the onset of an infection are both values unreliable.

Intestinal absorption of vitamin C is by an active, sodium-dependent, energy-requiring, carrier-mediated transport mechanism (33) and as intake increases, the tissues become progressively more saturated. The physiologically efficient, renal-tubular reabsorption mechanism retains vitamin C in the tissues up to a whole-body content of ascorbate of about 20 mg/kg body weight (30). However, under steady-state conditions, as intake rises from around 100 mg/day there is an increase in urinary output so that at 1000 mg/day almost all absorbed vitamin C is excreted (34, 35).

7.4 Populations at risk for vitamin C deficiency

The populations at risk of vitamin C deficiency are those for whom the fruit and vegetable supply is minimal. Epidemics of scurvy are associated with famine and war, when people are forced to become refugees and food supply is small and irregular. Persons in whom the total body vitamin C content is saturated (i.e. 20 mg/kg body weight) can subsist without vitamin C for approximately 2 months before the appearance of clinical signs, and as little as 6.5–10 mg/day of vitamin C will prevent the appearance of scurvy. In general, vitamin C status will reflect the regularity of fruit and vegetable consumption; however, socioeconomic conditions are also factors as intake is determined not just by availability of food, but by cultural preferences and cost.

In Europe and the United States an adequate intake of vitamin C is indicated by the results of various national surveys (*36–38*). In Germany and the United Kingdom, the mean dietary intakes of vitamin C in adult men and women were 75 and 72 mg/day (*36*), and 87 and 76 mg/day (*37*), respectively. In addition, a recent survey of elderly men and women in the United Kingdom reported vitamin C intakes of 72 (SD, 61) and 68 (SD, 60) mg/day, respectively (*39*). In the United States, in the third National Health and Nutrition Examination Survey (*38*), the median consumption of vitamin C from foods during the years 1988–91 was 73 and 84 mg/day in men and women, respectively. In all of these studies there was a wide variation in vitamin C intake. In the United States 25–30% of the population consumed less than 2.5 servings of fruit and vegetables daily. Likewise, a survey of Latin American children suggested that less than 15% consumed the recommended intake of fruits and vegetables (*40*). It is not possible to relate servings of fruits and vegetables to an exact amount of vitamin C, but the WHO dietary goal of 400 g/day (*41*), aimed at providing sufficient vitamin C to meet the 1970 FAO/WHO guidelines—that is, approximately 20–30 mg/day—and lower the risk of chronic disease. The WHO goal has been roughly translated into the recommendation of five portions of fruits and vegetables per day (*42*).

Reports from India show that the available supply of vitamin C is 43 mg/capita/day, and in the different states of India it ranges from 27 to 66 mg/day. In one study, low-income children consumed as little as 8.2 mg/day of vitamin C in contrast to a well-to-do group of children where the intake was 35.4 mg/day (*43*). Other studies done in developing countries found plasma vitamin C concentrations lower than those reported for developed countries, for example, 20–27 μmol/l for apparently healthy adolescent boys and girls in China and 3–54 μmol/l (median, 14 μmol/l) for similarly aged Gambian nurses (*44, 45*), although values obtained in a group of adults from a rural district in northern Thailand were quite acceptable (median, 44 μmol/l; range, 17–118 μmol/l) (*46*). However, it is difficult to assess the extent to which subclinical infections are lowering the plasma vitamin C concentrations seen in such countries.

Claims for a positive association between vitamin C consumption and health status are frequently made, but results from intervention studies are inconsistent. Low plasma concentrations are reported in patients with diabetes (47) and infections (48) and in smokers (49), but the relative contribution of diet and stress to these situations is uncertain (see Chapter 8 on antioxidants). Epidemiological studies indicate that diets with a high vitamin C content have been associated with lower cancer risk, especially for cancers of the oral cavity, oesophagus, stomach, colon, and lung (39, 50–52). However, there appears to be no effect of consumption of vitamin C supplements on the development of colorectal adenoma and stomach cancer (52–54), and data on the effect of vitamin C supplementation on coronary heart disease and cataract development are conflicting (55–74). Currently there is no consistent evidence from population studies that heart disease, cancers, or cataract development are specifically associated with vitamin C status. This of course does not preclude the possibility that other components in vitamin C-rich fruits and vegetables provide health benefits, but it is not yet possible to isolate such effects from other factors such as lifestyle patterns of people who have a high vitamin C intake.

7.5 Dietary sources of vitamin C and limitations to vitamin C supply

Ascorbate is found in many fruits and vegetables (75). Citrus fruits and juices are particularly rich sources of vitamin C but other fruits including cantaloupe and honeydew melons, cherries, kiwi fruits, mangoes, papaya, strawberries, tangelo, tomatoes, and water melon also contain variable amounts of vitamin C. Vegetables such as cabbage, broccoli, Brussels sprouts, bean sprouts, cauliflower, kale, mustard greens, red and green peppers, peas, and potatoes may be more important sources of vitamin C than fruits, given that the vegetable supply often extends for longer periods during the year than does the fruit supply.

In many developing countries, the supply of vitamin C is often determined by seasonal factors (i.e. the availability of water, time, and labour for the management of household gardens and the short harvesting season of many fruits). For example, mean monthly ascorbate intakes ranged from 0 to 115 mg/day in one Gambian community in which peak intakes coincided with the seasonal duration of the mango crop and to a lesser extent with orange and grapefruit harvests. These fluctuations in dietary ascorbate intake were closely reflected by corresponding variations in plasma ascorbate (11.4–68.4 μmol/l) and human milk ascorbate (143–342 μmol/l) (76).

Vitamin C is very labile, and the loss of vitamin C on boiling milk provides one dramatic example of a cause of infantile scurvy. The vitamin C content of food is thus strongly influenced by season, transport to market, length of time on the shelf and in storage, cooking practices, and the chlorination of the water used in cooking. Cutting or bruising of produce releases ascorbate oxidase. Blanching techniques inactivate the oxidase enzyme and help to preserve ascorbate; lowering the pH of a food will similarly achieve this, as in the preparation of sauerkraut (pickled cabbage). In contrast, heating and exposure to copper or iron or to mildly alkaline conditions destroys the vitamin, and too much water can leach it from the tissues during cooking.

It is important to realize that the amount of vitamin C in a food is usually not the major determinant of a food's importance for supply, but rather regularity of intake. For example, in countries where the potato is an important staple food and refrigeration facilities are limited, seasonal variations in plasma ascorbate are due to the considerable deterioration in the potato's vitamin C content during storage; the content can decrease from 30 to 8 mg/100 g over 8–9 months (77). Such data illustrate the important contribution the potato can make to human vitamin C requirements even though the potato's vitamin C concentration is low.

An extensive study has been made of losses of vitamin C during the packaging, storage, and cooking of blended foods (i.e. maize and soya-based relief foods). Data from a United States international development programme show that vitamin C losses from packaging and storage in polythene bags of such relief foods are much less significant than the 52–82% losses attributable to conventional cooking procedures (78).

7.6 Evidence used to derive recommended intakes of vitamin C

7.6.1 Adults

At saturation the whole body content of ascorbate in adult males is approximately 20 mg/kg, or 1500 mg. Clinical signs of scurvy appear when the whole-body content falls below 300–400 mg, and the last signs disappear when the body content reaches about 1000 mg (28, 30). Human studies have also established that ascorbate in the whole body is catabolized at an approximate rate of 3% per day (2.9% per day, SD, 0.6) (29).

There is a sigmoidal relationship between intake and plasma concentrations of vitamin C (79). Below intakes of 30 mg/day, plasma concentrations are around 11 μmol/l. Above this intake, plasma concentrations increase steeply to 60 μmol/l and plateau at around 80 μmol/l, which represents the renal threshold. Under near steady-state conditions, plateau concentrations of vitamin C are achieved by intakes in excess of 200 mg/day (Figure 7.1) (34).

FIGURE 7.1

Plasma vitamin C concentrations achieve steady state at intakes in excess of 200 mg/day

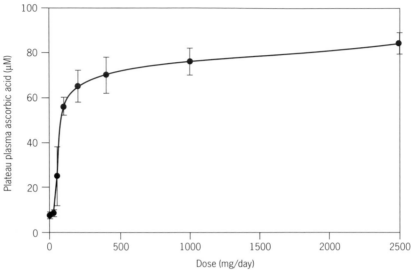

Source: reference (34).

At low doses dietary vitamin C is almost completely absorbed, but over the range of usual dietary intakes (30–180 mg/day), absorption may decrease to 75% because of competing factors in the food (35, 80).

A body content of 900 mg falls halfway between tissue saturation (1500 mg) and the point at which clinical signs of scurvy appear (300–400 mg). Assuming an absorption efficiency of 85%, and a catabolic rate of 2.9%, the average intake of vitamin C can be calculated as:

$$900 \times 2.9/100 \times 100/85 = 30.7 \text{ mg/day.}$$

This value can be rounded to 30 mg/day. The recommended nutrient intake (RNI) would therefore be:

$$900 \times (2.9 + 1.2)/100 \times 100/85 = 43.4 \text{ mg/day.}$$

This can be rounded to 45 mg/day.

An RNI of 45 mg would achieve 50% saturation in the tissues in 97.5% of adult males. An intake of 45 mg vitamin C will produce a plasma ascorbate concentration near the base of the steep slope of the diet-plasma dose response curve (Figure 7.1). No turnover studies have been done in women, but from the smaller body size and whole body content of women, requirements might be expected to be lower. However, in depletion studies plasma concentrations fell more rapidly in women than in men (*81*). It would seem prudent, therefore, to make the same recommendation for non-pregnant, non-lactating women as for men. Thus, an intake of 45 mg/day will ensure that measurable amounts of ascorbate will be present in the plasma of most people and will be available to supply tissue requirements for metabolism or repair at sites of depletion or damage. A whole-body content of around 900 mg of vitamin C would provide at least one month's safety interval, even for a zero intake, before the body content falls to 300 mg (*82*).

The Sheffield (*27*) and Iowa studies (*28*) referred to earlier indicated that the minimum amount of vitamin C needed to cure scurvy in men is less than 10 mg/day. This level however, is not sufficient to provide measurable amounts of ascorbate in plasma and leukocyte cells, which will remain low. As indicated above, no studies have been done on women and minimum requirements to protect non-pregnant and non-lactating women against scurvy might be slightly lower than those for men. Although 10 mg/day will protect against scurvy, this amount provides no safety margin against further losses of ascorbate. The mean requirement is therefore calculated by interpolation between 10 and 45 mg/day, at an intake of 25–30 mg/day.

7.6.2 Pregnant and lactating women

During pregnancy there is a moderate increased need for vitamin C, particularly during the last trimester. Eight mg/day of vitamin C is reported to be sufficient to prevent scorbutic signs in infants aged 4–17 months (*83*). Therefore, an extra 10 mg/day throughout pregnancy should enable reserves to accumulate to meet the extra needs of the growing fetus in the last trimester.

During lactation, however, 20 mg/day of vitamin C is secreted in milk. For an assumed absorption efficiency of 85%, maternal needs will require an extra 25 mg per day. It is therefore recommended that the RNI should be set at 70 mg/day to fulfil the needs of both the mother and infant during lactation.

7.6.3 Children

As mentioned above, 8 mg/day of vitamin C is sufficient to prevent scorbutic signs in infants (*83*). The mean concentration of vitamin C in mature human milk is estimated to be 40 mg/l (SD, 10) (*84*), but the amount of vitamin C in human milk appears to reflect maternal dietary intake and not the infant's needs (*82, 83, 85*). The RNI for infants aged 0–6 months is therefore set, somewhat arbitrarily, at 25 mg/day, and the RNI is gradually increased as children get older.

7.6.4 Elderly

Elderly people frequently have low plasma ascorbate values and intakes lower than those in younger people, often because of problems of poor dentition or mobility (*86*). Elderly people are also more likely to have underlying sub-clinical diseases, which can also influence plasma ascorbate concentrations (see Chapter 8 on antioxidants). It has been suggested, however, that the requirements of elderly people do not differ substantially from those of younger people in the absence of pathology which may influence absorption or renal functioning (*82*). The RNIs for the elderly are therefore the same as those for adults (45 mg/day).

7.6.5 Smokers

Kallner et al. (*87*) reported that the turnover of vitamin C in smokers was 50% greater than that in non-smokers. However, there is no evidence that the health of smokers would be influenced in any way by increasing their RNI. The Expert Consultation therefore found no justification for making a separate RNI for smokers.

7.7 Recommended nutrient intakes for vitamin C

Table 7.1 presents a summary of the discussed RNIs for vitamin C by group.

TABLE 7.1
Recommended nutrient intakes (RNIs) for vitamin C, by group

Group	RNI (mg/day)[a]
Infants and children	
0–6 months	25
7–12 months	30[b]
1–3 years	30[b]
4–6 years	30[b]
7–9 years	35[b]
Adolescents	
10–18 years	40[b]
Adults	
19–65 years	45
65+ years	45
Pregnant women	55
Lactating women	70

[a] Amount required to half saturate body tissues with vitamin C in 97.5% of the population. Larger amounts may often be required to ensure an adequate absorption of non-haem iron.
[b] Arbitrary values.

7.8 Toxicity

The potential toxicity of excessive doses of supplemental vitamin C relates to intraintestinal events and to the effects of metabolites in the urinary system. Intakes of 2–3 g/day of vitamin C produce unpleasant diarrhoea from the osmotic effects of the unabsorbed vitamin in the intestinal lumen in most people (88). Gastrointestinal disturbances can occur after ingestion of as little as 1 g because approximately half of this amount would not be absorbed at this dose (35).

Oxalate is an end-product of ascorbate catabolism and plays an important role in kidney stone formation. Excessive daily amounts of vitamin C produce hyperoxaluria. In four volunteers who received vitamin C in doses ranging from 5 to 10 g/day, mean urinary oxalate excretion approximately doubled from 50 to 87 mg/day (range, 60–126 mg/day) (89). However, the risk of oxalate stone formation may become significant at high intakes of vitamin C (>1 g) (90), particularly in subjects with high amounts of urinary calcium (89).

Vitamin C may precipitate haemolysis in some people, including those with glucose-6-phosphate dehydrogenase deficiency (91), paroxysmal nocturnal haemaglobinuria (92), or other conditions where increased risk of red cell haemolysis may occur or where protection against the removal of the products of iron metabolism may be impaired, as in people with the haptoglobin Hp2-2 phenotype (93). Of these, only the haptoglobin Hp2-2 condition was associated with abnormal vitamin C metabolism (lower plasma ascorbate than expected) and only in cases where intake of vitamin C was provided mainly from dietary sources.

On the basis of the above, the Consultation agreed that 1 g of vitamin C appears to be the advisable upper limit of dietary intake per day.

7.9 Recommendations for future research

Research is needed to gain a better understanding of the following:

- functions of endogenous gastric ascorbate and its effect on iron absorption;
- functional measurements of vitamin C status which reflect the whole-body content of vitamin C and which are not influenced by infection;
- reasons for the vitamin C uptake by granulocytes which is associated with infection.

References

1. Stewart CP, Guthrie D, eds. *Lind's treatise on scurvy*. Edinburgh, University Press, 1953.
2. Nishikimi M et al. Cloning and chromosomal mapping of the human non-

functional gene for L-gulono-gamma-lactone oxidase, the enzyme for L-ascorbic acid biosynthesis missing in man. *Journal of Biological Chemistry*, 1994, 269:13685–13688.

3. Levine M. New concepts in the biology and biochemistry of ascorbic acid. *New England Journal of Medicine*, 1986, 314:892–902.

4. Englard S, Seifter S. The biochemical functions of ascorbic acid. *Annual Review of Nutrition*, 1986, 6:365–406.

5. Wondrack LM, Hsu CA, Abbott MT. Thymine 7-hydroxylase and pyrimidine deoxyribonucleoside 2'-hydroxylase activities in *Rhodotorula glutinis*. *Journal of Biological Chemistry*, 1978, 253:6511–6515.

6. Stubbe JA. Identification of two alpha keto glutarate-dependent dioxygenases in extracts of *Rhodotorula glutinis* catalyzing deoxyuridine hydroxylation. *Journal of Biological Chemistry*, 1985, 260:9972–9975.

7. Prockop DJ, Kivirikko KI. Collagens: molecular biology, diseases, and potential for therapy. *Annual Review of Biochemistry*, 1995, 64:403–434.

8. Peterkofsky B. Ascorbate requirement for hydroxylation and secretion of pro-collagen: relationship to inhibition of collagen synthesis in scurvy. *American Journal of Clinical Nutrition*, 1991, 54(Suppl.):S1135–S1140.

9. Kivirikko KI, Myllyla R. Post-translational processing of procollagens. *Annals of the New York Academy of Sciences*, 1985, 460:187–201.

10. Rebouche CJ. Ascorbic acid and carnitine biosynthesis. *American Journal of Clinical Nutrition*, 1991, 54(Suppl.):S1147–S1152.

11. Dunn WA et al. Carnitine biosynthesis from gamma-butyrobetaine and from exogenous protein-bound 6-*N*-trimethyl-L-lysine by the perfused guinea pig liver. Effect of ascorbate deficiency on the in situ activity of gamma-butyrobetaine hydroxylase. *Journal of Biological Chemistry*, 1984, 259:10764–10770.

12. Levine M et al. Ascorbic acid and in situ kinetics: a new approach to vitamin requirements. *American Journal of Clinical Nutrition*, 1991, 54(Suppl.): S1157–S1162.

13. Kaufman S. Dopamine-beta-hydroxylase. *Journal of Psychiatric Research*, 1974, 11:303–316.

14. Eipper B et al. Peptidylglycine alpha amidating monooxygenase: a multifunctional protein with catalytic, processing, and routing domains. *Protein Science*, 1993, 2:489–497.

15. Eipper B, Stoffers DA, Mains RE. The biosynthesis of neuropeptides: peptide alpha amidation. *Annual Review of Neuroscience*, 1992, 15:57–85.

16. Lindblad B, Lindstedt G, Lindstedt S. The mechanism of enzymic formation of homogentisate from *p*-hydroxyphenyl pyruvate. *Journal of the American Chemical Society*, 1970, 92:7446–7449.

17. Schorah CJ et al. Gastric juice ascorbic acid: effects of disease and implications for gastric carcinogenesis. *American Journal of Clinical Nutrition*, 1991, 53(Suppl.):S287–S293.

18. Correa P. Human gastric carcinogenesis: a multistep and multifactorial process. First American Cancer Society Award Lecture on Cancer Epidemiology and Prevention. *Cancer Research*, 1992, 52:6735–6740.

19. Byers T, Guerrero N. Epidemiologic evidence for vitamin C and vitamin E in cancer prevention. *American Journal of Clinical Nutrition*, 1995, 62(Suppl.): S1385–S1392.

20. Jialal I, Grundy SM. Preservation of the endogenous antioxidants in low

density lipoprotein by ascorbate but not probucol during oxidative modification. *Journal of Clinical Investigation*, 1991, 87:597–601.

21. Stokes PL et al. Folate metabolism in scurvy. *American Journal of Clinical Nutrition*, 1975, 28:126–129.

22. Hallberg L, Brune M, Rossander-Hulthen L. Is there a physiological role of vitamin C in iron absorption. *Annals of the New York Academy of Sciences*, 1987, 498:324–332.

23. Hallberg L et al. Deleterious effects of prolonged warming of meals on ascorbic acid content and iron absorption. *American Journal of Clinical Nutrition*, 1982, 36:846–850.

24. Hallberg L. Wheat fiber, phytates and iron absorption. *Scandinavian Journal of Gastroenterology*, 1987, 129(Suppl.):S73–S79.

25. McLaren DS. *A colour atlas of nutritional disorders*. London, Wolfe Medical Publications, 1992.

26. Bartley W, Krebs HA, O'Brien JRP. *Vitamin C requirements of human adults.* London, Her Majesty's Stationery Office, 1953 (Medical Research Council Special Report Series No. 280).

27. Krebs NA, Peters RA, Coward KH. Vitamin C requirement of human adults: experimental study of vitamin C deprivation in man. *Lancet*, 1948, 254:853–858.

28. Baker EM et al. Metabolism of ascorbic-1–14C acid in experimental human scurvy. *American Journal of Clinical Nutrition*, 1969, 22:549–558.

29. Baker EM et al. Metabolism of 14C- and 3H-labeled L-ascorbic acid in human scurvy. *American Journal of Clinical Nutrition*, 1971, 24:444–454.

30. Kallner A, Hartmann D, Hornig D. Steady-state turnover and body pool of ascorbic acid in man. *American Journal of Clinical Nutrition*, 1979, 32:530–539.

31. Moser U, Weber F. Uptake of ascorbic acid by human granulocytes. *International Journal of Vitamin and Nutrition Research*, 1984, 54:47–53.

32. Lee W et al. Ascorbic acid status: biochemical and clinical considerations. *American Journal of Clinical Nutrition*, 1998, 48:286–290.

33. McCormick DB, Zhang Z. Cellular assimilation of water-soluble vitamins in the mammal: riboflavin, B6, biotin and C. *Proceedings of the Society of Experimental Biology and Medicine*, 1993, 202:265–270.

34. Levine M et al. Vitamin C pharmacokinetics in healthy volunteers: evidence for a Recommended Dietary Allowance. *Proceedings of the National Academy of Sciences*, 1996, 93:3704–3709.

35. Graumlich J et al. Pharmacokinetic model of ascorbic acid in humans during depletion and repletion. *Pharmaceutical Research*, 1997, 14:1133–1139.

36. Arab L, Schellenberg B, Schlierf G. Nutrition and health. A survey of young men and women in Heidelberg. *Annals of Nutrition and Metabolism*, 1982, 26:1–77.

37. Gregory JR et al. *The Dietary and Nutritional Survey of British Adults.* London, Her Majesty's Stationery Office, 1990.

38. Interagency Board for Nutrition Monitoring and Related Research. *Third report on nutrition monitoring in the United States*. Washington, DC, Government Printing Office, 1995.

39. Finch S et al. *National diet and nutrition survey: people aged 65 years and over. Volume 1. Report of the diet and nutrition survey*. London, Her Majesty's Stationery Office, 1998.

40. Basch CE, Syber P, Shea S. 5-a-day: dietary behavior and the fruit and vegetable intake of Latino children. *American Journal of Public Health*, 1994, 84:814–818.

41. *Diet, nutrition and the prevention of chronic diseases. Report of a WHO Study Group*. Geneva, World Health Organization, 1990 (WHO Technical Report Series, No. 797).

42. Williams C. Healthy eating: clarifying advice about fruit and vegetables. *British Medical Journal*, 1995, 310:1453–1455.

43. Narasinga Rao BS. Dietary intake of antioxidants in relation to nutrition profiles of Indian population groups. In: Ong ASH, Niki E, Packer L, eds. *Nutrition, lipids, health and disease*. Champaign, IL, The American Oil Chemists' Society Press, 1995:343–353.

44. Chang-Claude JC. *Epidemiologic study of precancerous lesions of the oesophagus in young persons in a high-incidence area for oesophageal cancer in China* [dissertation]. Heidelberg, Heidelberg University, 1991.

45. Knowles J et al. Plasma ascorbate concentrations in human malaria [abstract]. *Proceedings of the Nutrition Society*, 1991, 50:66.

46. Thurnham DI et al. Influence of malaria infection on peroxyl-radical trapping capacity in plasma from rural and urban Thai adults. *British Journal of Nutrition*, 1990, 64:257–271.

47. Jennings PE et al. Vitamin C metabolites and microangiography in diabetes mellitus. *Diabetes Research*, 1987, 6:151–154.

48. Thurnham DI. β-Carotene, are we misreading the signals in risk groups? Some analogies with vitamin C. *Proceedings of the Nutrition Society*, 1994, 53:557–569.

49. Faruque O et al. Relationship between smoking and antioxidant status. *British Journal of Nutrition*, 1995, 73:625–632.

50. Yong L et al. Intake of vitamins E, C, and A and risk of lung cancer. *American Journal of Epidemiology*, 1997, 146:231–243.

51. Byers T, Mouchawar J. Antioxidants and cancer prevention in 1997. In: Paoletti R et al., eds. *Vitamin C: the state of the art in disease prevention sixty years after the Nobel Prize*. Milan, Springer, 1998:29–40.

52. Schorah CJ. Vitamin C and gastric cancer prevention. In: Paoletti R et al., eds. *Vitamin C: the state of the art in disease prevention sixty years after the Nobel Prize*. Milan, Springer, 1998:41–49.

53. Blot WJ et al. Nutrition intervention trials in Linxian, China: supplementation with specific vitamin/mineral combinations, cancer incidence, and disease-specific mortality in the general population. *Journal of the National Cancer Institute*, 1993, 85:1483–1492.

54. Greenberg ER et al. A clinical trial of antioxidant vitamins to prevent colorectal adenoma. *New England Journal of Medicine*, 1994, 331:141–147.

55. Rimm EB et al. Vitamin E consumption and the risk of coronary heart disease in men. *New England Journal of Medicine*, 1993, 328:1450–1456.

56. Sahyoun NR, Jacques PF, Russell RM. Carotenoids, vitamins C and E, and mortality in an elderly population. *American Journal of Epidemiology*, 1996, 144:501–511.

57. Jha P et al. The antioxidant vitamins and cardiovascular disease: a critical review of the epidemiologic and clinical trial data. *Annals of Internal Medicine*, 1995, 123:860–872.

58. Losonczy KG, Harris TB, Havlik RJ. Vitamin E and vitamin C supplement use and risk of all cause and coronary heart disease mortality in older persons:

the established populations for epidemiologic studies of the elderly. *American Journal of Clinical Nutrition*, 1996, 64:190–196.

59. Enstrom JE, Kanim LE, Klein MA. Vitamin C intake and mortality among a sample of the United States population. *Epidemiology*, 1992, 3:194–202.

60. Enstrom JE, Kanim LE, Breslow L. The relationship between vitamin C intake, general health practices, and mortality in Alameda County, California. *American Journal of Public Health*, 1986, 76:1124–1130.

61. Seddon JM et al. Dietary carotenoids, vitamins A, C, and E, and advanced age-related macular degeneration. *Journal of the American Medical Association*, 1994, 272:1413–1420 (erratum published in *Journal of the American Medical Association*, 1995, 273:622).

62. Riemersma RA et al. Risk of angina pectoris and plasma concentrations of vitamins A, C, and E and carotene. *The Lancet*, 1991, 337:1–5.

63. Gey KF et al. Increased risk of cardiovascular disease at suboptimal plasma concentrations of essential antioxidants: an epidemiological update with special attention to carotene and vitamin C. *American Journal of Clinical Nutrition*, 1993, 57(Suppl.):S787–S797.

64. Kushi LH et al. Dietary antioxidant vitamins and death from coronary heart disease in postmenopausal women. *New England Journal of Medicine*, 1996, 334:1156–1162.

65. Simon JA, Hudes ES, Browner WS. Serum ascorbic acid and cardiovascular disease prevalence in US adults. *Epidemiology*, 1998, 9:316–321.

66. Jacques PF et al. Antioxidant status in persons with and without senile cataract. *Archives of Ophthalmology*, 1988, 106:337–340.

67. Robertson JM, Donner AP, Trevithick JR. A possible role for vitamins C and E in cataract prevention. *American Journal of Clinical Nutrition*, 1991, 53(Suppl.):S346–S351.

68. Leske MC, Chylack LT, Wu S. The lens opacities case/control study: risk factors for cataract. *Archives of Opthalmology*, 1991, 109:244–251.

69. Italian-American Cataract Study Group. Risk factors for age-related cortical, nuclear, and posterior sub-capsular cataracts. *American Journal of Epidemiology*, 1991, 133:541–553.

70. Goldberg J et al. Factors associated with age-related macular degeneration. An analysis of data from the first National Health and Nutrition Examination Survey. *American Journal of Epidemiology*, 1988, 128:700–710.

71. Vitale S et al. Plasma antioxidants and risk of cortical and nuclear cataract. *Epidemiology*, 1993, 4:195–203.

72. Hankinson SE et al. Nutrient intake and cataract extraction in women: a prospective study. *British Medical Journal*, 1992, 305:335–339.

73. Mares-Perlman JA. Contribution of epidemiology to understanding relationships of diet to age-related cataract. *American Journal of Clinical Nutrition*, 1997, 66:739–740.

74. Jacques PF et al. Long-term vitamin C supplement use and prevalence of early age-related lens opacities. *American Journal of Clinical Nutrition*, 1997, 66:911–916.

75. Haytowitz D. Information from USDA's Nutrient Data Book. *Journal of Nutrition*, 1995, 125:1952–1955.

76. Bates CJ, Prentice AM, Paul AA. Seasonal variations in vitamins A, C, riboflavin and folate intakes and status of pregnant and lactating women in a rural Gambian community: some possible implications. *European Journal of Clinical Nutrition*, 1994, 48:660–668.

77. Paul AA, Southgate DAT. *McCance and Widdowson's the composition of foods*. London, Her Majesty's Stationery Office, 1978.
78. Committee on International Nutrition, Food and Nutrition Board. *Vitamin C fortification of food aid commodities: final report*. Washington, DC, National Academy Press, 1997.
79. Newton HMV et al. Relation between intake and plasma concentration of vitamin C in elderly women. *British Medical Journal*, 1983, 287:1429.
80. Melethil SL, Mason WE, Chiang C. Dose dependent absorption and excretion of vitamin C in humans. *International Journal of Pharmacology*, 1986, 31:83–89.
81. Blanchard J. Depletion and repletion kinetics of vitamin C in humans. *Journal of Nutrition*, 1991, 121:170–176.
82. Olson JA, Hodges RE. Recommended dietary intakes (RDI) of vitamin C in humans. *American Journal of Clinical Nutrition*, 1987, 45:693–703.
83. Irwin MI, Hutchins BK. A conspectus of research on vitamin C requirements in man. *Journal of Nutrition*, 1976, 106:821–879.
84. *Complementary feeding of young children in developing countries: a review of current scientific knowledge*. Geneva, World Health Organization, 1998 (WHO/NUT/98.1; http://whqlibdoc.who.int/hq/1998/WHO_NUT_98.1.pdf, accessed 24 June 2004).
85. Van Zoeren-Grobben D et al. Human milk vitamin content after pasteurisation, storage, or tube feeding. *Archives of Diseases in Childhood*, 1987, 62:161–165.
86. Department of Health and Social Security. *Nutrition and health in old age*. London, Her Majesty's Stationery Office, 1979 (Report on Health and Social Subjects, No. 16).
87. Kallner AB, Hartmann D, Hornig DH. On the requirements of ascorbic acid in man: steady state turnover and body pool in smokers. *American Journal of Clinical Nutrition*, 1981, 34:1347–1355.
88. Kubler W, Gehler J. On the kinetics of the intestinal absorption of ascorbic acid: a contribution to the calculation of an absorption process that is not proportional to the dose. *International Journal of Vitamin and Nutrition Research*, 1970, 40:442–453.
89. Schmidt K-H et al. Urinary oxalate excretion after large intakes of ascorbic acid in man. *American Journal of Clinical Nutrition*, 1981, 34:305–311.
90. Urivetzky M, Kessaris D, Smith AD. Ascorbic acid overdosing: a risk factor for calcium oxalate nephrolithiasis. *Journal of Urology*, 1992, 147:1215–1218.
91. Mehta JB, Singhal SB, Mehta BC. Ascorbic acid induced haemolysis in G-6-PD deficiency. *Lancet*, 1990, 336:944.
92. Iwamoto N et al. Haemolysis induced by ascorbic acid in paroxysmal nocturnal haemoglobinuria. *Lancet*, 1994, 343:357.
93. Langlois MR et al. Effect of haptoglobin on the metabolism of vitamin C. *American Journal of Clinical Nutrition*, 1997, 66:606–610.

8. Dietary antioxidants

8.1 Nutrients with an antioxidant role

The potential beneficial effects of antioxidants in protecting against disease have been used as an argument for recommending increasing intakes of several nutrients above those derived by conventional methods. If it is possible to quantify such claims, antioxidant properties should be considered in decisions concerning the daily requirements of these nutrients. This section examines metabolic aspects of the most important dietary antioxidants — vitamins C and E, the carotenoids, and several minerals — and tries to define the populations which may be at risk of inadequacy to determine whether antioxidant properties per se should be, and can be, considered in setting a requirement. In addition, pro-oxidant metabolism and the importance of iron are also considered.

Members of the Food and Nutrition Board of the National Research Council in the United States recently defined a dietary antioxidant as a substance in foods which significantly decreases the adverse effects of reactive oxygen species, reactive nitrogen species, or both on normal physiological function in humans (1). It is recognized that this definition is somewhat narrow because maintenance of membrane stability is also a feature of antioxidant function (2) and an important antioxidant function of both vitamin A (3) and zinc (4). However, it was decided to restrict consideration of antioxidant function in this document to nutrients which were likely to interact more directly with reactive species.

8.2 The need for biological antioxidants

It is now well established that free radicals, especially superoxide ($O_2^{\cdot -}$), nitric oxide ($NO^{\cdot}$), and other reactive species such as hydrogen peroxide (H_2O_2), are continuously produced in vivo (5–7). Superoxide in particular is produced by leakage from the electron transport chains within the mitochondria and microsomal P450 systems (8) or formed more deliberately, for example, by activated phagocytes as part of the primary immune defence in response to foreign substances or to combat infection by microorganisms (9). Nitric oxide is produced from L-arginine by nitric oxide synthases, and these enzymes are found in virtually every tissue of the mammalian body, albeit at widely different levels (7). Nitric oxide is a free radical but is believed to be essentially a beneficial metabolite and indeed it may react with lipid peroxides and function as an antioxidant (10). Nitric oxide also serves as a mediator whereby macrophages express cytotoxic activity against microorganisms and neoplastic cells (11). If nitric oxide is at a sufficiently high concentration, it can react rapidly with superoxide in the absence of a catalyst to form peroxynitrite. Peroxynitrite is a potentially damaging nitrogen species which can react through several different mechanisms, including the formation of an intermediate through a reaction with a hydroxyl radical (12).

To cope with potentially damaging reactive oxidant species (ROS), aerobic tissues contain endogenously produced antioxidant enzymes such as superoxide dismutase (SOD), glutathione peroxidase (GPx), and catalase as well as several exogenously acquired radical-scavenging substances such as vitamins E and C and the carotenoids (13). Under normal conditions, the high concentrations of SOD maintain superoxide concentrations at a level too low to allow the formation of peroxynitrite. It is also important to mention the antioxidant, reduced glutathione (GSH). GSH is ubiquitous in aerobic tissues, and although it is not a nutrient, it is synthesized from sulfhydryl-containing amino acids and is highly important in intermediary antioxidant metabolism (14).

Integrated antioxidant defences protect tissues and are presumably in equilibrium with continuously generated ROS to maintain tissues metabolically intact most of the time. Disturbances to the system occur when production of ROS is rapidly increased, for example, by excessive exercise, high exposure to xenobiotic compounds (such as an anaesthetic, pollutants, or unusual food), infection, or trauma. Superoxide production is increased by activation of NADPH oxidases in inflammatory cells or after the production of xanthine oxidase, which follows ischaemia. The degree of damage resulting from the temporary imbalance depends on the ability of the antioxidant systems to respond to the oxidant or pro-oxidant load. Fruits and vegetables are good sources of many antioxidants, and it is reported that diets rich in these foods are associated with a lower risk of the chronic diseases of cancer (15) and heart disease (16). Hence, it is believed that a healthful diet maintains the exogenous antioxidants at or near optimal levels thus reducing the risk of tissue damage. The most prominent representatives of dietary antioxidants are vitamin C, tocopherols, carotenoids, and flavonoids (17–19). Requirements for flavonoids are not being considered at this time, as work on this subject is still very much in its infancy. In contrast, several intervention studies have been carried out to determine whether supplements of the other nutrients can provide additional benefits against diseases such as those mentioned above.

The components of biological tissues are an ideal mixture of substrates for oxidation. Polyunsaturated fatty acids (PUFAs), transition metals, and oxygen are present in abundance but are prevented from reaction by cellular organization and structure. PUFAs are present in membranes but are always found with vitamin E. Transition metals, particularly iron, are bound to both transport and storage proteins; abundant binding sites on such proteins prevent overloading the protein molecule with metal ions. Tissue structures, however, break down during inflammation and disease, and free iron and other transition metals have been detected during these periods (20, 21).

Potentially damaging metabolites can arise from interactions between transition metals and the ROS described above. In particular, the highly reactive hydroxyl radical can be formed by the Fenton (reaction 1) and Haber-Weiss reactions (reaction 2; with an iron-salt catalyst) (22). Pathologic conditions greatly increase the concentrations of both superoxide and nitric oxide, and the formation of peroxynitrite has been demonstrated in macrophages, neutrophils, and cultured endothelium (reaction 3) (12, 23).

$$\text{Reaction 1:} \quad Fe^{2+} + H_2O_2 = Fe^{3+} + OH^{\cdot} + OH^{-}$$
$$\text{Reaction 2:} \quad O_2^{\cdot -} + H_2O_2 = O_2 + OH^{\cdot} + OH^{-}$$
$$\text{Reaction 3:} \quad NO + O_2^{\cdot -} = ONOO^{\cdot}$$

During inflammation or other forms of stress and disease, the body adopts new measures to counter potential pro-oxidant damage. The body alters the transport and distribution of iron by blocking iron mobilization and absorption, and stimulating iron uptake from plasma by liver, spleen, and macrophages (3, 24, 25). Nitric oxide has been shown to play a role in the coordination of iron traffic by mimicking the consequences of iron starvation and leading to the cellular uptake of iron (26). The changes accompanying disease are generally termed the acute-phase response and are, generally, protective (27). Some of the changes in plasma acute-phase reactants which affect iron at the onset of disease or trauma are shown in Table 8.1.

8.3 Pro-oxidant activity of biological antioxidants

Most biological antioxidants are antioxidants because when they accept an unpaired electron, the free radical intermediate formed has a relatively long half-life in the normal biological environment. The long half-life means that these intermediates remain stable for long enough to interact in a controlled fashion with other intermediates which prevent autoxidation, and the excess energy of the surplus electron is dissipated without damage to the tissues. Thus it is believed that the tocopheroxyl radical formed by oxidation of α-tocopherol is sufficiently stable to enable its reduction by vitamin C or

TABLE 8.1

Systems altered during disease which reduce risk of autoxidation

System	Changes in plasma	Physiologic objectives
Mobilization and metabolism of iron	Decrease in transferrin Increase in ferritin Increase in lactoferrin Increase in haptoglobin Decrease in iron absorption Movement of plasma iron from blood to storage sites	Reduce levels of circulating and tissue iron to reduce risk of free radical production and pro-oxidant damage Reduce level of circulating iron available for microbial growth
Positive acute phase proteins	Increase in antiproteinases Increase in fibrinogen	Restriction of inflammatory damage to diseased area
White blood cells	Variable increase in white blood cells of which 70% are granulocytes	Production of reactive oxygen species to combat infection Scavenge vitamin C to prevent interaction of vitamin C with free iron
Vitamin C metabolism	Uptake of vitamin C from plasma by stimulated granulocytes Reduction of plasma vitamin C in acute and chronic illness or stress-associated conditions Temporary fall in leukocyte vitamin C associated with acute stress	Reduce levels of vitamin C in the circulation—because it is a potential pro-oxidant in inflamed tissue—or where free iron may be present Facilitate movement of vitamin C to tissues affected by disease (e.g. lungs in smokers) Protect granulocytes and macrophages from oxidative damage

Sources: modified from Koj (28) and Thurnham (3, 29, 30).

GSH to regenerate the quinol (*31, 32*) rather than oxidizing surrounding PUFAs. Similarly, the oxidized forms of vitamin C, the ascorbyl free radical and dehydroascorbate, may be recycled back to ascorbate by GSH or the enzyme dehydroascorbate reductase (*13*). The ability to recycle these dietary antioxidants may be an indication of their physiological essentiality to function as antioxidants.

The biological antioxidant properties of the carotenoids depend very much on oxygen tension and concentration (*33, 34*). At low oxygen tension β-carotene acts as a chain-breaking antioxidant whereas at high oxygen tension it readily autoxidizes and exhibits pro-oxidant behaviour (*33*). Palozza (*34*) has reviewed much of the evidence and has suggested that β-carotene has antioxidant activity between 2 and 20 mmHg of oxygen tension, but at the oxygen tension in air or above (>150 mmHg) it is much less effective as an antioxidant and can show pro-oxidant activity as the oxygen tension increases. Palozza (*34*) also suggested that autoxidation reactions of β-carotene may be controlled by the presence of other antioxidants (e.g. vitamins E and C) or other carotenoids. There is some evidence that intake of large quantities of fat-soluble nutrients such as β-carotene and other carotenoids may cause them to compete with each other during absorption and lower plasma concentrations of other nutrients derived from the diet. However, a lack of other antioxidants is unlikely to explain the increased incidence of lung cancer that was observed in a α-tocopherol/β-carotene intervention study, because there was no difference in cancer incidence between the group which received both β-carotene and α-tocopherol and the groups which received one treatment only (*35*).

The free radical formed from a dietary antioxidant is potentially a pro-oxidant as is any other free radical. In biological conditions that deviate from the norm, there is always the potential for an antioxidant free radical to become a pro-oxidant if a suitable receptor molecule is present to accept the electron and promote the autoxidation (*36*). Mineral ions are particularly important pro-oxidants. For example, vitamin C will interact with both copper and iron to generate cuprous or ferrous ions, respectively, both of which are potent pro-oxidants (*29, 37*). Fortunately, mineral ions are tightly bound to proteins and are usually unable to react with tissue components unless there is a breakdown in tissue integrity. Such circumstances can occur in association with disease and excessive phagocyte activation, but even under these circumstances, there is rapid metabolic accommodation in the form of the acute-phase response to minimize the potentially damaging effects of an increase in free mineral ions in extracellular fluids (Table 8.1).

8.4 Nutrients associated with endogenous antioxidant mechanisms

Both zinc and selenium are intimately involved in protecting the body against oxidant stress. Zinc combined with copper is found in the cytoplasmic form of SOD whereas zinc and magnesium occur in the mitochondrial enzyme. Superoxide dismutase is present in all aerobic cells and is responsible for the dismutation of superoxide (reaction 4).

$$\text{Reaction 4:} \quad O_2^- + O_2^- + 2H^+ = H_2O_2 + O_2$$

Hydrogen peroxide is a product of this dismutation reaction and is removed by GPx, of which selenium is an integral component (reaction 5). To function effectively, this enzyme also needs a supply of hydrogen, which it obtains from reduced glutathione (GSH). Cellular concentrations of GSH are maintained by the riboflavin-dependent enzyme glutathione reductase.

$$\text{Reaction 5:} \quad H_2O_2 + 2GSH = GSSG + 2H_2O$$

Four forms of selenium-dependent GPx have been described, each with different activities in different parts of the cell (*38*). In addition, a selenium-dependent enzyme, thioredoxin reductase, was recently characterized in human erythrocytes. Thioredoxin reductase may be particularly important to the thyroid gland because it can cope with higher concentrations of peroxide and hydroperoxides generated in the course of thyroid hormone synthesis better than can GPx (*39*). It has been suggested that in combination with iodine deficiency, the inability to remove high concentrations of hydrogen peroxide may cause atrophy in the thyroid gland, resulting in myxedematous cretinism (*39*).

SOD and GPx are widely distributed in aerobic tissues and, if no catalytic metal ions are available, endogenously produced superoxide and hydrogen peroxide at physiological concentrations probably have limited, if any, damaging effects (*36*). SOD and GPx are of fundamental importance to the life of the cell, and their activity is not readily reduced by deficiencies in dietary intake of zinc and selenium. In contrast, enzyme activity can be stimulated by increased oxidant stress (e.g. ozone) (*40*). Activities of zinc-dependent enzymes have been shown to be particularly resistant to the influence of dietary zinc (*41*), and although erythrocyte GPx activity correlates with selenium when the intake is below 60–80 μg/day (*42*), there is no evidence of impaired clinical function at low GPx activities found in humans. Nevertheless, one selenium intervention study reported remarkably lower risks of several cancers in subjects taking supplements for 4.5 years at doses of 200 μg/day (*43*). The effects were so strong on total cancer mortality that the study was stopped prematurely. However, the subjects were patients with a history of basal or squamous cell carcinomas and were not typical of the general population (43). In addition, a prospective analysis of serum selenium in cancer patients (44) (1.72 µmol/l) found very little difference from concentrations in matched controls (1.63 µmol/l) although the difference was significant (45). Furthermore, areas with high selenium intakes have a lower cancer incidence than do those with low intakes, but the high selenium areas were the least industrialized (45).

8.5 Nutrients with radical-quenching properties

Vitamins C and E are the principal nutrients which possess radical-quenching properties. Both are powerful antioxidants, and the most important difference between these two compounds stems from their different solubility in biological fluids. Vitamin C is water-soluble and is therefore especially found in the aqueous fractions of the cell and in body fluids whereas vitamin E is highly lipophilic and is found in membranes and lipoproteins.

8.5.1 Vitamin E

Vitamin E falls into the class of conventional antioxidants which generally consist of phenols or aromatic amines (see Chapter 5). In the case of the four tocopherols that, together with the four tocotrienols constitute vitamin E, the initial step involves a very rapid transfer of phenolic hydrogen to the recipient free radical with the formation of a phenoxyl radical from vitamin E. The phenoxyl radical is resonance stabilized and is relatively unreactive towards lipid or oxygen. It does not therefore continue the chain (33, 46). However, the phenoxyl radical is no longer an antioxidant and to maintain the antioxidant properties of membranes, it must be recycled or repaired (i.e. reconverted to vitamin E) because the amount of vitamin E present in membranes can be several thousand-fold less than the amount of potentially oxidizable substrate (47). Water-soluble vitamin C is the popular candidate for this role (31), but thiols and particularly GSH can also function in this role in vitro (32, 48–50).

There are eight possible isomers of vitamin E, but α-tocopherol (5,7,8-trimethyltocol) is the most biologically important antioxidant in vivo (46). In plasma samples, more than 90% is present as α-tocopherol but there may be approximately 10% of γ-tocopherol. In foods such as margarine and soy products the γ form may be predominant whereas palm oil products are rich in the tocotrienols.

Vitamin E is found throughout the body in both cell and subcellular membranes. It is believed to be orientated with the quinol ring structure on the outer surface (i.e. in contact with the aqueous phase) to enable it to be maintained in its active reduced form by circulating reductants such as vitamin C (*31*). Within biological membranes, vitamin E is believed to intercalate with phospholipids and provide protection to PUFAs. PUFAs are particularly susceptible to free radical-mediated oxidation because of their methylene-interrupted double-bond structure. The amount of PUFAs in the membrane far exceeds the amount of vitamin E, and the tocopherol–PUFA ratios are highest in tissues where oxygen exposure is greatest and not necessarily where the PUFA content is highest (*47*).

Oxidation of PUFAs leads to disturbances in membrane structure and function and is damaging to cell function. Vitamin E is highly efficient at preventing the autoxidation of lipid and it appears that its primary, and possibly only, role in biological tissues is to perform this function (*46*). Autoxidation of lipid is initiated by a free radical abstracting hydrogen from PUFA to form a lipid radical (reaction 6), which is followed by a rearrangement of the double-bond structure to form a conjugated diene. In vitro the presence of minute amounts of peroxides and transition metals will stimulate the formation of the initial radical. Oxygen adds to the lipid radical to form a lipid peroxide (reaction 7), which then reacts with another lipid molecule to form a hydroperoxide and a new lipid radical (reaction 8). This process is shown in general terms below for the autoxidation of any organic molecule (RH), where the initial abstraction is caused by a hydroxyl radical (OH·).

$$\text{Reaction 6:} \quad RH + OH^{\cdot} = R^{\cdot} + H_2O$$
$$\text{Reaction 7:} \quad R^{\cdot} + O_2 = ROO^{\cdot}$$
$$\text{Reaction 8:} \quad ROO^{\cdot} + RH = ROOH + R^{\cdot}$$

Autoxidation or lipid peroxidation is represented by reactions 6 and 7. The process stops naturally when reaction between two radicals (reaction 9) occurs but initially this occurs less frequently than does reaction 8.

$$\text{Reaction 9:} \quad ROO^{\cdot} + ROO^{\cdot} = \text{non-radical products}$$

The presence of the chain-breaking antioxidant, vitamin E (ArOH), reacts in place of RH shown in reaction 8 and donates the hydrogen from the chromanol ring to form the hydroperoxide (reaction 10). The vitamin E radical (ArO·, tocopheroxyl radical) which is formed is fairly stable and therefore stops autoxidation. Hydroperoxides formed by lipid peroxidation can be released from membrane phospholipids by phospholipase A2 and then degraded by GPx in the cell cytoplasm (see Chapter 10 on selenium).

$$\text{Reaction 10:} \quad ROO^{\cdot} + ArOH = ArO^{\cdot} + ROOH$$

8.5.2 Vitamin C

Many, if not all of the biological properties of vitamin C are linked to its redox properties (see Chapter 7). For example, the consequences of scurvy, such as the breakdown of connective tissue fibres (*51*) and muscular weakness (*52*), are both linked to hydroxylation reactions in which ascorbate maintains loosely bound iron in the ferrous form to prevent its oxidation to the ferric form, which makes the hydroxylase enzymes inactive (*53*). Ascorbate exhibits similar redox functions in catecholamine biosynthesis (*53*) and in microsomal cytochrome P450 enzyme activity, although the latter may only be important in young animals (*54*). In the eye, vitamin C concentrations may be 50 times higher than in the plasma and may protect against the oxidative damage of light (*55*). Vitamin C is also present in the gonads, where it may play a critical role in sperm maturation (*56*). Spermatogenesis involves many more cell divisions than does oogenesis, resulting in an increased risk of mutation. Fraga et al. (*57*) reported that levels of sperm oxidized by nucleoside 8-OH-2'-deoxyguanosine (an indicator of oxidative damage to DNA) varied inversely with the intake of vitamin C (5–250 mg/day). No apparent effects on sperm quality were noted. Frei (*58*) also showed that vitamin C was superior to all other biological antioxidants in plasma in protecting lipids exposed ex vivo to a variety of sources of oxidative stress. The importance of vitamin C in stabilizing various plasma components such as folate, homocysteine, proteins and other micronutrients has not been properly evaluated. When blood plasma is separated from erythrocytes, vitamin C is the first antioxidant to disappear.

Vitamin C is a powerful antioxidant because it can donate a hydrogen atom and form a relatively stable ascorbyl free radical (i.e. L-ascorbate anion, see Figure 8.1). As a scavenger of ROS, ascorbate has been shown to be effective against the superoxide radical anion, hydrogen peroxide, the hydroxyl radical, and singlet oxygen (*59*, *60*). Vitamin C also scavenges reactive nitrogen oxide species to prevent nitrosation of target molecules (*61*). The ascorbyl free radical can be converted back to reduced ascorbate by accepting another hydrogen atom or it can undergo further oxidation to dehydroascorbate. Dehydroascorbate is unstable but is more fat soluble than ascorbate and is taken up 10–20 times more rapidly by erythrocytes, where it will be reduced back to ascorbate by GSH or NADPH from the hexose monophosphate shunt (*56*).

Thus, mechanisms exist to recycle vitamin C, which are similar to those for vitamin E. The existence of a mechanism to maintain plasma ascorbate in the reduced state means that the level of vitamin C necessary for optimal antioxidant activity is not absolute because the turnover will change in

FIGURE 8.1
Ascorbic acid and its oxidation products

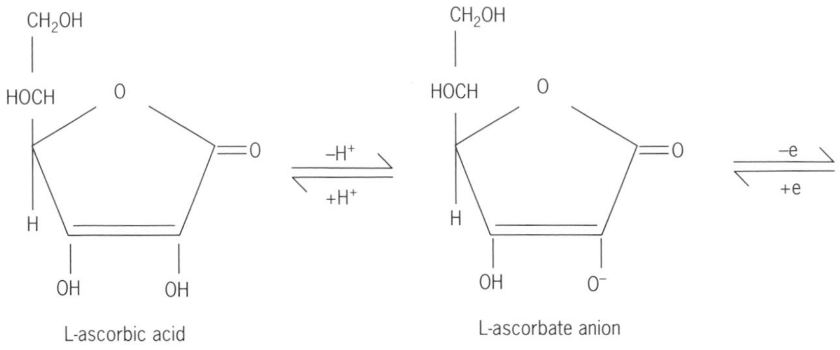

L-ascorbic acid   L-ascorbate anion

response to oxidant pressure. Recycling of vitamin C will depend on the reducing environment which exists in metabolically active cells. In atrophic tissues or tissues exposed to inflammation, cell viability may fail and with it, the ability to recycle vitamin C. In such an environment, the ability of newly released granulocytes (62) or macrophages (63) to scavenge vitamin C from the surrounding fluid may be invaluable for conservation of an essential nutrient as well as reducing the risk of ascorbate becoming a pro-oxidant through its ability to reduce iron (37).

8.5.3 β-Carotene and other carotenoids

Many hundreds of carotenoids are found in nature but relatively few are found in human tissues, the five main ones being β-carotene, lutein, lycopene, β-cryptoxanthin, and α-carotene (17, 18, 64). β-carotene is the main source of provitamin A in the diet. There are approximately 50 carotenoids with provitamin A activity, but β-carotene is the most important and is one of the most widely distributed carotenoids in plant species (64). Approximately 2–6 mg β-carotene is consumed by adults daily in developed countries (65, 66), probably along with similar amounts of lutein (67) and lycopene (66). Smaller amounts may be consumed in the developing world (68, 69). Consumption of β-cryptoxanthin, a provitamin A carotenoid found mainly in fruits (66), is small, but as bioavailability of carotenoids may be greater from fruits than from vegetables, its contribution to dietary intake and vitamin A status may be higher than the amount in the diet would predict.

β-Carotene has two six-membered carbon rings (β-ionone rings) separated by 18 carbon atoms in the form of a conjugated chain of double bonds. β-Carotene is unique in possessing two β-ionone rings in its structure, both of which are essential for vitamin A activity. The antioxidant properties of the carotenoids closely relate to the extended system of conjugated double bonds, which occupies the central part of carotenoid molecules, and to the various functional groups on the terminal ring structures (*33, 70, 71*). The reactive oxidant species scavenged by carotenoids are singlet oxygen and peroxyl radicals (*33, 72–74*). Carotenoids in general and lycopene specifically are very efficient at quenching singlet oxygen (*72, 73*). In this process the carotenoid absorbs the excess energy from singlet oxygen and then releases it as heat. Singlet oxygen is generated during photosynthesis; therefore, carotenoids are important for protecting plant tissues, but there is some evidence for an antioxidant role in humans. β-Carotene has been used in the treatment of erythropoietic protoporphyria (*75*) (a light-sensitive condition) with amounts in excess of 180 mg/day (*76*). It has been suggested that large amounts of dietary carotenes may provide some protection against solar radiation but results are equivocal. No benefit was reported when large amounts of β-carotene were used to treat individuals with a high risk of non-melanomatous skin cancer (*77*). However, two carotenoids—lutein (3,3′-dihydroxy α-carotene) and zeaxanthin (the 3,3′-dihydroxylated form of β-carotene)—are found specifically associated with the rods and cones in the eye (*78*) and may protect the retinal pigment epithelium against the oxidative effects of blue light (*79, 80*).

Burton and Ingold (*33*) were the first to draw attention to the radical-trapping properties of β-carotene. Using in vitro studies, they showed that β-carotene was effective in reducing the rate of lipid peroxidation at the low oxygen concentrations found in tissues. Because all carotenoids have the same basic structure, they should all have similar properties. Indeed, several authors suggest that the hydroxy-carotenoids are better radical-trapping antioxidants than is β-carotene (*81, 82*). It has also been suggested that because the carotenoid molecule is long enough to span the bilayer lipid membrane (*83*), the presence of oxy functional groups on the ring structures may facilitate similar reactivation of the carotenoid radical in a manner similar to that of the phenoxyl radical of vitamin E (*33*).

There is some evidence for an antioxidant role for β-carotene in immune cells. Bendich (*84*) suggested that β-carotene protects phagocytes from autoxidative damage; enhances T and B lymphocyte proliferative responses; stimulates effector T cell function; and enhances macrophage, cytotoxic T cell, and natural killer cell tumoricidal capacity. However, there are data which conflict with the evidence of the protective effects of β-carotene on the immune system (*85, 86*) and other data which have found no effect (*87*). An explanation for the discrepancy may reside in the type of subjects chosen: defences may be boosted in those at risk but it may not be possible to demonstrate any benefit in healthy subjects (*88*).

8.6 A requirement for antioxidant nutrients

Free radicals are a product of tissue metabolism, and the potential damage which they can cause is minimized by the antioxidant capacity and repair mechanisms within the cell. Thus in a metabolically active tissue cell in a healthy subject with an adequate dietary intake, damage to tissue will be minimal and most of the damage, if it does occur, will be repaired (*36*). Fruit and vegetables are an important dietary source of antioxidant nutrients, and it is now well established that individuals consuming generous amounts of these foods have a lower risk of chronic disease than those whose intake is small (*15*, *16*, *89*). These observations suggest that the antioxidant nutrient requirements of the general population can be met by a generous consumption of fruit and vegetables and the slogan "five portions a day" has been promoted to publicize this idea (*90*).

Occasionally, free radical damage may occur which is not repaired, and the risk of this happening may increase in the presence of infection or physical trauma. Such effects may exacerbate an established infection or may initiate irreversible changes leading to a state of chronic disease (e.g. a neoplasm or atherosclerotic lesions). Can such effects be minimized by a generous intake of dietary antioxidants in the form of fruit and vegetables or are supplements needed?

It is generally recognized that certain groups of people have an increased risk of free radical-initiated damage. Premature infants, for example, are at increased risk of oxidative damage because they are born with immature antioxidant status (*91–93*) and this may be inadequate for coping with high levels of oxygen and light radiation. People who smoke are exposed to free radicals inhaled in the tobacco smoke and have an increased risk of many diseases. People abusing alcohol need to develop increased metabolic capacity to handle the extra alcohol load. Similar risks may be faced by people working in environments where there are elevated levels of volatile solvents (e.g. petrol and cleaning fluids in distilleries and chemical plants). Car drivers and other people working in dense traffic may be exposed to elevated levels of exhaust fumes. Human metabolism can adapt to a wide range of xenobiotic substances, but metabolic activity may be raised as a result, leading to the consequent production of more ROS, which are potentially toxic to cell metabolism.

Of the above groups, smokers are the most widely accessible and this has made them a target for several large antioxidant-nutrient intervention studies.

In addition, smokers often display low plasma concentrations of carotenoids and vitamin C. However, no obvious benefits to the health of smokers have emerged from these studies and, in fact, β-carotene supplements were associated with an increased risk of lung cancer in two separate studies (35, 94) and with more fatal cardiac events in one of them (95). There was no effect on subsequent disease recurrences among other risk groups—identified by their already having had some non-malignant form of cancer, such as non-melanomatous skin cancer (77) or a colorectal adenoma (96)—after several years of elevated intakes of antioxidant nutrients. The use of β-carotene (77) or vitamin E alone or in combination with vitamin C (96) showed no benefits. Thus, the results of these clinical trials do not support the use of supplementation with antioxidant micronutrients as a means of reducing cancer or even cardiovascular rates, although in the general population toxicity from such supplements is very unlikely.

Some intervention trials, however, have been more successful in demonstrating a health benefit. Stich and colleagues (97, 98) gave large quantities of β-carotene and sometimes vitamin A to chewers of betel quids in Kerala, India, and to Canadian Inuits with pre-malignant lesions of the oral tract and witnessed reductions in leukoplakia and micronuclei from the buccal mucosa. Blot et al. (99) reported a 13% reduction in gastric cancer mortality in people living in Linxian Province, People's Republic of China, after taking a cocktail of β-carotene, vitamin E, and selenium. These studies are difficult to interpret because the subjects may have been marginally malnourished at the start and the supplements may have merely restored nutritional adequacy. However, correcting malnutrition is unlikely to be the explanation for the positive results of a selenium supplementation study conducted in the United States in patients with a history of basal or squamous cell cancers of the skin (43). Interestingly, the intervention with 200 μg/day of selenium for an average of 4.5 years had no effect on the recurrence of the skin neoplasms (relative risk [RR], 1.10; confidence interval, 0.95–1.28). However, analysis of secondary end-points showed significant reductions in total cancer mortality (RR, 0.5) and incidence (RR, 0.63) and in the incidences of lung, colorectal, and prostate cancers. The mean age of this group was 63 years and obviously they were not a normal adult population, but results of further studies are awaited with keen interest. In addition, results of the Cambridge Heart Antioxidant Study have provided some support for a beneficial effect of vitamin E in individuals who have had a myocardial infarction (100). Recruits to the study were randomly assigned to receive vitamin E (800 or 400 mg/day) or a placebo. Initial results of the trial suggested a significant reduction in non-fatal myocardial infarctions but a non-significant excess of cardiovascular deaths

(*100*). The trial officially ended in 1996, but mortality has continued to be monitored and the authors now report significantly fewer deaths in those who received vitamin E for the full trial (*101*) (see Chapter 5 on vitamin E). However, very recently results from the Medical Research Council/British Heart Foundation intervention study in 20 536 patients with heart disease were reported (102). Patients received vitamin E (600 mg), vitamin C (250 mg) and β-carotene (20 mg) or placebo daily for five years. There were no significant reductions in all cause mortality, or deaths due to vascular or non-vascular causes. Thus these antioxidant supplements provided no measurable health benefits for these patients.

In conclusion, some studies have shown that health benefits can be obtained by some people with an increased risk of disease from supplements of antioxidant nutrients. The amounts of supplements used, however, have been large and the effect possibly has been pharmacologic. Further work is needed to show whether more modest increases in nutrient intakes in healthy adult populations will delay or prevent the onset of chronic disease. Therefore, the available evidence regarding health benefits to be achieved by increasing intakes of antioxidant nutrients does not assist in setting nutrient requirements.

8.7 Recommendations for future research

If nutrient intakes are ever to be recommended on the basis of antioxidant properties then more research is needed to gain a better understanding of:

- The optimal plasma or tissue concentrations of nutrients to fully support interactions between antioxidant micronutrients like vitamins E and C, or vitamin E and Se to counter oxidant stress in the tissues.
- The mechanisms whereby micronutrients like vitamins A and C, and minerals iron and zinc are reduced at the time of oxidant stress and the physiological purposes of the changes.

The minimal concentrations of antioxidant nutrients in humans to prevent conversion of benign viruses to their more virulent forms as demonstrated by Beck and colleagues in mice (103).

References

1. Young VR et al. *Dietary reference intakes. Proposed definition and plan for review of dietary antioxidant and related compounds.* Washington, DC, National Academy Press, 1998.
2. Dormandy TL. An approach to free radicals. *Lancet*, 1983, 2:1010–1014.
3. Thurnham DI. Antioxidants and pro-oxidants in malnourished populations. *Proceedings of the Nutrition Society*, 1990, 48:247–259.
4. Shankar AH, Prasad AS. Zinc and immune function: the biological basis of

altered resistance to infection. *American Journal of Clinical Nutrition*, 1998, 68(Suppl.):S447–S463.

5. Halliwell B, Gutteridge JMC. *Free radicals in biology and medicine,* 2nd ed. Oxford, Clarendon Press, 1989.

6. Ames BN. Dietary carcinogens and anticarcinogens, oxygen radicals and degenerative diseases. *Science,* 1983, 221:1256–1264.

7. Moncada S, Higgs EA. Mechanisms of disease: the L-arginine-nitric oxide pathway. *New England Journal of Medicine,* 1993, 329:2002–2012.

8. Fridovich I. Superoxide radical: an endogenous toxicant. *Annual Review of Pharmacology and Toxicology,* 1983, 23:239–257.

9. Baboire MB. Oxygen microbial killing of phagocytes. *New England Journal of Medicine,* 1973, 298:659–680.

10. Hogg N et al. Inhibition of low-density lipoprotein oxidation by nitric oxide. *FEBS Letters,* 1993, 334:170–174.

11. Hibbs JBJ et al. Nitric oxide: a cytotoxic activated macrophage effector molecule. *Biochemical and Biophysical Research Communications,* 1988, 157:87–94.

12. Koppenol WH et al. Peroxynitrite, a cloaked oxidant formed by nitric oxide and superoxide. *Chemical Research in Toxicology,* 1992, 5:834–842.

13. Diplock AT et al. Functional food science and defence against reactive oxidative species. *British Journal of Nutrition,* 1998, 80(Suppl. 1):S77–S112.

14. Meister A. Glutathione metabolism and its selective modification. *Journal of Biological Chemistry,* 1988, 263:17 205–17 206.

15. Hennekens CH. Micronutrients and cancer prevention. *New England Journal of Medicine,* 1986, 315:1288–1289.

16. Van Poppel G et al. Antioxidants and coronary heart disease. *Annals of Medicine,* 1994, 26:429–434.

17. Thurnham DI. Carotenoids: functions and fallacies. *Proceedings of the Nutrition Society,* 1994, 53:77–87.

18. Rock CL, Jacob RA, Bowen PE. Update on the biological characteristics of the antioxidant micronutrients: vitamin C, vitamin E and the carotenoids. *Journal of the American Dietetic Association,* 1996, 96:693–702.

19. Hertog MGL et al. Dietary antioxidant flavonoids and risk of coronary heart disease: the Zutphen Elderly Study. *Lancet,* 1993, 342:1007–1011.

20. Chevion M et al. Copper and iron are mobilised following myocardial ischemia: possible predictive criteria for tissue injury. *Proceedings of the National Academy of Sciences,* 1993, 90:1102–1106.

21. Beare S, Steward WP. Plasma free iron and chemotherapy toxicity. *Lancet,* 1996, 347:342–343.

22. Halliwell B, Gutteridge JMC. Biologically relevant metal ion-dependent hydroxyl radical generation. An update. *FEBS Letters,* 1992, 307:108–112.

23. Carreras MC et al. Kinetics of nitric oxide and hydrogen peroxide production and formation of peroxynitrite during the respiratory burst of human neutrophils. *FEBS Letter,* 1994, 341:65–68.

24. Thurnham DI. Iron as a pro-oxidant. In: Wharton BA, Ashwell M, eds. *Iron, nutritional and physiological significance.* London, Chapman & Hall, 1995:31–41.

25. Weiss G, Wachter H, Fuchs D. Linkage of cell-mediated immunity to iron metabolism. *Immunology Today,* 1995, 16:495–500.

26. Pantopoulos K, Weiss G, Hentze MW. Nitric oxide and the post-transcriptional control of cellular iron traffic. *Trends in Cellular Biology,* 1994, 4:82–86.

27. Thompson D, Milford-Ward A, Whicher JT. The value of acute phase protein measurements in clinical practice. *Annals of Clinical Biochemistry*, 1992, 29:123–131.

28. Koj A. Biological functions of acute phase proteins. In: Gordon AH, Koj A, eds. *The acute phase response to injury and infection*. London, Elsevier, 1985:145–160.

29. Thurnham DI. β-Carotene, are we misreading the signals in risk groups? Some analogies with vitamin C. *Proceedings of the Nutrition Society*, 1994, 53:557–569.

30. Thurnham DI. Impact of disease on markers of micronutrient status. *Proceedings of the Nutrition Society*, 1997, 56:421–431.

31. Packer JE, Slater TF, Willson RL. Direct observations of a free radical interaction between vitamin E and vitamin C. *Nature*, 1979, 278:737–738.

32. Niki E et al. Regeneration of vitamin E from α-chromanoxyl radical by glutathione and vitamin C. *Chemistry Letters*, 1982, 27:789–792.

33. Burton GW, Ingold KU. β-Carotene: an unusual type of lipid antioxidant. *Science*, 1984, 224:569–573.

34. Palozza P. Pro-oxidant actions of carotenoids in biologic systems. *Nutrition Reviews*, 1998, 56:257–265.

35. Heinonen OP et al. The effect of vitamin E and beta carotene on the incidence of lung cancer and other cancers in male smokers. *New England Journal of Medicine*, 1994, 330:1029–1035.

36. Halliwell B, Gutteridge JMC, Cross CE. Free radicals, antioxidants, and human disease: where are we now? *Journal of Laboratory and Clinical Medicine*, 1992, 119:598–620.

37. Stadtman ER. Ascorbic acid and oxidative inactivation of proteins. *American Journal of Clinical Nutrition*, 1991, 54(Suppl.):S1125–S1128.

38. Arthur JR et al. Regulation of selenoprotein gene expression and thyroid hormone metabolism. *Transactions of the Biochemical Society*, 1996, 24:384–388.

39. Howie AF et al. Identification of a 57-kilodalton selenoprotein in human thyrocytes as thioredoxin reductase and evidence that its expression is regulated through the calcium phosphoinositol-signalling pathway. *Journal of Clinical Endocrinology and Metabolism*, 1998, 83:2052–2058.

40. Chow CK. Biochemical responses in lungs of ozone-tolerant rats. *Nature*, 1976, 260:721–722.

41. Aggett PJ, Favier A. Zinc. *International Journal of Vitamin and Nutrition Research*, 1993, 63:301–307.

42. Alfthan G et al. Selenium metabolism and platelet glutathione peroxidase activity in healthy Finnish men: effects of selenium yeast, selenite and selenate. *American Journal of Clinical Nutrition*, 1991, 53:120–125.

43. Clark LC et al. Effects of selenium supplementation for cancer prevention in patients with carcinoma of the skin. A randomised controlled trial. *Journal of the American Medical Association*, 1996, 276:1957–1963.

44. Willett WC et al. Prediagnostic serum selenium and risk of cancer. *Lancet*, 1983, 2:130–134.

45. Willett WC et al. Vitamins A, E and carotene: effects of supplementation on their plasma levels. *American Journal of Clinical Nutrition*, 1983, 38:559–566.

46. Burton GW, Ingold KU. Autoxidation of biological molecules. 1. The antiox-

idant activity of vitamin E and related chain-breaking phenolic antioxidants in vitro. *Journal of the American Chemistry Society*, 1981, 103:6472–6477.

47. Kornbrust DJ, Mavis RD. Relative susceptibility of microsomes from lung, heart, liver, kidney, brain and testes to lipid peroxidation: correlation with vitamin E content. *Lipids*, 1979, 15:315–322.

48. Wefers H, Sies H. The protection by ascorbate and glutathione against microsomal lipid peroxidation is dependent on vitamin E. *European Journal of Biochemistry*, 1988, 174:353–357.

49. McCay PB. Vitamin E: interactions with free radicals and ascorbate. *Annual Review of Nutrition*, 1985, 5:323–340.

50. Sies H, Murphy ME. The role of tocopherols in the protection of biological systems against oxidative damage. *Photochemistry and Photobiology*, 1991, 8:211–224.

51. Myllyla R, Kuutti-Savolainen E, Kivirikko KI. The role of ascorbate in the prolyl hydroxylase reaction. *Biochemical and Biophysical Research Communications*, 1978, 83:441–448.

52. Hulse JD, Ellis SR, Henderson LM. β-Hydroxylation of trimethyllysine by an α-ketoglutarate-dependent mitochondrial dioxygenase. *Journal of Biological Chemistry*, 1978, 253:1654–1659.

53. Bates CJ. The function and metabolism of vitamin C in man. In: Counsell JN, Hornig DH, eds. *Vitamin C—ascorbic acid*. London, Applied Science Publishers, 1981:1–22.

54. Zannoni VG, Lynch MM. The role of ascorbic acid in drug metabolism. *Drug Metabolism Review*, 1973, 2:57–69.

55. Koskela TK et al. Is the high concentration of ascorbic acid in the eye an adaptation to intense solar irradiation? *Investigative Ophthalmology and Visual Science*, 1989, 30:2265–2267.

56. Hornig DH. Distribution of ascorbic acid, metabolites and analogues in man and animals. *Annals of the New York Academy of Sciences*, 1975, 258:103–118.

57. Fraga CG et al. Ascorbic acid protects against endogenous oxidative DNA damage in human sperm. *Proceedings of the National Academy of Sciences*, 1991, 88:11 003–11 006.

58. Frei B. Ascorbic acid protects lipids in human plasma and low-density lipoprotein against oxidative damage. *American Journal of Clinical Nutrition*, 1991, 54(Suppl.):S1113–S1118.

59. Rose RC. The ascorbate redox potential of tissues: a determinant or indicator of disease? *News in Physiological Sciences*, 1989, 4:190–195.

60. Weber P, Bendich A, Schalch W. Vitamin C and human health—a review of recent data relevant to human requirements. *International Journal for Vitamin and Nutrition Research*, 1996, 66:19–30.

61. Tannenbaum SR, Wishnok JS, Leaf CD. Inhibition of nitrosamine formation by ascorbic acid. *American Journal of Clinical Nutrition*, 1991, 53(Suppl.):S247–S250.

62. Moser U, Weber F. Uptake of ascorbic acid by human granulocytes. *International Journal for Vitamin and Nutrition Research*, 1984, 54:47–53.

63. McGowen E et al. Ascorbic acid content and accumulation by alveolar macrophages from cigarette smokers and non-smokers. *Journal of Laboratory and Clinical Medicine*, 1984, 104:127–134.

64. Bendich A, Olson JA. Biological action of carotenoids. *FASEB Journal*, 1989, 3:1927–1932.

65. Gregory JR et al. *The dietary and nutritional survey of British adults.* London, Her Majesty's Stationery Office, 1990.
66. Chug-Ahuja JK et al. The development and application of a carotenoid database for fruits, vegetables, and selected multicomponent foods. *Journal of the American Dietetics Association*, 1993, 93:318–323.
67. Heinonen MI et al. Carotenoids in Finnish foods: vegetables, fruits, and berries. *Journal of Agricultural and Food Chemistry*, 1989, 37:655–659.
68. de Pee S, West C. Dietary carotenoids and their role in combatting vitamin A deficiency: a review of the literature. *European Journal of Clinical Nutrition*, 1996, 50:38–53.
69. *Carotenoids: views and expert opinions of an IARC Working Group on the Evaluation of Cancer Preventive Agents, Lyon, 10–16 December 1997.* Lyon, International Agency for Research on Cancer, 1998.
70. Stryker WS et al. The relation of diet, cigarette smoking, and alcohol consumption to plasma beta-carotene and alpha-tocopherol levels. *American Journal of Epidemiology*, 1988, 127:283–296.
71. Mathews-Roth MM et al. Carotenoid chromophore length and protection against photosensitization. *Photochemistry and Photobiology*, 1974, 19: 217–222.
72. Foote CS, Denny RW. Chemistry of singlet oxygen. VII. Quenching by β-carotene. *American Chemistry Society Journal*, 1968, 90:6233–6235.
73. Di Mascio P, Kaiser S, Sies H. Lycopene as the most efficient biological carotenoid singlet-oxygen quencher. *Archives of Biochemistry and Biophysics*, 1989, 274:532–538.
74. Palozza P, Krinsky NI. β-Carotene and α-tocopherol are synergistic antioxidants. *Archives of Biochemistry and Biophysics*, 1992, 297:184–187.
75. Mathews-Roth MM. Systemic photoprotection. *Dermatologic Clinics*, 1986, 4:335–339.
76. Mathews-Roth MM et al. Beta-carotene therapy for erythropoietic protoporphyria and other photosensitive diseases. *Archives of Dermatology*, 1977, 113:1229–1232.
77. Greenberg ER et al. A clinical trial of beta carotene to prevent basal-cell and squamous-cell cancers of the skin. *New England Journal of Medicine*, 1990, 323:789–795.
78. Bone RA et al. Analysis of macula pigment by HPLC: retinal distribution and age study. *Investigative Ophthalmology and. Visual Science*, 1988, 29:843–849.
79. Gerster H. Antioxidant protection of the ageing macula. *Age and Ageing*, 1991, 20:60–69.
80. Seddon AM et al. Dietary carotenoids, vitamin A, C, and E, and advanced age-related macular degeneration. *Journal of the American Medical Association*, 1994, 272:1413–1420.
81. Terao J. Antioxidant activity of β-carotene-related carotenoids in solution. *Lipids*, 1989, 24:659–661.
82. Chopra M, Thurnham DI. In vitro antioxidant activity of lutein. In: Waldron KW, Johnson IT, Fenwick GR, eds. *Food and cancer prevention*. London, Royal Society of Chemistry, 1993:123–129.
83. Edge R, McGarvey DJ, Truscott TG. The carotenoids as anti-oxidants. *Journal of Photochemistry and Photobiology* (Series B:Biology), 1997, 41:189–200.

84. Bendich A. Carotenoids and the immune response. *Journal of Nutrition*, 1989, 119:112–115.
85. Pool-Zobel BL et al. Consumption of vegetables reduces genetic damage in humans: first results of a human intervention trial with carotenoid-rich foods. *Carcinogenesis*, 1997, 18:1847–1850.
86. van Anterwerpen VL et al. Plasma levels of beta-carotene are inversely correlated with circulating neutrophil counts in young male cigarette smokers. *Inflammation*, 1995, 19:405–414.
87. Daudu PA et al. Effect of low β-carotene diet on the immune functions of adult women. *American Journal of Clinical Nutrition*, 1994, 60:969–972.
88. Krinsky NI. The evidence for the role of carotenoids in preventive health. *Clinical Nutrition*, 1988, 7:107–112.
89. Colditz GA et al. Increased green and yellow vegetable intake and lowered cancer deaths in an elderly population. *American Journal of Clinical Nutrition*, 1985, 41:32–36.
90. National Academy of Sciences. *Diet and health. Implications for reducing chronic disease.* Washington, DC, National Academy Press, 1989.
91. Sann L et al. Serum orosomucoid concentration in newborn infants. *European Journal of Pediatrics*, 1981, 136:181–185.
92. Kelly FJ et al. Time course of vitamin E repletion in the premature infant. *British Journal of Nutrition*, 1990, 63:631–638.
93. Moison RMW et al. Induction of lipid peroxidation by pulmonary surfactant by plasma of preterm babies. *Lancet*, 1993, 341:79–82.
94. Omenn GS et al. Effects of a combination of beta carotene and vitamin A on lung cancer and cardiovascular disease. *New England Journal of Medicine*, 1996, 334:1150–1155.
95. Rapola JM et al. Randomised trial of α-tocopherol and β-carotene supplements on incidence of major coronary events in men with previous myocardial infarction. *Lancet*, 1997, 349:1715–1720.
96. Greenberg ER et al. A clinical trial of antioxidant vitamins to prevent colorectal adenoma. *New England Journal of Medicine*, 1994, 331:141–147.
97. Stich HF et al. Remission of oral leukoplakias and micronuclei in tobacco/betel quid chewers treated with beta-carotene and with beta-carotene plus vitamin A. *International Journal of Cancer*, 1988; 42:195–199.
98. Stich HF, Hornby P, Dunn BP. A pilot beta-carotene intervention trial with Inuits using smokeless tobacco. *International Journal of Cancer*, 1985, 36:321–327.
99. Blot WJ et al. Nutrition intervention trials in Linxian, China: supplementation with specific vitamin/mineral combinations, cancer incidence, and disease specific mortality in the general population. *Journal of the National Cancer Institute*, 1993, 85:1483–1492.
100. Stephens NG et al. Randomised control trial of vitamin E in patients with coronary disease: Cambridge Heart Antioxidant Study (CHAOS). *Lancet*, 1996, 347:781–786.
101. Mitchinson MJ et al. Mortality in the CHAOS trial. *Lancet*, 1999, 353:381–382.
102. Heart Protection Study Group. MRC/BHF Heart Protection Study of antioxidant vitamin supplementation in 20536 high-risk individuals: a randomised placebo-controlled trial. *Lancet*, 2002, 360:23–33.
103. Beck MA. Selenium and host defence towards viruses. *Proceedings of the Nutrition Society*, 1999; 58:707–711.

9. Thiamine, riboflavin, niacin, vitamin B$_6$, pantothenic acid, and biotin

9.1 Introduction

The B-complex vitamins covered here are listed in Table 9.1 along with the physiological roles of the coenzyme forms and a brief description of clinical deficiency symptoms.

Rice and wheat are the staples for many populations of the world. Excessive refining and polishing of cereals removes considerable proportions of B vitamins contained in these cereals. Clinical manifestations of deficiency of some B vitamins—such as beriberi (cardiac and dry), peripheral neuropathies, pellagra, and oral and genital lesions (related to riboflavin deficiency)—were once major public health problems in some parts of the world. These manifestations have now declined, the decline being brought about not through programmes which distribute synthetic vitamins but through changes in the patterns of food availability and consequent changes in dietary practices.

Although many clinical manifestations of B-vitamin deficiencies have decreased, there is evidence of widespread subclinical deficiency of these vitamins (especially of riboflavin and pyridoxine). These subclinical deficiencies, although less dramatic in their manifestations, exert deleterious metabolic effects. Despite the progress in reduction of large-scale deficiency in the world, there are periodic reports of outbreaks of B-complex deficiencies which are linked to deficits of B vitamins in populations under various distress conditions.

Refugee and displaced population groups (20 million people by current United Nations estimates) are at risk for B-complex deficiency because most cereal foods used under emergency situations are not fortified with micronutrients (1). Recent reports have implicated the low B-complex content of diets as a factor in the outbreak of peripheral neuropathy and visual loss observed in the adult population of Cuba (2–4). This deficiency in Cuba resulted from the consequences of an economic blockade (4).

Because of the extensive literature pertaining to the study of the B-complex vitamins, the references cited here have been limited to those published after

TABLE 9.1
Physiologic roles and deficiency signs of B-complex vitamins

Vitamin	Physiologic roles	Clinical signs of deficiency
Thiamin (B₁)	Coenzyme functions in metabolism of carbohydrates and branched-chain amino acids	Beriberi, polyneuritis, and Wernicke-Korsakoff syndrome
Riboflavin (B₂)	Coenzyme functions in numerous oxidation and reduction reactions	Growth, cheilosis, angular stomatitis, and dermatitis
Niacin (nicotinic acid and nicotinamide)	Cosubstrate/coenzyme for hydrogen transfer with numerous dehydrogenases	Pellagra with diarrhoea, dermatitis, and dementia
Vitamin B₆ (pyridoxine, pyridoxamine, and pyridoxal)	Coenzyme functions in metabolism of amino acids, glycogen, and sphingoid bases	Nasolateral seborrhoea, glossitis, and peripheral neuropathy (epileptiform convulsions in infants)
Pantothenic acid	Constituent of coenzyme A and phosphopantetheine involved in fatty acid metabolism	Fatigue, sleep disturbances, impaired coordination, and nausea
Biotin	Coenzyme functions in bicarbonate-dependent carboxylations	Fatigue, depression, nausea, dermatitis, and muscular pains

the publication of the 1974 edition of the FAO/WHO *Handbook on human nutritional requirements* (5). Greater weight has been given to studies which used larger numbers of subjects over longer periods, more thoroughly assessed dietary intake, varied the level of the specific vitamin being investigated, and used multiple indicators, including those considered functional in the assessment of status. These indicators have been the main basis for ascertaining requirements. Although extensive, the bibliographic search of recently published reports presented in this chapter most likely underestimates the extent of B-complex deficiency given that many cases are not reported in the medical literature. Moreover, outbreaks of vitamin deficiencies in populations are usually not publicized because governments may consider the existence of these conditions to be politically sensitive information. Additional references are listed in the publication by the Food and Nutrition Board of the Institute of Medicine of the United States National Academy of Sciences (6).

9.2 Thiamine

9.2.1 Background
Deficiency

Thiamine (vitamin B₁, aneurin) deficiency results in the disease called beriberi, which has been classically considered to exist in dry (paralytic) and wet (oedematous) forms (*7, 8*). Beriberi occurs in human-milk-fed infants whose nursing mothers are deficient. It also occurs in adults with high carbohydrate intakes (mainly from milled rice) and with intakes of anti-thiamine factors, such as the bacterial thiaminases that are in certain ingested raw fish (*7*). Beriberi is still endemic in Asia. In relatively industrialized nations, the neurologic manifestations of Wernicke-Korsakoff syndrome are frequently associated with chronic alcoholism in conjunction with limited food consumption (*9*). Some cases of thiamine deficiency have been observed with patients who are hypermetabolic, are on parenteral nutrition, are undergoing chronic renal dialysis, or have undergone a gastrectomy. Thiamine deficiency has also been observed in Nigerians who ate silk worms, Russian schoolchildren (Moscow), Thai rural elderly, Cubans, Japanese elderly, Brazilian Xavante Indians, French Guyanese, south-east Asian schoolchildren who were infected with hookworm, Malaysian detention inmates, and people with chronic alcoholism.

Toxicity
Thiamine toxicity is not a problem because renal clearance of the vitamin is rapid.

Role in human metabolic processes
Thiamine functions as the coenzyme thiamine pyrophosphate (TPP) in the metabolism of carbohydrates and branched-chain amino acids. Specifically the Mg^{2+}-coordinated TPP participates in the formation of α-ketols (e.g. among hexose and pentose phosphates) as catalysed by transketolase and in the oxidation of α-keto acids (e.g. pyruvate, α-ketoglutarate, and branched-chain α-keto acids) by dehydrogenase complexes (*10, 11*). Hence, when there is insufficient thiamine, the overall decrease in carbohydrate metabolism and its interconnection with amino acid metabolism (via α-keto acids) has severe consequences, such as a decrease in the formation of acetylcholine for neural function.

9.2.2 Biochemical indicators
Indicators used to estimate thiamine requirements are urinary excretion, erythrocyte transketolase activity coefficient, erythrocyte thiamine, blood pyruvate and lactate, and neurologic changes. The excretion rate of the vitamin and its metabolites reflects intake, and the validity of the assessment of thiamine nutriture is improved with load test. Erythrocyte transketolase activity coefficient reflects TPP levels and can indicate rare genetic defects. Erythrocyte thiamine is mainly a direct measure of TPP but when combined with high

performance liquid chromatography (HPLC) separation can also provide a measure of thiamine and thiamine monophosphate.

Thiamine status has been assessed by measuring urinary thiamine excretion under basal conditions or after thiamine loading; transketolase activity; and free and phosphorylated forms in blood or serum (6, 9). Although overlap with baseline values for urinary thiamine was found with oral doses below 1 mg, a correlation of 0.86 between oral and excreted amounts was found by Bayliss et al. (12). The erythrocyte transketolase assay, in which an activity coefficient based on a TPP stimulation of the basal level is given, continues to be a main functional indicator (9), but some problems have been encountered. Gans and Harper (13) found a wide range of TPP effects when thiamine intakes were adequate (i.e. above 1.5 mg/day over a 3-day period). In some cases, the activity coefficient may appear normal after prolonged deficiency (14). This measure seemed poorly correlated with dietary intakes estimated for a group of English adolescents (15). Certainly, there are both interindividual and genetic factors affecting the transketolase (16). Baines and Davies (17) suggested that it is useful to determine erythrocyte TPP directly because the coenzyme is less susceptible to factors that influence enzyme activity; there are also methods for determining thiamine and its phosphate esters in whole blood (18).

9.2.3 Factors affecting requirements

Because thiamine facilitates energy utilization, its requirements have traditionally been expressed on the basis of energy intake, which can vary depending on activity levels. However, Fogelholm et al. (19) found no difference in activation coefficients for erythrocyte transketolase between a small group of skiers and a less physically active group of control subjects. Also, a study with thiamine-restricted Dutch males whose intake averaged 0.43 mg/day for 11 weeks did not reveal an association between short bouts of intense exercise and decreases in indicators of thiamine status (20). Alcohol consumption may interfere with thiamine absorption as well (9).

9.2.4 Evidence used to derive recommended intakes

Recommendations for infants are based on adequate food intake. Mean thiamine content of human milk is 0.21 mg/l (0.62 μmol/l) (21), which corresponds to 0.16 mg (0.49 μmol) thiamine per 0.75 l of secreted milk per day. The blood concentration for total thiamine averages 210 ± 53 nmol/l for infants up to 6 months but decreases over the first 12–18 months of life (22).

A study of 13–14-year-old children related dietary intake of thiamine to several indicators of thiamine status (15). Sauberlich et al. (23) concluded from a carefully controlled depletion–repletion study of seven healthy young men that 0.3 mg thiamine per 4184 kJ met their requirements. Intakes below this amount lead to irritability and other symptoms and signs of deficiency (24). Anderson et al. (25) reported thiamine intakes of 1.0 and 1.2 mg/day as minimal for women and men, respectively. Hoorn et al. (26) reported that 23% of 153 patients aged 65–93 years were deemed deficient based on a trans-ketolase activation coefficient greater than 1.27, which was normalized after thiamine administration. Nichols and Basu (27) found that only 57% of 60 adults aged 65–74 years had TPP effects of less than 14% and suggested that ageing may increase thiamine requirements.

An average total energy cost of 230 MJ has been estimated for pregnancy (28). With an intake of 0.4 mg thiamine/4184 kJ, this amounts to a total of 22 mg thiamine needed during pregnancy, or 0.12 mg/day when the additional thiamine need for the second and third trimesters (180 days) is included. Taking into account the increased need for thiamine because of an increased growth in maternal and fetal compartments and a small increase in energy utilization, an overall additional requirement of 0.3 mg/day is considered adequate (6).

It is estimated that lactating women transfer 0.2 mg thiamine to their infants through their milk each day. Therefore, an additional 0.1 mg is estimated as the need for the increased energy cost of about 2092 kJ/day associated with lactation (6).

9.2.5 Recommended nutrient intakes for thiamine

The recommendations for thiamine are given in Table 9.2.

TABLE 9.2
Recommended nutrient intakes for thiamine, by group

Group	Recommended nutrient intake (mg/day)
Infants and children	
0–6 months	0.2
7–12 months	0.3
1–3 years	0.5
4–6 years	0.6
7–9 years	0.9
Adolescents	
Females, 10–18 years	1.1
Males, 10–18 years	1.2
Adults	
Females, 19+ years	1.1
Males, 19+ years	1.2
Pregnant women	1.4
Lactating women	1.5

9.3 Riboflavin

9.3.1 Background

Deficiency

Riboflavin (vitamin B_2) deficiency results in the condition of hypo- or ariboflavinosis, with sore throat; hyperaemia; oedema of the pharyngeal and oral mucous membranes; cheilosis; angular stomatitis; glossitis; seborrheic dermatitis; and normochromic, normocytic anaemia associated with pure red cell cytoplasia of the bone marrow (8, 29). As riboflavin deficiency almost invariably occurs in combination with a deficiency of other B-complex vitamins, some of the symptoms (e.g. glossitis and dermatitis) may result from other complicating deficiencies. The major cause of hyporiboflavinosis is inadequate dietary intake as a result of limited food supply, which is sometimes exacerbated by poor food storage or processing. Children in developing countries will commonly demonstrate clinical signs of riboflavin deficiency during periods of the year when gastrointestinal infections are prevalent. Decreased assimilation of riboflavin also results from abnormal digestion, such as that which occurs with lactose intolerance. This condition is highest in African and Asian populations and can lead to a decreased intake of milk, as well as an abnormal absorption of the vitamin. Absorption of riboflavin is also affected in some other conditions, for example, tropical sprue, celiac disease, malignancy and resection of the small bowel, and decreased gastrointestinal passage time. In relatively rare cases, the cause of deficiency is inborn errors in which the genetic defect is in the formation of a flavoprotein (e.g. acyl-coenzyme A [coA] dehydrogenases). Also at risk are infants receiving phototherapy for neonatal jaundice and perhaps those with inadequate thyroid hormone. Some cases of riboflavin deficiency have been observed in Russian schoolchildren (Moscow) and south-east Asian schoolchildren (infected with hookworm).

Toxicity

Riboflavin toxicity is not a problem because of limited intestinal absorption.

Role in human metabolic processes

Conversion of riboflavin to flavin mononucleotide (FMN) and then to the predominant flavin, flavin adenine dinucleotide (FAD), occurs before these flavins form complexes with numerous flavoprotein dehydrogenases and oxidases. The flavocoenzymes (FMN and FASD) participate in oxidation–reduction reactions in metabolic pathways and in energy production via the respiratory chain (10, 11).

9.3.2 Biochemical indicators

Indicators used to estimate riboflavin requirements are urinary flavin excretion, erythrocyte glutathione reductase activity coefficient, and erythrocyte flavin. The urinary flavin excretion rate of the vitamin and its metabolites reflects intake; validity of assessment of riboflavin adequacy is improved with load test. Erythrocyte glutathione reductase activity coefficient reflects FAD levels; results are confounded by such genetic defects as glucose-6-phosphate dehydrogenase deficiency and heterozygous β-thalassemia. Erythrocyte flavin is largely a measure of FMN and riboflavin after hydrolysis of labile FAD and HPLC separation.

Riboflavin status has been assessed by measuring urinary excretion of the vitamin in fasting, random, and 24-hour specimens or by load return tests (amounts measured after a specific amount of riboflavin is given orally); measuring erythrocyte glutathione reductase activity coefficient; or erythrocyte flavin concentration (6, 9, 29). The HPLC method with fluorometry gives lower values for urinary riboflavin than do fluorometric methods, which measure the additive fluorescence of similar flavin metabolites (30). The metabolites can comprise as much as one third of total urinary flavin (31, 32) and in some cases may depress assays dependent on a biological response because certain catabolites can inhibit cellular uptake (33). Under conditions of adequate riboflavin intake (approximately 1.3 mg/day for adults), an estimated 120 µg (320 nmol) total riboflavin or 80 µg/g of creatinine is excreted daily (32).

The erythrocyte glutathione reductase assay, with an activity coefficient (AC) expressing the ratio of activities in the presence and absence of added FAD, continues to be used as a main functional indicator of riboflavin status, but some limitations in the technique have been noted. The reductase in erythrocytes from individuals with glucose-6-phosphate dehydrogenase deficiency (often present in blacks) has an increased avidity for FAD, which makes this test invalid (34). Sadowski (35) has set an upper limit of normality for the AC at 1.34 based on the mean value plus 2 standard deviations from several hundred apparently healthy individuals aged 60 years and over. Suggested guidelines for the interpretation of such enzyme ACs are as follows: less than 1.2, acceptable; 1.2–1.4, low; greater than 1.4, deficient (9). In general agreement with earlier findings on erythrocyte flavin, Ramsay et al. (36) found a correlation between cord blood and maternal erythrocyte deficiencies and suggested that values greater than 40 nmol/l could be considered adequate.

9.3.3 Factors affecting requirements

Several studies reported modest effects of physical activity on the erythrocyte glutathione reductase AC (*37–41*). A slight increase in the AC and decrease in urinary flavin of weight-reducing women (*39*) and older women undergoing exercise training (*41*) were "normalized" with 20% additional riboflavin. However, riboflavin supplementation did not lead to an increase in work performance when such subjects were not clinically deficient (*42–45*).

Bioavailability of riboflavin in foods, mostly as digestible flavocoenzymes, is excellent at nearly 95% (*6*), but absorption of the free vitamin is limited to about 27 mg per single meal or dose in an adult (*46*). No more than about 7% of food flavin is found as 8-α-FAD covalently attached to certain flavoprotein enzymes. Although some portions of the 8-α-(amino acid)-riboflavins are released by proteolysis of these flavoproteins, they do not have vitamin activity (*47*).

A lower fat–carbohydrate ratio may decrease the riboflavin requirements of the elderly (*48*). Riboflavin interrelates with other B vitamins, notably niacin, which requires FAD for its formation from tryptophan, and vitamin B₆, which requires FMN for conversion of the phosphates of pyridoxine and pyridoxamine to the coenzyme pyridoxal 5′-phosphate (PLP) (*49*). Contrary to earlier reports, no difference was seen in riboflavin status of women taking oral contraceptives when dietary intake was controlled by providing a single basic daily menu and meal pattern after 0.6 mg riboflavin/4184 kJ was given in a 2-week acclimation period (*50*).

9.3.4 Evidence used to derive recommended intakes

As reviewed by Thomas et al. (*51*), early estimates of riboflavin content in human milk showed changes during the postpartum period; more recent investigations of flavin composition of both human (*52*) and cow (*53*) milk have helped clarify the nature of the flavins present and provide better estimates of riboflavin equivalence. For human milk consumed by infants up to age 6 months, the riboflavin equivalence averages 0.35 mg/l (931 nmol/l) or 0.26 mg/0.75 l of milk/day (691 nmol/0.75 l of milk/day) (*6*). For low-income Indian women with erythrocyte glutathione reductase activity ratios averaging 1.80 and a milk riboflavin content of 0.22 mg/l, their breast-fed infants averaged AC ratios near 1.36 (*54*). Hence, a deficiency sufficient to reduce human-milk riboflavin content by one third can lead to a mild subclinical deficiency in infants.

Studies of riboflavin status in adults include those by Belko et al. (*38, 39*) in modestly obese young women on low-energy diets, by Bates et al. (*55*) on deficient Gambians, and by Kuizon et al. (*56*) on Filipino women. Most of a 1.7-mg dose of riboflavin given to healthy adults consuming at least this amount was largely excreted in the urine (*32*). Such findings corroborate earlier work indicating a relative saturation of tissue with intakes above 1.1 mg/day. Studies by Alexander et al. (*57*) on riboflavin status in the elderly show that doubling the estimated riboflavin intakes of 1.7 mg/day for women aged 70 years and over, with a reductase AC of 1.8, led to a doubling of urinary riboflavin from 1.6 μg to 3.4 μg/mg (4.2 to 9.0 nmol/mg) creatinine and a decrease in AC to 1.25. Boisvert et al. (*48*) obtained normalization of the glutathione reductase AC in elderly Guatemalans with approximately 1.3 mg/day of riboflavin, with a sharp increase in urinary riboflavin occurring at intakes above 1.0–1.1 mg/day.

Pregnant women have an increased erythrocyte glutathione reductase AC (*58, 59*). Kuizon et al. (*56*) found that riboflavin at 0.7 mg/4184 kJ was needed to lower the AC of four of eight pregnant women to 1.3 within 20 days, whereas only 0.41 mg/4184 kJ was needed for five of seven non-pregnant women. Maternal riboflavin intake was positively associated with fetal growth in a study of 372 pregnant women (*60*). The additional riboflavin requirement of 0.3 mg/day for pregnancy is an estimate based on increased growth in maternal and fetal compartments. For lactating women, an estimated 0.3 mg riboflavin is transferred in milk daily and, because utilization for milk production is assumed to be 70% efficient, the value is adjusted upward to 0.4 mg/day.

9.3.5 Recommended nutrient intakes for riboflavin

The recommendations for riboflavin are given in Table 9.3.

TABLE 9.3
Recommended nutrient intakes for riboflavin, by group

Group	Recommended nutrient intake (mg/day)
Infants and children	
0–6 months	0.3
7–12 months	0.4
1–3 years	0.5
4–6 years	0.6
7–9 years	0.9
Adolescents	
Females, 10–18 years	1.0
Males, 10–18 years	1.3
Adults	
Females, 19+ years	1.1
Males, 19+ years	1.3
Pregnant women	1.4
Lactating women	1.6

9.4 Niacin
9.4.1 Background
Deficiency

Niacin (nicotinic acid) deficiency classically results in pellagra, which is a chronic wasting disease associated with a characteristic erythematous dermatitis that is bilateral and symmetrical, a dementia after mental changes including insomnia and apathy preceding an overt encephalopathy, and diarrhoea resulting from inflammation of the intestinal mucous surfaces (8, 9, 61). At present, pellagra occurs endemically in poorer areas of Africa, China, and India. Its cause has been mainly attributed to a deficiency of niacin; however, its biochemical interrelationship with riboflavin and vitamin B₆, which are needed for the conversion of L-tryptophan to niacin equivalents (NEs), suggests that insufficiencies of these vitamins may also contribute to pellagra (62). Pellagra-like syndromes occurring in the absence of a dietary niacin deficiency are also attributable to disturbances in tryptophan metabolism (e.g. Hartnup disease with impaired absorption of the amino acid and carcinoid syndrome where the major catabolic pathway routes to 5-hydroxytryptophan are blocked) (61). Pellagra also occurs in people with chronic alcoholism (61). Cases of niacin deficiency have been found in people suffering from Crohn disease (61).

Toxicity

Although therapeutically useful in lowering serum cholesterol, administration of chronic high oral doses of nicotinic acid can lead to hepatotoxicity as well as dermatologic manifestations. An upper limit (UL) of 35 mg/day as proposed by the United States Food and Nutrition Board (6) was adopted by this Consultation.

Role in human metabolic processes

Niacin is chemically synonymous with nicotinic acid although the term is also used for its amide (nicotinamide). Nicotinamide is the other form of the vitamin; it does not have the pharmacologic action of the acid that is administered at high doses to lower blood lipids, but exists within the redox-active coenzymes, nicotinamide adenine dinucleotide (NAD) and its phosphate (NADP), which function in dehydrogenase–reductase systems requiring transfer of a hydride ion (10, 11). NAD is also required for non-redox adenosine diphosphate–ribose transfer reactions involved in DNA repair (63) and calcium mobilization. NAD functions in intracellular respiration and with enzymes involved in the oxidation of fuel substrates such as glyceraldehyde-3-phosphate, lactate, alcohol, 3-hydroxybutyrate, and pyruvate. NADP functions in reductive biosyntheses such as fatty acid and steroid syntheses and in the oxidation of glucose-6-phosphate to ribose-5-phosphate in the pentose phosphate pathway.

9.4.2 Biochemical indicators

Indicators used to estimate niacin requirements are urinary excretion, plasma concentrations of metabolites, and erythrocyte pyridine nucleotides. The excretion rate of metabolites—mainly N'-methyl-nicotinamide and its 2- and 4-pyridones—reflects intake of niacin and is usually expressed as a ratio of the pyridones to N'-methyl-nicotinamide. Concentrations of metabolites, especially 2-pyridone, are measured in plasma after a load test. Erythrocyte pyridine nucleotides measure NAD concentration changes.

Niacin status has been monitored by daily urinary excretion of methylated metabolites, especially the ratio of the 2-pyridone to N'-methyl-nicotinamide; erythrocyte pyridine nucleotides; oral dose uptake tests; erythrocyte NAD; and plasma 2-pyridone (6, 9). Shibata and Matsuo (64) found that the ratio of urinary 2-pyridone to N'-methyl-nicotinamide was as much a measure of protein adequacy as it was a measure of niacin status. Jacob et al. (65) found this ratio too insensitive to marginal niacin intake. The ratio of the 2-pyridone to N'-methyl-nicotinamide also appears to be associated with the clinical symptoms of pellagra, principally the dermatitic condition (66). In plasma, 2-pyridone levels change in reasonable proportion to niacin intake (65). As in the case of the erythrocyte pyridine nucleotides (nicotinamide coenzymes), NAD concentration decreased by 70% whereas NADP remained unchanged in adult males fed diets with only 6 or 10 mg NEs/day (67). Erythrocyte NAD provided a marker that was at least as sensitive as urinary metabolites of niacin in this study (67) and in a niacin depletion study of elderly subjects (68).

9.4.3 Factors affecting requirements

The biosynthesis of niacin derivatives on the pathway to nicotinamide coenzymes stems from tryptophan, an essential amino acid found in protein, and as such, this source of NE increases niacin intake. There are several dietary, drug, and disease factors that reduce the conversion of tryptophan to niacin (61), such as the use of oral contraceptives (69). Although a 60-to-1 conversion factor represents the average for human utilization of tryptophan as an NE, there are substantial individual differences (70, 71). There is also an interdependence of enzymes within the tryptophan-to-niacin pathway where vitamin B$_6$ (as pyridoxal phosphate) and riboflavin (as FAD) are functional.

Further, riboflavin (as FMN) is required for the oxidase that forms coenzymic PLP from the alcohol and amine forms of phosphorylated vitamin B_6 (*49*).

9.4.4 Evidence used to derive recommended intakes

Niacin content of human milk is approximately 1.5 mg/l (12.3 µmol/l) and the tryptophan content is 210 mg/l (1.0 mmol/l) (*21*). Hence, the total content is approximately 5 mg NEs/l or 4 mg NEs/0.75 l secreted daily in human milk. Recent studies (*64, 70*) together with those reported in the 1950s suggest that 12.5 mg NEs, which corresponds to 5.6 mg NEs/4184 kJ, is minimally sufficient for niacin intake in adults.

For pregnant women, where 230 MJ is the estimated energy cost of pregnancy, calculated needs above those of non-pregnant women are 5.6 mg NEs/4186 kJ (1000 kcal) × 230 000 kJ (55 000 kcal), or 308 mg NEs for the entire pregnancy or 1.7 mg NEs/day (308 mg NEs/180 days) for the second and third trimester, which is about a 10% increase. In addition, about 2 mg NEs/day is required for growth in maternal and fetal compartments (*6*).

For lactating women, an estimated 1.4 mg preformed niacin is secreted daily, and an additional requirement of less than 1 mg is needed to support the energy expenditure of lactation. Hence, 2.4 mg NEs/day is the additional requirement for lactating women.

9.4.5 Recommended nutrient intakes for niacin

The recommendations for niacin are given in Table 9.4.

9.5 Vitamin B₆

9.5.1 Background

Deficiency

A deficiency of vitamin B_6 alone is uncommon because it usually occurs in association with a deficit in other B-complex vitamins (*72*). Early biochemical changes include decreased levels of plasma pyridoxal 5′-phosphate (PLP) and urinary 4-pyridoxic acid. These are followed by decreases in synthesis of transaminases (aminotransferases) and other enzymes of amino acid metabolism such that there is an increased presence of xanthurenate in the urine and a decreased glutamate conversion to the anti-neurotransmitter γ-aminobutyrate. Hypovitaminosis B_6 may often occur with riboflavin deficiency, because riboflavin is needed for the formation of the coenzyme PLP. Infants are especially susceptible to insufficient intakes, which can lead to epileptiform convulsions. Skin changes include dermatitis with cheilosis and glossitis. Moreover, there is usually a decrease in circulating lymphocytes and

TABLE 9.4
Recommended nutrient intakes for niacin, by group

Group	Recommended nutrient intake (mgNEs/day)
Infants and children	
0–6 months	2[a]
7–12 months	4
1–3 years	6
4–6 years	8
7–9 years	12
Adolescents	
10–18 years	16
Adults	
Females, 19+ years	14
Males, 19+ years	16
Pregnant women	18
Lactating women	17

NEs, niacin equivalents.
[a] Preformed.

sometimes a normocytic, microcytic, or sideroblastic anaemia as well (9). The sensitivity of such systems as sulfur amino acid metabolism to vitamin B_6 availability is reflected in homocysteinaemia. A decrease in the metabolism of glutamate in the brain, which is found in vitamin B_6 insufficiency, reflects a nervous system dysfunction. As is the case with other micronutrient deficiencies, vitamin B_6 deficiency results in an impairment of the immune system. Of current concern is the pandemic-like occurrence of low vitamin B_6 intakes in many people who eat poorly (e.g. people with eating disorders). Vitamin B_6 deficiency has also been observed in Russian schoolchildren (Moscow), south-east Asian schoolchildren (infected with hookworm), elderly Europeans (Dutch), and in some individuals with hyperhomocysteinaemia or who are on chronic haemodialysis. Several medical conditions can also affect vitamin B_6 metabolism and thus lead to deficiency symptoms.

Toxicity

Use of high doses of pyridoxine for the treatment of pre-menstrual syndrome, carpal tunnel syndrome, and some neurologic diseases has resulted in neurotoxicity. A UL of 100 mg/day as proposed by the United States Food and Nutrition Board (6) was adopted by this Consultation.

Role in human metabolic processes

There are three natural vitamers (different forms of the vitamin) of vitamin B_6, namely pyridoxine, pyridoxamine, and pyridoxal. All three must be phosphorylated and the 5′-phosphates of the first two vitamers are oxidized to the functional PLP, which serves as a carbonyl-reactive coenzyme to a number of enzymes involved in the metabolism of amino acids. Such enzymes include aminotransferases, decarboxylases, and dehydratases; δ-aminolevulinate synthase in haem biosynthesis; and phosphorylase in glycogen breakdown and sphingoid base biosynthesis (10, 11).

9.5.2 Biochemical indicators

Indicators used to estimate vitamin B_6 requirements are PLP, urinary excretion, erythrocyte aminotransferases activity coefficients, tryptophan catabolites, erythrocyte and whole blood PLP, and plasma homocysteine. PLP is the major form of vitamin B_6 in all tissues and the plasma PLP concentration reflects liver PLP. Plasma PLP changes fairly slowly in response to vitamin intake. The excretion rate of vitamin B_6 and particularly its catabolite, 4-pyridoxate, reflects intake. Erythrocyte aminotransferases for aspartate and alanine reflect PLP levels and show large variations in activity coefficients. The urinary excretion of xanthurenate, a tryptophan catabolite, is typically used after a tryptophan load test.

Vitamin B_6 status is most appropriately evaluated by using a combination of the above indicators, including those considered as direct indicators (e.g. vitamer concentration in cells or fluids) and those considered to be indirect or functional indicators (e.g. erythrocyte aminotransferase saturation by PLP or tryptophan metabolites) (9). Plasma PLP may be the best single indicator because it appears to reflect tissue stores (73). Kretsch et al. (74) found that diets containing less than 0.05 mg vitamin B_6 given to 11 young women led to abnormal electroencephalograph patterns in two of the women and a plasma PLP concentration of approximately 9 nmol/l. Hence, a level of about 10 nmol/l is considered sub-optimal. A plasma PLP concentration of 20 nmol/l has been proposed as an index of adequacy (6) based on recent findings (73, 75). Plasma PLP levels have been reported to fall with age (6, 76). Urinary 4-pyridoxic acid level responds quickly to changes in vitamin B_6 intake (73) and is therefore of questionable value in assessing status. However, a value higher than 3 µmol/day, achieved with an intake of approximately 1 mg/day, has been suggested to reflect adequate intake (77). Erythrocyte aminotransferases for aspartate and alanine are commonly measured before and after addition of PLP to ascertain amounts of apoenzymes, the proportion of which increases with vitamin B_6 depletion. Values of 1.5–1.6 for the aspartate aminotransferase and approximately 1.2 for the alanine aminotransferase have been suggested as being adequate (9, 77). Catabolites from tryptophan and methionine have also been used to assess vitamin B$_6$ status. In a review of the relevant literature, Leklem (77) suggested that a 24-hour urinary excretion of less than 65 μmol xanthurenate after a 2-g oral dose of tryptophan indicates normal vitamin B$_6$ status.

9.5.3 Factors affecting requirements

A recent review by Gregory (78) confirms that bioavailability of vitamin B$_6$ in a mixed diet is about 75% (79), with approximately 8% of this total contributed by pyridoxine β-D-glucoside, which is about half as effectively utilized (78) as free B$_6$ vitamers or their phosphates. The amine and aldehyde forms of vitamin B$_6$ are probably about 10% less effective than pyridoxine (80). Despite the involvement of PLP with many enzymes affecting amino acid metabolism, there seems to be only a slight effect of dietary proteins on vitamin B$_6$ status (81). Several studies have reported decreases in indicators of vitamin B$_6$ status in women receiving oral contraceptives (82, 83), but this probably reflects hormonal stimulation of tryptophan catabolism rather than any deficiency of vitamin B$_6$ per se. Subjects with pre-eclampsia or eclampsia have plasma PLP levels lower than those of healthy pregnant women (84, 85).

9.5.4 Evidence used to derive recommended intakes

The average intake of vitamin B$_6$ for infants, based on human-milk content, is 0.13 mg/l/day (86) or 0.1 mg/0.75 l/day. With an average maternal dietary intake of vitamin B$_6$ of 1.4 mg/day, human milk was found to contain 0.12 mg/l, and plasma PLP of nursing infants averaged 54 nmol/l (87). Extrapolation on the basis of metabolic body size, weight, and growth suggests 0.3 mg/day as an adequate intake for infants 6–12 months of age (6). Information on vitamin B$_6$ requirements for children is limited, but Heiskanen et al. (88) found an age-related decrease in erythrocyte PLP and an increase in the aspartate aminotransferase activation. However, this age-related decrease in erythrocyte PLP may accompany normal growth and health rather than reflect real deficiency.

In a review of earlier studies of men with various protein intakes, Linkswiler (89) concluded that normalization of a tryptophan load test required 1.0–1.5 mg vitamin B$_6$. Miller et al. (90) found that 1.6 mg vitamin B$_6$ led to plasma PLP levels above 30 nmol/l for young men with various protein intakes. From several investigations of young women (91–94), a requirement closer to 1.0–1.2 mg vitamin B$_6$ could be estimated.

Limited studies of the elderly indicate that requirements may be somewhat higher, at least to maintain plasma PLP above the 20-nmol level (*95, 96*), which is the proposed index of adequacy.

During pregnancy, indicators of vitamin B_6 status decrease, especially in the third trimester (*85, 97, 98*). It is not clear, however, whether this is a normal physiological phenomenon. For a maternal body store of 169 mg and fetal plus placental accumulation of 25 mg vitamin B_6, about 0.1 mg/day is needed, on average, over gestation (*6*). With additional allowances for the increased metabolic need and weight of the mother and assuming about 75% bioavailability, an additional average requirement of 0.25 mg in pregnancy can be estimated. Because most of this need is in the latter stages of pregnancy and vitamin B_6 is not stored to any significant extent, an extra 0.5 mg/day of vitamin B_6 may be justified to err on the side of safety.

For lactation, it may be prudent to add 0.6 mg vitamin B_6 to the base requirement for women because low maternal intakes could lead to a compromised vitamin B_6 status in the infant (*99*).

9.5.5 Recommended nutrient intakes for vitamin B₆

The recommendations for vitamin B_6 are given in Table 9.5.

TABLE 9.5
Recommended nutrient intakes for vitamin B₆, by group

Group	Recommended nutrient intake (mg/day)
Infants and children	
0–6 months	0.1
7–12 months	0.3
1–3 years	0.5
4–6 years	0.6
7–9 years	1.0
Adolescents	
Females, 10–18 years	1.2
Males, 10–18 years	1.3
Adults	
Females, 19–50 years	1.3
Males, 19–50 years	1.3
Females, 51+ years	1.5
Males, 51+ years	1.7
Pregnant women	1.9
Lactating women	2.0

9.6 Pantothenate
9.6.1 Background
Deficiency

The widespread occurrence of releasable pantothenic acid in food makes a dietary deficiency unlikely (8, 9, 100, 101). If a deficiency occurs, it is usually accompanied by deficits of other nutrients. The use of experimental animals, an antagonistic analogue (ω-methylpantothenate) given to humans, and more recently, the feeding of semi-synthetic diets virtually free of pantothenate (102), have all helped to define signs and symptoms of deficiency. Subjects become irascible; develop postural hypotension; have rapid heart rate on exertion; suffer epigastric distress with anorexia and constipation; experience numbness and tingling of the hands and feet ("burning feet" syndrome); and have hyperactive deep tendon reflexes and weakness of finger extensor muscles. Some cases of pantothenate deficiency have been observed in patients with acne and other dermatitic conditions.

Toxicity

Toxicity is not a problem with pantothenate, as no adverse effects have been observed (6).

Role in human metabolic processes

Pantothenic acid is a component of CoA, a cofactor that carries acyl groups for many enzymatic processes, and of phosphopantetheine within acyl carrier proteins, a component of the fatty acid synthase complex (10, 11). The compounds containing pantothenate are most especially involved in fatty acid metabolism and the pantothenate-containing prosthetic group additionally facilitates binding with appropriate enzymes.

9.6.2 Biochemical indicators

Indicators used to estimate pantothenate requirements are urinary excretion and blood levels. Excretion rate reflects intake. Whole blood, which contains the vitamin itself and pantothenate-containing metabolites, has a general correlation with intake; erythrocyte levels, however, seem more meaningful than plasma or serum levels.

Relative correspondence to pantothenate status has been reported for urinary excretion and for blood content of both whole blood and erythrocytes (6, 9). Fry et al. (102) reported a decline in urinary pantothenate levels from approximately 3 to 0.8 mg/day (13.7–3.6 μmol/day) in young men fed a deficient diet for 84 days. Urinary excretion for a typical American diet was found to be 2.6 mg/day (12 μmol/day) (79). Pantothenate intake estimated for adolescents was significantly correlated with pantothenate in urine (103). Whole-blood pantothenate fell from 1.95 to 1.41 µg/ml (8.8 to 6.4 µmol/l) when six adult males were fed a pantothenate-free diet (102). Whole-blood content corresponded to intake (103), and the range in whole blood was reported to be 1.57–2.66 µg/ml (7.2–12.1 µmol/l) (104). There is an excellent correlation of whole-blood concentrations of pantothenate with the erythrocyte con-centration, with an average value being 334 ng/ml (1.5 µmol/l) (103). The lack of sufficient population data, however, suggests the current use of an adequate intake rather than a recommended intake as a suitable basis for recommendations.

9.6.3 Factors affecting requirements

A measurement of urinary excretion of pantothenate after feeding a formula diet containing both bound and free vitamin indicates that approximately 50% of the pantothenate present in natural foods may be bioavailable (79).

9.6.4 Evidence used to derive recommended intakes

Infant requirements are based on an estimation of the pantothenic acid content of human milk, which according to reported values is at least 2.2 mg/l (21, 105). For a reported average human-milk intake of 0.75 l/day (106–108) these values suggest that 1.7 mg/day is an adequate intake by younger (0–6 months) infants. Taking into consideration growth and body size, 1.8 mg/day may be extrapolated for older (7–12 months) infants (105).

The studies of Eissenstat et al. (103) of adolescents suggest that intakes of less than 4 mg/day were sufficient to maintain blood and urinary pantothenate. Kathman and Kies (109) found a range of pantothenate intake of 4 mg/day to approximately 8 mg/day in 12 adolescents who were 11–16 years old. The usual pantothenate intake for American adults has been reported to be 4–7 mg/day (102, 109–111). Hence, around 5 mg/day is apparently adequate.

For pregnancy, there is only one relatively recent study that found lower blood pantothenate levels but no difference in urinary excretion in pregnant women compared with non-pregnant controls (112).

During lactation, blood pantothenate concentrations were found to be significantly lower at 3 months postpartum (112). Given a loss of 1.7 mg/day (7.8 µmol/day) through milk supply and lower maternal blood concentrations corresponding to intakes of about 5–6 mg/day, the recommended intake for a lactating woman may be increased to 7 mg/day.

9.6.5 Recommended nutrient intakes for pantothenic acid

The recommendations for pantothenate are given in Table 9.6.

TABLE 9.6
Recommended nutrient intakes for pantothenate, by group

Group	Recommended nutrient intake (mg/day)
Infants and children	
0–6 months	1.7
7–12 months	1.8
1–3 years	2.0
4–6 years	3.0
7–9 years	4.0
Adolescents	
10–18 years	5.0
Adults	
Females, 19+ years	5.0
Males, 19+ years	5.0
Pregnant women	6.0
Lactating women	7.0

9.7 Biotin

9.7.1 Background

Deficiency

Biotin deficiency in humans has been clearly documented with prolonged consumption of raw egg whites, which contain biotin-binding avidin. Biotin deficiency has also been observed in cases of parenteral nutrition with solutions lacking biotin given to patients with short-gut syndrome and other causes of malabsorption (9, 113, 114). Some cases of biotin deficiency have been noted in infants with intractable nappy dermatitis and in those fed special formulas. Dietary deficiency in otherwise normal people is probably rare. Some patients have multiple carboxylase deficiencies and there are occasional biotinidase deficiencies. Clinical signs of deficiency include dermatitis of an erythematous and seborrheic type; conjunctivitis; alopecia; and central nervous system abnormalities such as hypotonia, lethargy, and developmental delay in infants, and depression, hallucinations, and paresthesia of the extremities in adults.

Toxicity

Toxicity is not a problem because of the limited intestinal absorption of biotin.

Role in human metabolic processes

Biotin functions as a coenzyme within several carboxylases after its carboxyl functional group becomes amide linked to the ε-amino of specific lysyl residues of the apoenzymes (10, 11). In humans and other mammals, biotin operates within four carboxylases. Three of the four biotin-dependent carboxylases are mitochondrial (pyruvate carboxylase, methylcrotonyl-CoA carboxylase, and propionyl-CoA carboxylase) whereas the fourth (acetyl-CoA carboxylase) is found in both mitochondria and the cytosol. In all these cases, biotin serves as a carrier for the transfer of active bicarbonate into a substrate to generate a carboxyl product.

9.7.2 Biochemical indicators

Indicators used to estimate biotin requirements are urinary excretion of biotin and excretion of 3-hydroxyisovalerate. The excretion rate of the vitamin and its metabolites in urine is assessed by avidin-based radioimmunoassay with HPLC. Excretion of 3-hydroxyisovalerate inversely reflects the activity of β-methylcrotonyl-CoA carboxylase, which is involved in leucine metabolism.

Both indicators, urinary excretion of biotin as assessed with an avidin-based radioimmunoassay with HPLC, and 3-hydroxyisovalerate excretion have been used to assess status (115). The isolation and chemical identification of more than a dozen metabolites of biotin established the main features of its function in microbes and mammals (116, 117). Zempleni et al. have quantified the major biotin metabolites (118). Both biotin and bis-norbiotin excretions were found to decline in parallel in individuals on a diet containing raw egg whites (115). In these individuals the levels of urinary 3-hydroxyisovalerate, which increase as a result of decreased activity of β-methylcrotonyl-CoA carboxylase and altered leucine metabolism, rose from a normal mean of 112 to 272 μmol/24 hours. Decreased excretion of biotin, abnormally increased excretion of 3-hydroxyisovalerate, or both have been associated with overt cases of biotin deficiency (119–124). The lack of sufficient population data, however, suggests the current use of an adequate intake rather than a recommended intake as a suitable basis for recommendations.

9.7.3 Evidence used to derive recommended intakes

The biotin content of human milk is estimated to be approximately 6 μg/l (24 nmol/l) based on several studies (125–127) that report values ranging from about 4 to 7 μg/l (16.4–28.9 nmol/l). Hence, the estimated intake of biotin for an infant consuming 0.75 l of human milk per day is 5 μg/day during the first half-year and for older infants (7–12 months of age) is perhaps 6 μg/day.

Requirements for children and adults have been extrapolated as follows (6):

Adequate intake for child or adult = (adequate intake young infant)

$$\times (\text{weight adult or child/weight infant})^{0.75}$$

For pregnancy, there are at present insufficient data to justify an increase in the adequate intake, although Mock et al. (128) reported decreased urinary biotin and 3-hydroxyisovalerate in a large fraction of seemingly healthy pregnant women.

For lactating women, the intake of biotin may need to be increased by an additional 5 µg/day to cover the losses due to breastfeeding.

9.7.4 Recommended nutrient intakes for biotin

The recommendations for biotin are given in Table 9.7.

9.8 General considerations for B-complex vitamins

9.8.1 Notes on suggested recommendations

For the six B-complex vitamins considered here, recommendations for infants are based largely on the composition and quantity of human milk consumed, and are thus considered to be adequate intakes. Younger infants (0–6 months) are considered to derive adequate intake from milk alone; recommendations for older infants (7–12 months) are adjusted by metabolic scaling such that a factor—weight of 7–12 month-old infant/weight of 0–6 month-old infant)$^{0.75}$—is multiplied by the recommendation for the younger infant (6). Recommendations have been given to use the higher (7–12 months) level of B-vitamin requirements for all infants in the first year of life.

TABLE 9.7
Recommended nutrient intakes for biotin, by group

Group	Recommended nutrient intake (µg/day)
Infants and children	
0–6 months	5
7–12 months	6
1–3 years	8
4–6 years	12
7–9 years	20
Adolescents	
10–18 years	25
Adults	
Females, 19+ years	30
Males, 19+ years	30
Pregnant women	30
Lactating women	35

For most of the B vitamins, there is little or no direct information that can be used to estimate the amounts required by children and adolescents. Hence, an extrapolation from the adult level is used where a factor—(weight of child/weight of adult)$^{0.75}$ × (1 + growth factor)—is multiplied by the adult recommendation (6).

For all but one of the B-complex vitamins covered here, data are not sufficient to justify altering recommendations for the elderly. Only vitamin B₆ has altered recommendations for the elderly. However, for pregnancy and lactation, increased maternal needs related to increases in energy and replacement of secretion losses are considered.

9.8.2 Dietary sources of B-complex vitamins

A listing of some food sources that provide good and moderate amounts of the vitamins considered in this chapter is given in Table 9.8.

9.9 Recommendations for future research

In view of the issues raised in this chapter on B-complex vitamins, the following recommendations are given:

- Actual requirements of B-complex vitamins are least certain for children, adolescents, pregnant and lactating women, and the elderly, and as such, deserve further study.
- Studies need to include graded levels of the vitamin above and below current recommendations and should consider or establish clearly defined cut-off values for clinical adequacy and inadequacy and be conducted for periods of time sufficient for ascertaining equilibrium dynamics.

TABLE 9.8
Dietary sources of water-soluble B vitamins[a]

Vitamin	Good-to-moderate dietary sources
Thiamine (B₁)	Pork, organ meats, whole grains, and legumes
Riboflavin (B₂)	Milk and dairy products, meats, and green vegetables
Niacin (nicotinic acid and nicotinamide)	Liver, lean meats, grains, and legumes (can be formed from tryptophan)
Vitamin B₆ (pyridoxine, pyridoxamine, and pyridoxal)	Meats, vegetables, and whole-grain cereals
Pantothenic acid	Animal tissues, whole-grain cereals, and legumes (widely distributed)
Biotin	Liver, yeast, egg, yolk, soy flour, and cereals

[a] Not including vitamin B₁₂.

- For status indicators, additional functional tests would be useful for riboflavin (e.g. the activity of FMN-dependent pyridoxine [pyridoxamine] 5′-phosphate oxidase in erythrocytes), niacin (e.g. sensitive blood measures, especially of NAD), and perhaps pantothenate.
- The food content and bioavailability of pantothenate and biotin need further investigation to establish the available and preferred food sources reasonable for different populations.

Primary efforts should now be in the arena of public health and nutrition education with emphasis on directing people and their governments to available and healthful foods; the care necessary for their storage and preparation; and achievable means for adjusting intake with respect to age, sex, and health status.

References

1. *Report on the nutrition situation of refugees and displaced populations.* Geneva, United Nations Administrative Committee on Coordination, Subcommittee on Nutrition, 1998 (Refugee Nutrition Information System, 25).
2. Sadun A et al. Epidemic optic neuropathy in Cuba: eye findings. *Archives of Ophthalmology*, 1994, 112:691–699.
3. Ordunez-Garcia O et al. Cuban epidemic neuropathy, 1991–1994: history repeats itself a century after the "amblyopia of the blockade". *American Journal of Public Health*, 1996, 86:738–743.
4. Hedges R et al. Epidemic optic and peripheral neuropathy in Cuba: a unique geopolitical public health problem. *Survey of Ophthalmology*, 1997, 41:341–353.
5. Passmore R, Nicol BM, Narayana Rao M. *Handbook on human nutritional requirements.* Geneva, World Health Organization, 1974 (WHO Monograph Series, No. 61).
6. Food and Nutrition Board. *Dietary reference intakes for thiamin, riboflavin, niacin, vitamin B$_6$, folate, vitamin B$_{12}$, pantothenic acid, biotin, and choline.* Washington, DC, National Academy Press, 1998.
7. McCormick DB. Thiamin. In: Shils ME, Young VR, eds. *Modern nutrition in health and disease*, 6th ed. Philadelphia, PA, Lea & Febiger, 1988:355–361.
8. McCormick DB. Vitamin, Structure and function of. In: Meyers RA, ed. *Encyclopedia of molecular biology and molecular medicine, Vol. 6.* Weinheim, VCH (Verlag Chemie), 1997:244–252.
9. McCormick DB, Greene HL. Vitamins. In: Burtis VA, Ashwood ER, eds. *Tietz textbook of clinical chemistry*, 2nd ed. Philadelphia, PA, WB Saunders, 1994:1275–1316.
10. McCormick DB. Coenzymes, Biochemistry of. In: Meyers RA, ed. *Encyclopedia of molecular biology and molecular medicine, Vol. 1.* Weinheim, VCH (Verlag Chemie), 1996:396–406.
11. McCormick DB. Coenzymes, Biochemistry. In: Dulbecco R, ed. *Encyclopedia of human biology*, 2nd ed. San Diego, CA, Academic Press, 1997:847–864.
12. Bayliss RM et al. Urinary thiamine excretion after oral physiological doses of

the vitamin. *International Journal of Vitamin and Nutrition Research*, 1984, 54:161–164.

13. Gans DA, Harper AE. Thiamin status of incarcerated and nonincarcerated adolescent males: dietary intake and thiamin pyrophosphate response. *American Journal of Clinical Nutrition*, 1991, 53:1471–1475.

14. Schrijver J. Biochemical markers for micronutrient status and their interpretation. In: Pietrzik K, ed. *Modern lifestyles, lower energy intake and micronutrient status*. Heidelberg, Springer-Verlag, 1991:55–85.

15. Bailey AL et al. Thiamin intake, erythrocyte transketolase (EC 2.2.1.1) activity and total erythrocyte thiamin in adolescents. *British Journal of Nutrition*, 1994, 72:111–125.

16. Singleton CK et al. The thiamin-dependent hysteretic behavior of human transketolase: implications for thiamine deficiency. *Journal of Nutrition*, 1995, 125:189–194.

17. Baines M, Davies G. The evaluation of erythrocyte thiamin diphosphate as an indicator of thiamin status in man, and its comparison with erythrocyte transketolase activity measurements. *Annals of Clinical Biochemistry*, 1988, 25:698–705.

18. Gerrits J et al. Determination of thiamin and thiamin phosphates in whole blood by reversed-phase liquid chromatography with precolumn derivatization. In: McCormick DB, Suttie JW, Wagner C, eds. *Methods in enzymology. Vitamins and coenzymes*. San Diego, CA, Academic Press, 1997, 279:74–82.

19. Fogelholm M et al. Dietary intake and thiamin, iron, and zinc status in elite Nordic skiers during different training periods. *International Journal of Sport Nutrition*, 1992, 2:351–365.

20. van der Beek EJ et al. Thiamin, riboflavin and vitamin B6: impact of restricted intake on physical performance in man. *Journal of American College of Nutrition*, 1994, 13:629–640.

21. Committee on Nutrition. Composition of human milk: normative data. In: Forbes GB, Woodruff CW, eds. *Pediatric nutrition handbook*, 2nd ed. Elk Grove Village, IL, American Academy of Pediatrics, 1985:363–368.

22. Wyatt DT, Nelson D, Hillman RE. Age-dependent changes in thiamin concentrations in whole blood and cerebrospinal fluid in infants and children. *American Journal of Clinical Nutrition*, 1991, 53:530–536.

23. Sauberlich HE et al. Thiamin requirement of the adult human. *American Journal of Clinical Nutrition*, 1979, 32:2237–2248.

24. Wood B et al. A study of partial thiamin restriction in human volunteers. *American Journal of Clinical Nutrition*, 1980, 33:848–861.

25. Anderson SH, Charles TJ, Nicol AD. Thiamine deficiency at a district general hospital: report of five cases. *Quarterly Journal of Medicine*, 1985, 55:15–32.

26. Hoorn RK, Flikweert JP, Westerink D. Vitamin B-1, B-2 and B-6 deficiencies in geriatric patients, measured by coenzyme stimulation of enzyme activities. *Clinica Chemica Acta*, 1975, 61:151–162.

27. Nichols HK, Basu TK. Thiamin status of the elderly: dietary intake and thiamin pyrophosphate response. *Journal of American College of Nutrition*, 1994, 13:57–61.

28. Food and Nutrition Board. *Nutrition during pregnancy. Part I. Weight gain. Part II. Nutrient supplements*. Washington, DC, National Academy Press, 1990.

29. McCormick DB. Riboflavin. In: Shils ME, Olson JA, Shike M, eds. *Modern nutrition in health and disease*, 8th ed. Philadelphia, PA, Lea & Febiger, 1994:366–375.

30. Smith MD. Rapid method for determination of riboflavin in urine by high-performance liquid chromatography. *Journal of Chromatography*, 1980, 182:285–291.

31. Chastain JL, McCormick DB. Flavin catabolites: identification and quantitation in human urine. *American Journal of Clinical Nutrition*, 1987, 46:830–834.

32. Roughead ZK, McCormick DB. Urinary riboflavin and its metabolites: effects of riboflavin supplementation in healthy residents of rural Georgia (USA). *European Journal of Clinical Nutrition*, 1991, 45:299–307.

33. Aw T-Y, Jones DP, McCormick DB. Uptake of riboflavin by isolated rat liver cells. *Journal of Nutrition*, 1983, 113:1249–1254.

34. Nichoalds GE. Riboflavin. Symposium in laboratory medicine. In: Labbae RF, ed. *Symposium on Laboratory Assessment of Nutritional Status. Clinics in Laboratory Medicine Series, Vol. 1*. Philadelphia, PA, WB Saunders, 1981, 1:685–698.

35. Sadowski JA. Riboflavin. In: Hartz SC, Russell RM, Rosenberg IH, eds. *Nutrition in the elderly. The Boston Nutritional Status Survey*. London, Smith-Gordon, 1992:119–125.

36. Ramsay VP et al. Vitamin cofactor saturation indices for riboflavin, thiamine, and pyridoxine in placental tissue of Kenyan women. *American Journal of Clinical Nutrition*, 1983, 37:969–973.

37. Belko AZ et al. Effects of exercise on riboflavin requirements of young women. *American Journal of Clinical Nutrition*, 1983, 37:509–517.

38. Belko AZ et al. Effects of aerobic exercise and weight loss on riboflavin requirements of moderately obese, marginally deficient young women. *American Journal of Clinical Nutrition*, 1984, 40:553–561.

39. Belko AZ et al. Effects of exercise on riboflavin requirements: biological validation in weight reducing women. *American Journal of Clinical Nutrition*, 1985, 41:270–277.

40. Soares MJ et al. The effect of exercise on the riboflavin status of adult men. *British Journal of Nutrition*, 1993, 69:541–551.

41. Winters LR et al. Riboflavin requirements and exercise adaptation in older women. *American Journal of Clinical Nutrition*, 1992, 56:526–532.

42. Powers HJ et al. Bicycling performance in Gambian children: effects of supplements of riboflavin or ascorbic acid. *Human Nutrition and Clinical Nutrition*, 1987, 41:59–69.

43. Prasad AP et al. Functional impact of riboflavin supplementation in urban school children. *Nutrition Research*, 1990, 10:275–281.

44. Tremblay A et al. The effects of a riboflavin supplementation on the nutritional status and performance of elite swimmers. *Nutrition Research*, 1984, 4:201–208.

45. Weight LM, Myburgh KH, Noakes TD. Vitamin and mineral supplementation: effect on the running performance of trained athletes. *American Journal of Clinical Nutrition*, 1988, 47:192–195.

46. Zempleni J, Galloway JR, McCormick DB. Pharmacokinetics of orally and intravenously administered riboflavin in healthy humans. *American Journal of Clinical Nutrition*, 1996, 63:54–66.

47. Chia CP, Addison R, McCormick DB. Absorption, metabolism, and excre-

tion of 8a-(amino acid)-riboflavins in the rat. *Journal of Nutrition*, 1978, 108:373–381.

48. Boisvert WA et al. Riboflavin requirement of healthy elderly humans and its relationship to macronutrient composition of the diet. *Journal of Nutrition*, 1993, 123:915–925.

49. McCormick DB. Two interconnected B vitamins: riboflavin and pyridoxine. *Physiological Reviews*, 1989, 69:1170–1198.

50. Roe DA et al. Factors affecting riboflavin requirements of oral contraceptive users and nonusers. *American Journal of Clinical Nutrition*, 1982, 35:495–501.

51. Thomas MR et al. The effects of vitamin C, vitamin B6, vitamin B12, folic acid, riboflavin, and thiamin on the breast milk and maternal status of well-nourished women at 6 months postpartum. *American Journal of Clinical Nutrition*, 1980, 33:2151–2156.

52. Roughead ZK, McCormick DB. Flavin composition of human milk. *American Journal of Clinical Nutrition*, 1990, 52:854–857.

53. Roughead ZK, McCormick DB. A qualitative and quantitative assessment of flavins in cow's milk. *Journal of Nutrition*, 1990, 120:382–388.

54. Bamji MS et al. Enzymatic evaluation of riboflavin status of infants. *European Journal of Clinical Nutrition*, 1991, 45:309–313.

55. Bates CJ et al. Riboflavin status of adolescent vs. elderly Gambian subjects before and during supplementation. *American Journal of Clinical Nutrition*, 1989, 50:825–829.

56. Kuizon MD et al. Riboflavin requirement of Filipino women. *European Journal of Clinical Nutrition*, 1992, 46:257–264.

57. Alexander M et al. Relation of riboflavin nutriture in healthy elderly to intake of calcium and vitamin supplements: evidence against riboflavin supplementation. *American Journal of Clinical Nutrition*, 1984, 39:540–546.

58. Bates CJ et al. Riboflavin status in Gambian pregnant and lactating women and its implications for recommended dietary allowances. *American Journal of Clinical Nutrition*, 1981, 34:928–935.

59. Vir SC, Love AH, Thompson W. Riboflavin status during pregnancy. *American Journal of Clinical Nutrition*, 1981, 34:2699–2705.

60. Badart-Smook A et al. Fetal growth is associated positively with maternal intake of riboflavin and negatively with maternal intake of linoleic acid. *Journal of the American Dietetic Association*, 1997, 97:867–870.

61. McCormick DB. Niacin. In: Shils ME, Young VR, eds. *Modern nutrition in health and disease*, 6th ed. Philadelphia, PA, Lea & Febiger, 1988:370–375.

62. Carpenter KJ, Lewin WJ. A re-examination of the composition of diets associated with pellagra. *Journal of Nutrition*, 1985, 115:543–552.

63. Berger NA. Poly (ADP-ribose) in the cellular response to DNA damage. *Radiation Research*, 1985, 101:4–15.

64. Shibata K, Matsuo H. Effect of supplementing low protein diets with the limiting amino acids on the excretion of N'-methylnicotinamide and its pyridones in rat. *Journal of Nutrition*, 1989, 119:896–901.

65. Jacob RA et al. Biochemical markers for assessment of niacin status in young men: urinary and blood levels of niacin metabolites. *Journal of Nutrition*, 1989, 119:591–598.

66. Dillon JC et al. The urinary metabolites of niacin during the course of pellagra. *Annals of Nutrition and Metabolism*, 1992, 36:181–185.

67. Fu CS et al. Biochemical markers for assessment of niacin status in young

men: levels of erythrocyte niacin coenzymes and plasma tryptophan. *Journal of Nutrition*, 1989, 119:1949–1955.

68. Ribaya-Mercado JD et al. Effect of niacin status on gastrointestinal function and serum lipids [abstract]. *FASEB Journal*, 1997, 11:179.

69. Rose DP, Braidman IP. Excretion of tryptophan metabolites as affected by pregnancy, contraceptive steroids, and steroid hormones. *American Journal of Clinical Nutrition*, 1971, 24:673–683.

70. Patterson JI et al. Excretion of tryptophan-niacin metabolites by young men: effects of tryptophan, leucine, and vitamin B6 intakes. *American Journal of Clinical Nutrition*, 1980, 33:2157–2167.

71. Horwitt MK, Harper AE, Henderson LM. Niacin-tryptophan relationships for evaluating niacin equivalents. *American Journal of Clinical Nutrition*, 1981, 34:423–427.

72. McCormick DB. Vitamin B_6. In: Shils ME, Young VR, eds. *Modern nutrition in health and disease*, 6th ed. Philadelphia, PA, Lea & Febiger, 1988:376–382.

73. Liu A et al. Relationship between body store of vitamin B6 and plasma pyridoxal-P clearance: metabolic balance studies in humans. *Journal of Laboratory and Clinical Medicine*, 1985, 106:491–497.

74. Kretsch MJ, Sauberlich HE, Newbrun E. Electroencephalographic changes and periodontal status during short-term vitamin B-6 depletion of young, nonpregnant women. *American Journal of Clinical Nutrition*, 1991, 53:1266–1274.

75. Bailey AL, Wright AJA, Southon S. Pyridoxal-5-phosphate determination in human plasma by high performance liquid chromatography: how appropriate are cut-off values for vitamin B6 deficiency? *European Journal of Clinical Nutrition*, 1999, 53:448–455.

76. Hamfelt A, Tuvemo T. Pyridoxal phosphate and folic acid concentration in blood and erythrocyte aspartate aminotransferase activity during pregnancy. *Clinica Chemica Acta*, 1972, 41:287–298.

77. Leklem JE. Vitamin B-6: a status report. *Journal of Nutrition*, 1990, 120(Suppl. 11):S1503–S1507.

78. Gregory JF III. Bioavailability of vitamin B-6. *European Journal of Clinical Nutrition*, 1997, 51(Suppl. 1):S43–S48.

79. Tarr JB, Tamura T, Stokstad EL. Availability of vitamin B_6 and pantothenate in an average American diet in man. *American Journal of Clinical Nutrition*, 1981, 34:1328–1337.

80. Wozenski JR, Leklem JE, Miller LT. The metabolism of small doses of vitamin B-6 in men. *Journal of Nutrition*, 1980, 110:275–285.

81. Pannemans DLE, van den Berg H, Westerterp KR. The influence of protein intake on vitamin B-6 metabolism differs in young and elderly humans. *Journal of Nutrition*, 1994, 124:1207–1214.

82. Shane B, Contractor SF. Assessment of vitamin B_6 status. Studies on pregnant women and oral contraceptive users. *American Journal of Clinical Nutrition*, 1975, 28:739–747.

83. Rose DP. Oral contraceptives and vitamin B6. In: *Human vitamin B_6 requirements. Proceedings of a workshop: Letterman Army Institute of Research, Presidio of San Francisco, California, June 11–12 1976*. Washington, DC, National Academy Press, 1978:193–201.

84. Brophy MH, Siiteri PK. Pyridoxal phosphate and hypertensive disorders of pregnancy. *American Journal of Obstetrics and Gynecology*, 1975, 121:1075–1079.

85. Shane B, Contractor SF. Vitamin B$_6$ status and metabolism in pregnancy. In: Tryfiates GP, ed. *Vitamin B6 metabolism and role in growth*. Westport, CT, Food & Nutrition Press, 1980:137–171.

86. West KD, Kirksey A. Influence of vitamin B6 intake on the content of the vitamin in human milk. *American Journal of Clinical Nutrition*, 1976, 29:961–969.

87. Andon MB et al. Dietary intake of total and glycosylated vitamin B-6 and the vitamin B-6 nutritional status of unsupplemented lactating women and their infants. *American Journal of Clinical Nutrition*, 1989, 50:1050–1058.

88. Heiskanen K et al. Vitamin B-6 status during childhood: tracking from 2 months to 11 years of age. *Journal of Nutrition*, 1995, 125:2985–2992.

89. Linkswiler HM. Vitamin B6 requirements of men. In: *Human vitamin B$_6$ requirements. Proceedings of a workshop: Letterman Army Institute of Research, Presidio of San Francisco, California, June 11–12 1976*. Washington, DC, National Academy Press, 1978:279–290.

90. Miller LT, Leklem JE, Shultz TD. The effect of dietary protein on the metabolism of vitamin B-6 in humans. *Journal of Nutrition*, 1985, 115:1663–1672.

91. Brown RR et al. Urinary 4-pyridoxic acid, plasma pyridoxal phosphate, and erythrocyte aminotransferase levels in oral contraceptive users receiving controlled intakes of vitamin B6. *American Journal of Clinical Nutrition*, 1975, 28:10–19.

92. Kretsch MJ et al. Vitamin B-6 requirement and status assessment: young women fed a depletion diet followed by a plant- or animal-protein diet with graded amounts of vitamin B-6. *American Journal of Clinical Nutrition*, 1995, 61:1091–1101.

93. Hansen CM, Leklem JE, Miller LT. Vitamin B-6 status of women with a constant intake of vitamin B-6 changes with three levels of dietary protein. *Journal of Nutrition*, 1996, 126:1891–1901.

94. Hansen CM, Leklem JE, Miller LT. Changes in vitamin B-6 status indicators of women fed a constant protein diet with varying levels of vitamin B-6. *American Journal of Clinical Nutrition*, 1997, 66:1379–1387.

95. Ribaya-Mercado JD et al. Vitamin B-6 requirements of elderly men and women. *Journal of Nutrition*, 1991, 121:1062–1074.

96. Selhub J et al. Vitamin status and intake as primary determinants of homocysteinemia in an elderly population. *Journal of the American Medical Association*, 1993, 270:2693–2698.

97. Cleary RE, Lumeng L, Li T-K. Maternal and fetal plasma levels of pyridoxal phosphate at term: adequacy of vitamin B6 supplementation during pregnancy. *American Journal of Obstetrics and Gynecology*, 1975, 121:25–28.

98. Lumeng L et al. Adequacy of vitamin B6 supplementation during pregnancy: a prospective study. *American Journal of Clinical Nutrition*, 1976, 29:1376–1383.

99. Borschel MW. Vitamin B6 in infancy: requirements and current feeding practices. In: Raiten DJ, ed. *Vitamin B-6 metabolism in pregnancy, lactation and infancy*. Boca Raton, FL, CRC Press, 1995:109–124.

100. McCormick DB. Pantothenic acid. In: Shils ME, Young VR, eds. *Modern nutrition in health and disease*, 6th ed. Philadelphia, PA, Lea & Febiger, 1988:383–387.

101. Plesofsky-Vig N. Pantothenic acid and coenzyme A. In: Shils ME, Olson JA, Shike M, eds. *Modern nutrition in health and disease*, 8th ed. Philadelphia, PA, Lea & Febiger, 1994:395–401.

102. Fry PC, Fox HM, Tao HG. Metabolic response to a pantothenic acid deficient diet in humans. *Journal of Nutritional Science and Vitaminology*, 1976, 22:339–346.

103. Eissenstat BR, Wyse BW, Hansen RG. Pantothenic acid status of adolescents. *American Journal of Clinical Nutrition*, 1986, 44:931–937.

104. Wittwer CT et al. Enzymes for liberation of pantothenic acid in blood: use of plasma pantetheinase. *American Journal of Clinical Nutrition*, 1989, 50:1072–1078.

105. Picciano MF. Vitamins in milk. A. Water-soluble vitamins in human milk. In: Jensen RG, ed. *Handbook of milk composition*. San Diego, CA, Academic Press, 1995.

106. Butte NF et al. Human milk intake and growth in exclusively breast-fed infants. *Journal of Pediatrics*, 1984, 104:187–195.

107. Allen JC et al. Studies in human lactation: milk composition and daily secretion rates of macronutrients in the first year of lactation. *American Journal of Clinical Nutrition*, 1991, 54:69–80.

108. Heinig MJ et al. Energy and protein intakes of breast-fed and formula-fed infants during the first year of life and their association with growth velocity: the DARLING Study. *American Journal of Clinical Nutrition*, 1993, 58:152–161.

109. Kathman JV, Kies C. Pantothenic acid status of free living adolescent and young adults. *Nutrition Research*, 1984, 4:245–250.

110. Srinivasan V et al. Pantothenic acid nutritional status in the elderly—institutionalized and noninstitutionalized. *American Journal of Clinical Nutrition*, 1981, 34:1736–1742.

111. Bul NL, Buss DH. Biotin, pantothenic acid and vitamin E in the British household food supply. *Human Nutrition: Applied Nutrition*, 1982, 36A:125–129.

112. Song WO, Wyse BW, Hansen RG. Pantothenic acid status of pregnant and lactating women. *Journal of the American Dietetic Association*, 1985, 85:192–198.

113. McCormick DB. Biotin. In: Shils ME, Young VR, eds. *Modern nutrition in health and disease*, 6th ed. Philadelphia, PA, Lea & Febiger, 1988:436–439.

114. Mock DM. Biotin. In: Ziegler EE, Filer LJ Jr, eds. *Present knowledge in nutrition*, 7th ed. Washington, DC, International Life Sciences Institute, The Nutrition Foundation, 1996:220–235.

115. Mock NI et al. Increased urinary excretion of 3-hydroxyisovaleric acid and decreased urinary excretion of biotin are sensitive early indicators of decreased status in experimental biotin deficiency. *American Journal of Clinical Nutrition*, 1997, 65:951–958.

116. McCormick DB, Wright LD. The metabolism of biotin and analogues. In: Florkin M, Stotz EH, eds. *Comprehensive biochemistry, Vol. 21*. Amsterdam, Elsevier, 1971:81–110.

117. McCormick DB. Biotin. In: Hegsted M, ed. *Present knowledge in nutrition*, 4th ed. Washington, DC, The Nutrition Foundation, 1976:217–225.

118. Zempleni J, McCormick DB, Mock DM. Identification of biotin sulfone, bisnorbiotin methylketone, and tetranorbiotin-l-sulfoxide in human urine. *American Journal of Clinical Nutrition*, 1997, 65:508–511.

119. Mock DM et al. Biotin deficiency: an unusual complication of parenteral alimentation. *New England Journal of Medicine*, 1981, 304:820–823.

120. Kien CL et al. Biotin-responsive in vivo carboxylase deficiency in two siblings with secretory diarrhea receiving total parenteral nutrition. *Journal of Pediatrics*, 1981, 99:546–550.

121. Gillis J et al. Biotin deficiency in a child on long-term TPN. *Journal of Parenteral and Enteral Nutrition*, 1982, 6:308–310.

122. Mock DM et al. Biotin deficiency complicating parenteral alimentation: diagnosis, metabolic repercussions, and treatment. *Journal of Pediatrics*, 1985, 106:762–769.

123. Lagier P et al. Zinc and biotin deficiency during prolonged parenteral nutrition in infants. *Presse Médicale*, 1987, 16:1795–1797.

124. Carlson GL et al. Biotin deficiency complicating long-term parenteral nutrition in an adult patient. *Clinical Nutrition*, 1995, 14:186–190.

125. Holland B et al. *McCance & Widdowson's the composition of foods*. 5th revised and extended edition. London, Her Majesty's Stationery Office, 1991.

126. Salmenpera L et al. Biotin concentrations in maternal plasma and milk during prolonged lactation. *International Journal of Vitamin and Nutrition Research*, 1985, 55:281–285.

127. Hirano M et al. Longitudinal variations of biotin content in human milk. *International Journal for Vitamin and Nutrition Research*, 1992, 62:281–282.

128. Mock DM et al. Biotin status assessed longitudinally in pregnant women. *Journal of Nutrition*, 1997, 127:710–716.

10. Selenium

10.1 Role of selenium in human metabolic processes

Our understanding of the significance of selenium in the nutrition of human subjects has grown rapidly during the past 20 years (1, 2). Demonstrations of its essentiality to rats and farm animals were followed by appreciation that the development of selenium-responsive diseases often reflected the distribution of geochemical variables which restricted the entry of the element from soils into food chains. Such findings were the stimulus to in-depth investigations of the regional relevance of selenium in human nutrition (3). These studies have now yielded an increased understanding of the complex metabolic role of this trace nutrient. Selenium has been implicated in the protection of body tissues against oxidative stress, maintenance of defences against infection, and modulation of growth and development.

The selenium content of normal adult humans can vary widely. Values from 3 mg in New Zealanders to 14 mg in some Americans reflect the profound influence of the natural environment on the selenium contents of soils, crops, and human tissues. Approximately 30% of tissue selenium is contained in the liver, 15% in kidney, 30% in muscle, and 10% in blood plasma. Much of tissue selenium is found in proteins as selenoanalogues of sulfur amino acids; other metabolically active forms include selenotrisulphides and other acid-labile selenium compounds. At least 15 selenoproteins have now been characterized. Examples are given in Table 10.1.

Functionally, there appear to be at least two distinct families of selenium-containing enzymes. The first includes the glutathione peroxidases (4) and thioredoxin reductase (5), which are involved in controlling tissue concentrations of highly reactive oxygen-containing metabolites. These metabolites are essential at low concentrations for maintaining cell-mediated immunity against infections but highly toxic if produced in excess. The role of selenium in the cytosolic enzyme, glutathione peroxidase (GSHPx), was first illustrated in 1973. During stress, infection, or tissue injury, selenoenzymes may protect against the damaging effects of hydrogen peroxide or oxygen-rich free radicals. This family of enzymes catalyses the destruction of

TABLE 10.1
A selection of characterized selenoproteins

Protein	Selenocysteine residues	Tissue distribution
Cytosolic GSHPx	1	All, including thyroid
Phospholipid hydroperoxide GSHPx	1	All, including thyroid
Gastrointestinal GSHPx	1	Gastrointestinal tract
Extracellular GSHPx	1	Plasma, thyroid
Thioredoxin reductase	1 or 2	All, including thyroid
Iodothyronine-deiodinase (type 1)	1	Liver, kidneys, and thyroid
Iodothyronine-deiodinase (type 2)	1	Central nervous system, and pituitary
Iodothyronine-deiodinase (type 3)	1	Brown adipose tissue, central nervous system, and placenta
Selenoprotein P	10	Plasma
Selenoprotein W	1	Muscle
Sperm capsule selenoprotein	3	Sperm tail

GSHPx, glutathione peroxidase.

hydrogen peroxide or lipid hydroperoxides according to the following general reactions:

$$H_2O_2 + 2GSH \rightarrow 2H_2O + GSSG$$
$$ROOH + 2GSH \rightarrow ROH + H_2O + GSSG$$

where GSH is glutathione and GSSG is its oxidized form. At least four forms of GSHPx exist; they differ both in their tissue distribution and in their sensitivity to selenium depletion (*4*). The GSHPx enzymes of liver and blood plasma fall in activity rapidly at early stages of selenium deficiency. In contrast, a form of GSHPx associated specifically with phospholipid-rich tissue membranes is preserved against selenium deficiency and is believed to have broader metabolic roles (e.g. in prostaglandin synthesis) (*6*). In concert with vitamin E, selenium is also involved in the protection of cell membranes against oxidative damage. (See also Chapter 8 on antioxidants.)

The selenoenzyme thioredoxin reductase is involved in disposal of the products of oxidative metabolism (*5*). It contains two selenocysteine groups per molecule and is a major component of a redox system with a multiplicity of functions, among which is the capacity to degrade locally excessive and potentially toxic concentrations of peroxide and hydroperoxides likely to induce cell death and tissue atrophy (*6*).

Another group of selenoproteins are the iodothyronine deiodinases essential for the conversion of thyrocin or tetraiodothyronine (T_4) to its physiologically active form tri-iodothyronine (T_3) (*7*). Three members of this family of iodothyronines differing in tissue distribution and sensitivity to selenium deficiency have been characterized (see Table 10.1). The consequences of a low selenium status on physiologic responses to a shortage of iodine are complex. The influence of a loss of selenium-dependent iodothyronine deiodinase differs in its severity depending on whether a target tissue needs a preformed supply of T_3 (e.g. via plasma) or whether, as with the brain, pituitary gland, and placenta, it can rely upon local synthesis of T_3 from T_4. Despite this, marked changes in the T_3–T_4 ratio as a consequence of a reduced selenium status (when iodine supplies are also marginal) indicate the modifying influence of selenium on thyroid hormone balance in both animal models and human subjects. The possible significance of this can be anticipated from the fact that whereas thyroid weights increase typically by 50% in rats offered an iodine-deficient diet, thyroid weight is increased 154% by diets concurrently deficient in both selenium and iodine (see also section 10.2.5).

Between 60% and 80% of selenium in human plasma is accounted for by a well-characterized fraction designated selenoprotein P, the function of which has yet to be determined. It is thought to be a selenium storage protein because there is limited evidence that it also has an antioxidant role. At least 10 other selenoproteins exist, including one which is a component of the mitochondrial capsule of sperm cells, damage to which may account for the development of sperm abnormalities during selenium deficiency. Other aspects of the function and metabolism of selenium are reviewed elsewhere (8, 9).

10.2 Selenium deficiency

10.2.1 Non-endemic deficiencies of selenium

Biochemical evidence of selenium depletion (e.g. a decline in blood GSHPx activity) is not uncommon in subjects maintained on parenteral or enteral feeding for long periods (10, 11). Low selenium contents of some infant formulae have been reported to reduce infant serum selenium and GSHPx values to levels down to one fifth of normal in 5–8-month-old infants (12, 13). The low selenium content of many older infant formulae would have not only been insufficient to meet infant requirements (12) but when used to supplement breast milk would have diluted the total selenium intake from maternal plus fortified milk. For this reason it has been recommended that formula milks should provide at least 10 µg selenium/day to complement the maternal supply of selenium (13, 14).

Clinical manifestations of deficiency arising from such situations are uncommon and poorly defined. They include muscular weakness and myalgia with, in several instances, the development of congestive heart failure. In at least one instance such pathologic signs have developed as a consequence of a generally inadequate diet providing selenium at less than 10 µg/day. The

2-year-old subject in question recovered rapidly after selenium administration (*15*). With this last exception, virtually all of the above reports describe observations in subjects under close medical supervision. This may well be relevant to the scarcity of consistent pathological findings (*16*).

10.2.2 Keshan disease

Keshan disease was first described in the Chinese medical literature more than 100 years ago, but not until 40 years after its widespread occurrence in 1935 was it discovered that selenium deficiency was an important factor in its etiology (*3*). Endemic in children aged 2–10 years and in women of childbearing age, this disease has a geographic distribution covering localities from north-east to south-west China. Typical manifestations are fatigue after even mild exercise, cardiac arrhythmia and palpitations, loss of appetite, cardiac insufficiency, cardiomegaly, and congestive heart failure. Pathological changes include a multifocal myocardial necrosis and fibrosis. The coronary arteries are essentially unaffected. Ultrastructural studies show that membranous organelles, such as mitochondria or sarcolemma, are affected earliest. The disease has a marked seasonal fluctuation in incidence (*3*) and may appear after only 3 months exposure to conditions in localities known to be associated with a high risk of myocarditis (*3*, *8*). Once the disease is established, selenium is of little or no therapeutic value. However, prophylaxis consisting of oral administration of selenium 3 months before the periods of highest anticipated risk is highly effective.

Although geographic similarities in the distribution of Keshan disease and the selenium- and vitamin E-responsive white muscle disease in animals first prompted successful investigation of the relevance of a low selenium status, evidence has grown steadily that the disease is multifactorial in origin. The strongest suspicions have fallen on the development of a viral myocarditis probably attributable to enhancement of the virulence of a coxsackie virus during its passage through selenium-deficient host tissues (*17*). Although other nutritional variables such as a marginal vitamin E status may also be involved, the finding of extremely low selenium contents in staple crops of affected areas and convincing demonstrations of the prophylactic effectiveness of selenium administration leave no doubt that selenium deficiency is the primary factor (*3*, *18*).

Recent studies indicate that geochemical variables have an important influence on the distribution of Keshan disease. Acid soils high in organic matter and iron oxide content appear to be responsible for fixing selenium in forms that are poorly absorbed by staple crops which, in the instance of cereal grains, typically have a selenium content of less than $0.01\,\mu g/g$ (*19*). Similar geochemical conditions are believed to be associated with reports of selenium-responsive disorders resembling Keshan disease in the Transbaikalia region of southern Siberia. In that region, dietary intakes of selenium are inadequate to maintain blood GSHPx activity; biochemical indicators of tissue peroxidative damage are elevated until selenium therapy is initiated (8).

10.2.3 Kaschin-Beck disease

A selenium-responsive bone and joint disease (osteoarthropathy) has been detected in children aged 5–13 years in China and less extensively in southeast Siberia. The disease is characterized by joint necrosis—epiphyseal degeneration of the arm and leg joints resulting in structural shortening of the fingers and long bones with consequent growth retardation and stunting (3, 20). Although not identical to Keshan disease, Kaschin-Beck disease also occurs in areas where the availability of soil selenium for crop growth is low. The selenium contents of hair and of whole blood are abnormally low and the blood content of GSHPx is reduced. Although the disease is ameliorated by selenium therapy, other factors such as the frequent presence of mycotoxins in cereal grains grown in the area may be involved. A spontaneous decrease in incidence from 1970 (44%) to 1980 (14%) to 1986 (1%) has been attributed to general improvements in the nutritional status of Chinese rural communities (20).

10.2.4 Selenium status and susceptibility to infection

As mentioned previously, expression of the cardiac lesions of Keshan disease probably involve not only the development of selenium deficiency but also infection with a coxsackie virus (strain CVB 3/0), initially non-virulent, but after passage through a selenium deficient subject, becoming virulent and myopathogenic. The enhancement of virulence of this RNA virus involves modifications to the nucleotide sequence of the phenotype which resemble the wild-type virulent strain CVB 3/20 (17). These modifications were found to be maintained and expressed during subsequent passage of the virus through experimental animals with a normal selenium status (21).

The enhancement of the virulence of a virus due to a selenium deficiency (resulting from either a nutritional challenge or an increased metabolic demand on tissue selenium deposits) does not appear to be unique to the coxsackie viruses. The early preclinical stages of development of human immunodeficiency virus (HIV) infection are accompanied by a very marked decline in plasma selenium. Subclinical malnutrition assumes increased significance during the development of acquired immune deficiency syndrome (AIDS). However, for the nutrients affected, there are strong indications that only the

and Kaschin-Beck disease in China reflects the distribution of soils from which selenium is poorly available to rice, maize, wheat, and pasture grasses (Table 10.2b). Cereal crop selenium contents of 3–7 ng/g are not uncommon (3). It has been suggested that <10 ng/g for grain selenium and <3 ng/g for water-soluble soil selenium could be used as indexes to define deficient areas (19). Fluctuations in the selenium status of many communities in northern Europe reflect the intrinsically low selenium content of glacial soils in this region and the extent to which selenium supplementation of fertilizers has been successful in increasing the selenium content of cereal grains, milk, and other animal products. Deliberate importation of cereals from areas with relatively high available selenium in soil has also occurred or been recommended in some areas of Finland, New Zealand, and the United Kingdom after steady declines in the selenium status of some communities were noted. Conversely, low-selenium grains are being selected in parts of China, India, and Venezuela to reduce the risks of selenosis.

TABLE 10.2
The selenium contents of foods and diets

a) Typical ranges of selenium concentrations (ng/g fresh weight) in food groups

Food group	India (43)	United States (33)	International compilation (8)
Cereals and cereal products	5–95	10–370	10–550
Meat, meat products, and eggs	40–120	100–810	10–360
Fish and marine	280–1080	400–1500	110–970
Fish and freshwater	—	—	180–680
Pulses	10–138	—	—
Dairy products	5–15	10–130	1–170
Fruits and vegetables	1–7	1–60	1–20

b) Typical distribution of selenium in dietary constituents (µg/day) in selected countries

Food group	China (18) Keshan-disease area	China (18) Disease-free area	India (43) Low-income vegetarian diets	India (43) Low-income conventional diets	Finland (44)	United Kingdom (45)
Total diet	7.7	16.4	27.4	52.5	30.0	31.0
Cereals and cereal products	5.4	11.6	15.7	21.1	2.8	7.0
Pulses	—	—	3.9	3.6	1.1	—
Meat and eggs	0.6	2.2	—	3.7	9.2	10.0
Fish			—	18.4	9.5	4.0
Dairy products			6.9	4.8	6.5	3.0
Fruits and vegetables	1.7	2.6	0.9	0.9	0.5	6.0
Other	—	—	—	—	1.1	3.0

Comprehensive data summarizing the selenium contents of staple foods are available elsewhere (e.g. reference *44*). Reports from the United Nations Food and Agricultural Organization (FAO) and the International Atomic Energy Agency (IAEA) provide representative data on daily total selenium intakes for more than 40 countries (*8*). The great influence of dietary and geographic variables on selenium status is evident from recent summaries of data describing national and regional differences in the selenium content of human and formula milks, of diets of adults, and of human serum (see Tables 10.3–10.5).

TABLE 10.3
Geographic differences in the selenium intakes of infants[a]

Country or area	Selenium intake (µg/day)[b]	Reference
Human milk		
Australia	9.4 ± 3.6	46
Austria	8.8–9.8	13
Belgium	8.4	47
Burundi	4.7 ± 0.8	48
Chile	14.1 ± 2.6	49
China, Keshan disease area	2.0	18
China, seleniferous area	199	18
Finland	4.0–7.6	50
Germany	19.3	51
Hungary	9.6 ± 3.7	49
India	14.1 ± 3.6	49
New Zealand, North Island	8.1–10.2	52
New Zealand, South Island	5.3	53
Philippines	22.9 ± 4.1	49
Sweden	10.6 ± 2.3	49
The Former Yugoslav Republic of Macedonia	6.0 ± 1.3	49
United States, east coast	8.8–11.4	54
United States, unspecified	12.3	55
Zaire	12.3 ± 3.6	49
Infant formula		
Austria	3.6	13
Belgium	2.0	47
Germany	6.5–6.8	51
New Zealand	3.3	56
New Zealand, selenium fortified	11.3	56
Spain	6.6	19
United Kingdom	4.9 (2.3–8.2)	47
United States, 1982	5.9 (4.2–8.1)	57
United States, 1997	11.7–18.3	58
International reference value	13.9	59

[a] Assumed age 6 months; assumed human milk or infant formula intake 750 ml per day (*60*).
[b] Mean ± standard deviation (SD) or range.

TABLE 10.4
Geographic differences in the selenium intakes of adults

Country or area	Selenium intake (μg/day)[a]	Reference(s)
Canada	98.0–224.0	61
China, Kaschin-Beck disease area	2.6–5.0	20
China, Keshan disease area	3.0–11.0	62, 63
China, disease-free area	13.3 ± 3.1	18
China, seleniferous area	1338.0	64
Finland, before selenium fertilization	26.0	65–67
Finland, after selenium fertilization	56.0	65–67
France	47.0	68
Germany	38.0–48.0	69
India, conventional diets	48.0	43
India, vegan diets, low income	27.0	43
Italy	41.0	63
New Zealand, low-selenium area	11.0 ± 3.0	64, 70
Slovakia	27.0 ± 8.0	71
Sweden, vegan diets	10.0	64
Sweden, south, conventional diets	40.0 ± 4.0	72
United Kingdom, 1974	60.0	38
United Kingdom, 1985	43.0	38
United Kingdom, 1994	32.0	38
United Kingdom, 1995	33.0	45
United States	80.0 ± 37.0	54
Males	90.0 ± 14.0	73
Females	74.0 ± 12.0	73
United States, seleniferous area	216.0	64
Venezuela	80.0–500.0	74

[a] Mean ± standard error or range.

TABLE 10.5
Representative mean serum selenium concentrations from selected studies

Country or area	Sample serum selenium concentration (μmol/l)[a]
Pathologic subjects	
Keshan disease (China)	0.15–0.25
Kaschin-Beck disease (China)	0.22 ± 0.03
Myxedematous cretins (Zaire)	0.26 ± 0.12
HIV and AIDS	0.36–0.54
Normal subjects	
Bulgaria	0.66–0.72
Hungary	0.71 ± 0.13
New Zealand	0.69
Norway	1.52–1.69
Serbia and Croatia	0.63–0.85
United States, Maryland	1.69–2.15
United States, South Dakota	2.17–2.50
Proposed reference ranges for healthy subjects	0.5–2.5; 0.67–2.04

HIV, human immunodeficiency virus; AIDS, acquired immune deficiency syndrome.
Source: 8, 18, 23, 25, 33, 75–78.
[a] Range of mean or mean ± standard error.

10.4 Absorption and bioavailability

Selenium compounds are generally very efficiently absorbed by humans, and selenium absorption does not appear to be under homeostatic control (*79*). For example, absorption of the selenite form of selenium is greater than 80% whereas that of selenium as selenomethionine or as selenate may be greater than 90% (*79, 80*). Therefore, the rate-limiting step determining the overall availability of dietary selenium is not likely to be its absorption but rather its conversion within tissues to its metabolically active forms (e.g. its incorporation into GSHPx or 5'-deiodinase) (*40*). A number of depletion–repletion experiments have been carried out on animals to estimate the bioavailability of selenium in human foods (*81*). Based on the restoration of GSHPx activity in depleted rats, the bioavailability of selenium in wheat is quite good, usually 80%, or better. The selenium in Brazil nuts and beef kidney also appears readily available (90% or more by most criteria). The selenium in tuna seems to be less available (perhaps only 20–60% of that absorbed from selenite) than selenium from certain other seafoods (e.g. shrimp, crab, and Baltic herring). The selenium in a variety of mushrooms appears to be of uniformly low availability to rats.

Data on the nutritional bioavailability of selenium to humans are sparse. A supplementation study carried out on Finnish men of relatively low selenium status showed that selenate selenium was as effective as the selenium in seleniferous wheat in increasing platelet GSHPx activity (*82*). The wheat selenium, however, increased plasma selenium levels more than did selenate selenium; and once the supplements were withdrawn, platelet GSHPx activity declined less in the group given wheat. This study showed the importance of estimating not only short-term availability but also long-term retention and the convertibility of tissue selenium stores into biologically active forms.

10.5 Criteria for assessing selenium requirements

Levander (*83*) convincingly illustrated the impracticability of assessing selenium requirements from input–output balance data because the history of selenium nutrition influences the proportion of dietary selenium absorbed, retained, or excreted. Because of the changing equilibria with selenium intake, experiments yield data which are of limited value for estimating minimal requirements. Estimates of selenium requirements for adults range from 7.4 to 80.0 µg/day, these values having been derived from Chinese and North American studies, respectively. Such discrepancies reflect differences in the usual daily selenium intakes of the experimental subjects and the extent to which they were changed experimentally. This situation, not unique to selenium, emphasizes the importance of basing requirement estimates on functional criteria derived from evidence describing the minimum levels of intake which, directly or indirectly, reflect the normality of selenium-dependent processes.

New opportunities for the development of biochemical indexes of selenium adequacy have yet to be exploited. Until this is done, the most suitable alternative is to monitor changes in the relationship between serum selenium and dietary selenium supply, taking advantage of the relatively constant proportionality in the fraction of serum selenium to functionally significant GSHPx (84).

A detailed review of 36 reports describing serum selenium values in healthy subjects indicated that they ranged from a low of 0.52 μmol/l in Serbia to a high of 2.5 μmol/l in Wyoming and South Dakota in the United States (75). It was suggested that mean values within this range derived from 7502 apparently healthy individuals should be regarded tentatively as a standard for normal reference. This survey clearly illustrated the influence of crop management on serum selenium level; in Finland and New Zealand, selenium fortification of fertilizers for cereals increased serum selenium from 0.6 to 1.5 μmol/l. The data in Table 10.5 also include representative mean serum selenium values (range, 0.15–0.54 μmol/l) in subjects with specific diseases known to be associated with disturbances in selenium nutrition or metabolism. These data are derived from studies of Keshan disease, Kaschin-Beck disease, and specific studies of cretinism, hypothyroidism, and HIV and AIDS where clinical outcome or prognosis has been related to selenium status.

The present Consultation adopted a virtually identical approach to derive its estimates of basal requirements for selenium (Se_R^{basal}) as the earlier WHO/FAO/IAEA assessment (85). As yet, there are no published reports suggesting that the basal estimates using serum selenium or GSHPx activity as criteria of adequacy are invalid. Some modification was, however, considered necessary to estimate population minimum intakes with adequate allowance for the variability (CV) associated with estimates of the average selenium intakes from the typical diets of many communities. In the WHO/FAO/IAEA report (85), a CV of 16% was assumed for conventional diets and 12.5% for the milk-based diets of infants to limit the risks of inadequacy arising from unexpectedly low selenium contents. More recent studies suggest that the variability of selenium intake from diets for which the selenium content has been predicted rather than measured may be substantially greater than previously estimated (Tables 10.3 and 10.4).

10.6 Recommended selenium intakes

10.6.1 Adults

Because balance techniques are inappropriate for determining selenium requirements, previous estimates of selenium requirements have been based on epidemiological evidence derived from areas of China endemic or non-endemic for Keshan disease (18, 85). These comprehensive biochemical and clinical studies showed that Keshan disease did not occur in regions where the mean intake of selenium by adult males or females was greater than 19.1 or 13.3 µg/day, respectively. Although these intakes were sufficient to eliminate clinical evidence of myocarditis and other signs of Keshan disease, other studies showed that they were inadequate to restore erythrocyte or plasma selenium concentrations or GSHPx activities to levels indicative of reserves.

In one study adult male subjects, initially of low selenium status, were given a carefully monitored diet providing selenium at 11 µg/day together with supplements of selenomethionine given orally which provided 0, 10, 30, 60, or 90 µg/day. Starting at overtly deficient levels, total daily selenium intakes of above 41 µg/day were found sufficient to increase plasma GSHPx substantially and to saturate plasma activity in 60-kg male subjects within 5–8 months. It was estimated that satisfactory levels of plasma selenium (>80 µmol/l) and of GSHPx activity (>0.3 mmol NADPH oxidized/min/l or approximately two thirds of plasma saturation activity) indicative of adequate selenium reserves would be attained after intakes of approximately 27 µg/day by 65-kg male subjects (85). Such criteria which satisfy the definition of average normative requirements for selenium ($Se_R^{normative}$), have been used as the basis for calculating recommended nutrient intake (RNI) values in this report after interpolating estimates of average requirements by allowing for differences in weight and basal metabolic rate of age groups up to 65 years and adding a 25% increase (2 × assumed standard deviation) to allow for individual variability in the estimates of RNI (Table 10.6).

10.6.2 Infants

The estimates of the RNI for infants (Table 10.6) are compatible with estimates of the international reference range of the selenium content of breast milk (18.5 µg/l; see Table 10.3); with data from an extensive international survey of breast milk selenium conducted by WHO and IAEA (49); and with more recent WHO data (60) on the milk consumption of exclusively human-milk-fed infants in developed and developing countries. Data from the WHO/IAEA survey (49) suggest that the human milk from all six countries included in the survey met the RNI of selenium for infants aged 0–6 months. In two of six countries, Hungary and Sweden, the selenium content

TABLE 10.6
Recommended nutrient intakes for selenium, by group

| Group | Assumed weight[a] (kg) | Average normative requirement[b] | | RNI (μg/day)[c] |
		$Se_R^{normative}$ (kg/day)	$Se_R^{normative}$ (total/day)	
Infants and children				
0–6 months	6	0.85	5.1	6
7–12 months	9	0.91	8.2	10
1–3 years	12	1.13	13.6	17
4–6 years	19	0.92	17.5	22
7–9 years	25	0.68	17.0	21
Adolescents				
Females, 10–18 years	49	0.42	20.6	26
Males, 10–18 years	51	0.50	22.5	32
Adults				
Females,				
19–65 years	55	0.37	20.4	26
65+ years	54	0.37	20.2	25
Males,				
19–65 years	65	0.42	27.3	34
65+ years	64	0.41	26.2	33
Pregnant women				
2nd trimester				28
3rd trimester				30
Lactating women				
0–6 months postpartum				35
7–12 months postpartum				42

[a] Weight interpolated from reference (86).
[b] Derived from WHO/FAO/IAEA values by interpolation (85).
[c] Recommended nutrient intake (RNI) derived from the average $Se_R^{normative}$ + 2 × assumed standard deviation (of 12.5%).

of human milk was marginal with respect to the RNI for infants aged 7–12 months.

Data from Austria (*12*), Germany (*13*, *87*), the United States (*88*), and elsewhere suggest that infant formula may contain selenium in amounts insufficient to meet the RNI or recommended dietary allowance for infants. Lombeck et al. (*13*) in an extensive study showed that cow-milk-based formula may well provide less than one third of the selenium of human milk. Estimates of selenium intake by 2-month-old infants were 7.8 μg/day from formula compared with 22.4 μg/day from human milk. Levander (*88*) has suggested that infant formulas should provide a minimum of 10 μg/day but not more than 45 μg/day. This recommendation may well have been implemented judging from recent increases in the selenium content of infant formulas (*58*).

10.6.3 Pregnant and lactating women

Data from balance experiments are not sufficiently consistent for defining the increase in selenium needed to support fetal growth and development during pregnancy. For this reason the European Union Scientific Committee for Food (89), the United Kingdom Committee on Medical Aspects of Food Policy (90), and the Netherlands Food and Nutrition Council (91) have suggested that the component of selenium needed for human pregnancy is obtained by an adaptive increase in the efficiency of absorption of dietary selenium rather than by an increased dietary demand.

Others, contesting this view, have attempted to predict the increase of dietary selenium needed for pregnancy by factorial estimation of the likely quantity of selenium incorporated into the tissues of the fetus (60, 85). Such estimates have assumed that the total products of conception amount to 4.6–6 kg lean tissue with a protein content of approximately 18.5–20%. If, as appears to be a reasonable assumption, the selenium content of this protein resembles that of a skeletal muscle, growth of these tissues could account for between 1.0 and 4.5 µg/day of selenium depending on whether the analyses reflect consumption of diets from a low-selenium (but non-pathogenic) environment such as that found in New Zealand (52, 53) or from a region with relatively high selenium intakes, such as the United States (see Table 10.3) (54, 55). Typically such estimates have assumed an 80% absorption and utilization of dietary selenium from which it would appear reasonable to estimate that allowing for a variability of estimates (CV, 12.5%), an increase of 2 µg/day would be appropriate for the second trimester and 4 µg/day would be appropriate for the third trimester of pregnancy (see Table 10.6).

As is evident from Table 10.3 the selenium content of human milk is sensitive to changes in maternal dietary selenium. The increase of maternal dietary selenium needed to meet requirements for lactation has been estimated from the estimated RNI for infants aged 0–6 months and 7–12 months. For the period 0–6 months it is estimated that the infant must receive 6 µg/day of selenium from human milk; assuming that the selenium of maternal milk is used with an efficiency of 80% and given a SD of 12.5%, the increase of maternal dietary selenium required to produce this will be:

$$6 \times \frac{100}{80} + (2 \times SD) = 9\,\mu g/day.$$

The corresponding increase needed to meet the infant RNI of 10 µg/day for infants aged 7–12 months will be 16 µg/day. Added to the non-pregnancy maternal RNI of 26 µg/day, the total RNI for lactating women during the first 6 months postpartum will be 35 µg/day and for months 7–12 will be 42 µg/day (Table 10.6).

As implied by the data in Tables 10.2–10.4, agricultural growing practices, geologic factors, and social deprivation enforcing the use of an abnormally wide range of dietary constituents may significantly modify the variability of dietary selenium intakes. If accumulated experience suggests that the CV of selenium intake may be 40% or more, and tabulated rather than analysed data are used to predict the dietary intake of selenium, the selenium allowances may have to be increased accordingly (85).

10.7 Upper limits

A comprehensive account of the clinically significant biochemical manifestations of chronic and acute intoxication from selenium arising from high concentrations in food, drinking water, and the environment was published jointly by WHO, the United Nations Environment Programme, and the International Labour Organization (ILO) (79). Common clinical features are hair loss and structural changes in the keratin of hair and nails, the development of icteroid skin, and gastrointestinal disturbances (92, 93). An increased incidence of nail dystrophy has been associated with consumption of high-selenium foods supplying more than 900 µg/day. These foods were grown in selenium-rich (seleniferous) soil from specific areas in China (94). A positive association between dental caries and urinary selenium output under similar circumstances has also been reported (95, 96).

Levander (33) stresses that the signs and symptoms of human overexposure to selenium are not well defined. Furthermore, sensitive biochemical markers of impending selenium intoxication have yet to be developed. In their absence, it is suggested that the upper tolerable nutrient intake level (UL) for selenium should be set, provisionally, at 400 µg/day for adults. It is noteworthy that a maximum tolerable dietary concentration of 2 mg/kg dry diet has been proposed for all classes of domesticated livestock and has proved satisfactory in use (97). This suggests that the proposed UL of 400 µg/day for human subjects provides a fully adequate margin of safety. The UL for children and for pregnant or lactating women has yet to be determined.

10.8 Comparison with other estimates

Compared with WHO/FAO/IAEA (85), European Union (89), United Kingdom (90), and United States (86) recommendations, the present proposals represent a significant decrease in the suggested need for selenium. Reasons for this are the following:

- Current recommendations are based on a high weight range that do not reflect realities in many developing countries. Thus, there is a need to derive recommendations which are applicable for a proportionally lower weight range than that utilized in most developed countries.
- The decision, accepted by WHO, FAO, and IAEA (*85*), that it is neither essential nor desirable to maintain selenium status at a level which fully saturates blood GSHPx activity when, based on current evidence, this is not an advantage for health.
- The decision to present estimates as RNIs which, although including an allowance for individual variability, do not provide for the possibility that foods may often differ widely in selenium content according to their geographic sources.

The lower requirements presented in this report are physiologically justifiable and will only give rise to concern if there are grounds for serious uncertainty as to the predictability of dietary selenium intake.

Food commodity inputs are changing rapidly and in some instances, unpredictably. Under most circumstances, it will be unreasonable to expect that the often marked influence of geographic variability on the supply of selenium from cereals and meats can be taken into account. Changes in trade patterns with respect to the sources of cereals and meats are already having significant influences on the selenium nutrition of consumer communities (*38, 72*). Such evidence fully justifies the warning to allow for a high intrinsic variability of dietary selenium content when estimating selenium requirements of populations for which the principal sources of this micronutrient are unknown.

10.9 Recommendations for future research

Relationships between selenium status and pathologically relevant biochemical indexes of deficiency merit much closer study with the object of providing more reliable and earlier means of detecting a suboptimal status.

Indications that a suboptimal selenium status may have much wider significance in influencing disease susceptibility must be pursued. Such studies must cover both the impact of selenium deficiency on protection against oxidative damage during tissue trauma and its genetic implication for viral virulence.

We lack knowledge of the influence of soil composition on the selenium content of cereals and animal tissues. Chinese experience with respect to the dramatic influence of soil iron and low pH on selenium availability may well be relevant to extensive tracts of lateritic soils in Africa and elsewhere. There are grounds for the belief that factors in common for selenium and iodine may influence their supply and availability from soils into the human food chain. FAO should be encouraged to develop studies relevant to the influence of soil conditions on the supply of these two metabolically interdependent elements which affect human health.

The early detection of selenium toxicity (selenosis) is hindered by a lack of suitable biochemical indicators. Effective detection and control of selenosis in many developing countries awaits the development of improved specific diagnostic techniques.

References

1. Levander OA. Selenium. In: Mertz W, ed. *Trace elements in human and animal nutrition.* 5th ed. Orlando, FL, Academic Press, 1986:209–279.
2. Arthur JR, Beckett GJ. Neometabolic roles for selenium. *Proceedings of the Nutrition Society*, 1994, 53:615–624.
3. Ge K, Yang G. The epidemiology of selenium deficiency in the etiological study of endemic diseases in China. *American Journal of Clinical Nutrition*, 1993, 57(Suppl.):S259–S263.
4. Arthur JR et al. Regulation of selenoprotein gene expression and thyroid hormone metabolism. *Transactions of the Biochemical Society*, 1996, 24:384–388.
5. Howie AF et al. Identification of a 57-kilodalton selenoprotein in human thyrocytes as thioredoxin reductase. *Journal of Clinical Endocrinology and Metabolism*, 1998, 83:2052–2058.
6. Mairrino M et al. Reactivity of phospholipid hydroperoxide glutathione peroxidase with membrane and lipoprotein lipid hydroperoxides. *Free Radical Research Communications*, 1991, 12:131–135.
7. Arthur J. Selenium biochemistry and function. In: Fischer PWF et al., eds. *Trace elements in man and animals—9. Proceedings of the Ninth International Symposium on Trace Elements in Man and Animals.* Ottawa, NRC Research Press, 1997:1–5.
8. Reilly C. *Selenium in food and health.* London, Blackie Academic and Professional, 1996.
9. Anikina LV. Selenium-deficient cardiomyopathy (Keshan disease). In: Burk RF, ed. *Fifth International Symposium on Selenium in Biology and Medicine.* Nashville, TN, Vanderbilt University, 1992:122.
10. Brennan MF, Horwitz GD. Total parenteral nutrition in surgical patients. *Advances in Surgery*, 1984, 17:1–7.
11. van Rij AM et al. Selenium deficiency in total parenteral nutrition. *American Journal of Clinical Nutrition*, 1979, 32:2076–2085.
12. Rossipal E, Tiran B. Selenium and glutathione peroxidase levels in healthy infants and children in Austria and the influence of nutrition regimens on these levels. *Nutrition*, 1995, 11(Suppl. 5):S573–S575.
13. Lombeck I et al. Selenium content of human milk, cows milk and cows milk infant formulas. *European Journal of Pediatrics*, 1975, 139–145.
14. Okada A et al. Trace element metabolism in parenteral and enteral nutrition. *Nutrition*, 1995, 11:106–113.
15. Collip PJ, Chen SY. Cardiomyopathy and selenium deficiency in a two year old girl. *New England Journal of Medicine*, 1981, 304:1304–1305.

16. Lombeck I et al. Selenium intake of infants and young children, healthy children and dietetically treated patients with phenylketonuria. *European Journal of Pediatrics*, 1984, 143:99–102.

17. Levander OA, Beck MA. Interacting nutritional and infectious ecologies of Keshan disease. *Biological Trace Element Research*, 1997, 56:5–21.

18. Yang G-Q et al. Human selenium requirements in China. In: Combs GF et al., eds. *Selenium in biology and medicine*. New York, NY, AVI Van Nostrand, 1984:589–607.

19. Johnson CC et al. *Studies of selenium distribution in soil, grain, drinking water and human hair samples from the Keshan disease belt of Zhangjiakou district, Henei Province, China*. Nottingham, British Geological Survey, 1996 (Overseas Geology Series, Technical Report WC/96/52).

20. Li J-Y et al. Distribution of selenium in the microenvironment related to Kaschin-Beck disease. In: Combs GF et al., eds. *Selenium in biology and medicine*. New York, NY, AVI Van Nostrand, 1984:911–925.

21. Beck MA. The influence of antioxidant nutrients on viral infection. *Nutrition Reviews*, 1998, 56(Suppl.):S140–S146.

22. Baum MK, Shor-Posner G. Micronutrient status in relationship to mortality in HIV-1 disease. *Nutrition Reviews*, 1998, 56(Suppl.):S135–S139.

23. Baum MK et al. High risk of HIV-related mortality is associated with selenium deficiency. *Journal of Acquired Immune Deficiency Syndrome and Human Retrovirology*, 1997, 15:370–374.

24. Cirelli A, Ciardi M, DeSimone C. Serum selenium concentration and disease progress in patients with HIV infection. *Clinical Biochemistry*, 1991, 24:211–214.

25. Dworkin BM. Selenium deficiency in HIV infection and the acquired immunodeficiency syndrome (AIDS). *Chemico-Biological Interactions*, 1994, 91:181–186.

26. Taylor EW, Nadimpalli RG, Ramanathan CS. Genomic structures of viral agents in relation to the synthesis of selenoproteins. *Biological Trace Element Research*, 1997, 56:63–91.

27. Zazzo JF et al. Is nonobstructive cardiomyopathy in AIDS a selenium deficiency-related disease? *Journal of Parenteral and Enteral Nutrition*, 1988, 12:537–538.

28. Kavanaugh-McHugh AL, Ruff A, Pearlman A. Selenium deficiency and cardiomyopathy in acquired immunodeficiency syndrome. *Journal of Parenteral and Enteral Nutrition*, 1991, 15:347–349.

29. Ramanathan CS, Taylor EW. Computational genomic analysis of hemorrhagic fever viruses. Viral selenoproteins as a potential factor in pathogenesis. *Biological Trace Element Research*, 1997, 56:93–106.

30. Serfass RE, Ganther HE. Defective microbial activity in glutathione peroxidase deficient neutrophils of selenium deficient rats. *Nature*, 1975, 225:640–641.

31. Boyne R, Arthur JR. The response of selenium deficient mice to *Candida albicans* infection. *Journal of Nutrition*, 1986, 116:816–822.

32. Ip C, Sinha DK. Enhancement of mammary tumorigenesis by dietary selenium deficiency in rats with a high polyunsaturated fat intake. *Cancer Research*, 1981, 41:31–34.

33. Levander OA. A global view of human selenium nutrition. *Annual Review of Nutrition*, 1987, 7:227–250.

34. Birt DF, Pour PM, Pelling JC. The influence of dietary selenium on colon,

pancreas, and skin tumorigenesis. In: Wendel A, ed. *Selenium in biology and medicine*. Berlin, Springer-Verlag, 1989:297–304.

35. Arthur JR, Nicol F, Beckett GJ. Selenium deficiency thyroid hormone metabolism and thyroid hormone deiodinases. *American Journal of Clinical Nutrition*, 1993, 57(Suppl.):S236–S239.

36. Corrilain B et al. Selenium and the thyroid: how the relationship was established. *American Journal of Clinical Nutrition*, 1993, 57(Suppl.):S244–S248.

37. Olivieri O et al. Selenium, zinc and thyroid hormones in healthy subjects. Low T3/T4 ratio in the elderly is related to impaired selenium status. *Biological Trace Element Research*, 1996, 51:31–41.

38. MacPherson A et al. Loss of Canadian wheat imports lowers selenium intake and status of the Scottish population. In: Fischer PWF et al., eds. *Trace elements in man and animals – 9. Proceedings of the Ninth International Symposium on Trace Elements in Man and Animals*. Ottawa, NRC Research Press, 1997:203–205.

39. Vanderpas JB et al. Selenium deficiency mitigates hypothyroxinimia in iodine deficient subjects. *American Journal of Clinical Nutrition*, 1993, 57(Suppl.):S271–S275.

40. Contempre B et al. Selenium deficiency and thyroid fibrosis. A key role for macrophages and TGF-beta. *Molecular and Cellular Enyzmology*, 1996, 124:7–15.

41. Ma T, Guo J, Wang F. The epidemiology of iodine deficiency diseases in China. *American Journal of Clinical Nutrition*, 1993, 57(Suppl.):S264–S266.

42. Contempre B et al. Selenium and iodine in thyroid function: the combined deficiency in the etiology of the involution of the thyroid leading to myxoedematous cretinism. In: Browerman LE et al., eds. *Thyroid and trace elements. 6th Thyroid Symposium*. Eggenberg, Barmhersige Brudes, 1996:35–39.

43. Mahalingam TR et al. Studies on some trace and minor elements in blood. A survey of the Kalpakkam (India) population. Part III. Studies on dietary intake and its correlation to blood levels. *Biological Trace Element Research*, 1997, 57:223–238.

44. Varo P, Koivistoinen P. Mineral element composition of Finnish foods. XII. General discussion and nutritional evaluation. *Acta Agricultura Scandinavica*, 1980, 22(Suppl.):S165–S171.

45. *United Kingdom dietary intake of selenium*. London, Her Majesty's Stationery Office, 1997 (MAFF Food Surveillance Information Sheet, No. 126).

46. Cumming FJ, Fardy JJ, Woodward DR. Selenium and human lactation in Australia: milk and blood selenium levels in lactating women and selenium intake of their breast-fed infants. *Acta Paediatrica*, 1992, 81:1058–1061.

47. Sumar S, Kondza B, Foster LH. Selenium levels in preterm infant formulae and breast milk from the United Kingdom: a study of estimated intakes. In: Fischer PWF et al., eds. *Trace elements in man and animals—9. Proceedings of the Ninth International Symposium on Trace Elements in Man and Animals*. Ottawa, NRC Research Press, 1997:282–283.

48. Robberecht H, Benemariya H, Dellstra H. Daily dietary intake of copper, zinc and selenium of exclusively breast fed infants of middle-class women in Burundi, Africa. *Biological Trace Element Research*, 1995, 49:151–159.

49. *Minor and trace elements in milk: report of a joint WHO/IAEA collaborative study*. Geneva, World Health Organization, 1989.

50. Kumpulainen J et al. Longitudinal study on the dietary selenium intake of

exclusively breast fed infants and their mothers in Finland. *International Journal of Vitamin and Nutrition Research*, 1983, 53:420–426.

51. Lombeck I et al. Selenium content of human milk, cow's milk and cow's milk infant formulas. *European Journal of Paediatrics*, 1975, 129:139–145.

52. Millar KR, Sheppard AD. α-Tocopherol and selenium levels in human and cow's milk. *New Zealand Journal of Science*, 1972, 15:3–15.

53. Williams MMF. Selenium and glutathione peroxidase in mature human milk. *Proceedings of the University of Otago Medical School, Dunedin*, 1983, 61:20–21.

54. Levander OA, Moser PB, Morris VC. Dietary selenium intake and selenium concentrations of plasma, erythrocytes, and breast milk in pregnant and post-partum lactating and nonlactating women. *American Journal of Clinical Nutrition*, 1987, 46:694–698.

55. Shearer TR, Hadjimarkos DM. Geographic distribution of selenium in human milk. *Archives of Environmental Health*, 1975, 30:230–233.

56. Darlow BA et al. Selenium status of New Zealand infants fed either a selenium supplemented or a standard formula. *Journal of Paediatrics and Child Health*, 1995, 31:339–344.

57. Smith A, Picciano MF, Milner JA. Selenium intakes and status of human milk formula fed infants. *American Journal of Clinical Nutrition*, 1982, 35:521–526.

58. Lonnerdal B. Effects of milk and milk components on calcium, magnesium, and trace element absorption during infancy. *Physiological Reviews*, 1997, 77:643–669.

59. Iyengar V, Wooittiez J. Trace elements in human clinical specimens: evaluation of literature to identify reference values. *Clinical Chemistry*, 1988, 34:474–481.

60. *Complementary feeding of young children in developing countries: a review of current scientific knowledge.* Geneva, World Health Organization, 1998 (WHO/NUT/98.1).

61. Thomson JN, Erdody P, Smith DC. Selenium in Canadian foods and diets. *Journal of Nutrition*, 1975, 105:274–279.

62. Yang G et al. Endemic selenium intoxication of humans in China. *American Journal of Clinical Nutrition*, 1983, 37:872–881.

63. Luo XM et al. Selenium intake and metabolic balance of 10 men from a low selenium area of China. *American Journal of Clinical Nutrition*, 1985, 42:31–37.

64. Parr RM et al. *Human dietary intakes of trace elements: a global literature survey mainly for the period 1970–1991. I. Data listings and sources of information.* Vienna, International Atomic Energy Agency, 1992 (NAHRES 12).

65. Koivistoinen P, Varo P. Selenium in Finnish food. In: Combs GF et al., eds. *Selenium in biology and medicine.* New York, NY, Van Nostrand Reinhold, 1987:645–651.

66. Mutanen M et al. Comparison of chemical analysis and calculation method in estimating selenium content of Finnish diets. *Nutrition Research*, 1985, 5:693–697.

67. Mutanen M. Dietary intake and sources of selenium in young Finnish women. *Human Nutrition (Applied Nutrition)*, 1984, 38:265–269.

68. Simonoff M, Simonoff G. *Le selenium et la vie.* [*Selenium and life.*] Paris, Masson, 1991.

69. Oster O, Prellwitz W. The daily dietary selenium intake of West German adults. *Biological Trace Element Research*, 1989, 20:1–14.

70. Robinson MT, Thomason CD. Status of the food supply and residents of New

Zealand. In: Combs GF et al., eds. *Selenium in biology and medicine.* New York, NY, Van Nostrand Reinhold, 1987:631–644.

71. Kadrabova J, Madaric A, Ginter E. Determination of the daily selenium intake in Slovakia. *Biological Trace Element Research*, 1998, 61:277–286.

72. Abdulla MA, Behbehani A, Dashti H. Dietary intake and bioavailability of trace elements. *Biological Trace Element Research*, 1989, 21:173–178.

73. Levander OA, Morris VC. Dietary selenium levels needed to maintain balance in North American adults consuming self-selected diets. *American Journal of Clinical Nutrition*, 1984, 39:809–815.

74. Bratter P, Bratter N, Gwlik D. Selenium in human monitors related to the regional dietary intake levels in Venezuela. *Journal of Trace Elements and Electrolytes in Health and Disease*, 1993, 7:111–112.

75. Alfthan G, Neve J. Reference values for serum selenium in various areas evaluated according to the TRACY protocol. *Journal of Trace Elements in Medicine and Biology*, 1996, 10:77–87.

76. Diplock AT et al. Interaction of selenium and iodine deficiency diseases. In: Fischer PWF et al., eds. *Trace elements in man and animals—9. Proceedings of the Ninth International Symposium on Trace Elements in Man and Animals.* Ottawa, NRC Research Press, 1997:63–68.

77. Diplock AT. Indexes of selenium status in human populations. *American Journal of Clinical Nutrition*, 1993, 57(Suppl.):S256–S258.

78. Versieck J, Cornelis R. *Trace elements in human plasma or serum.* Boca Raton, FL, CRC Press, 1989.

79. *Selenium.* Geneva, World Health Organization, 1987 (Environmental Health Criteria, No. 58).

80. Patterson BH et al. Kinetic modelling of selenium in humans using stable isotope tracers. *Journal of Trace Elements and Electrolytes in Health and Disease*, 1993, 7:117–120.

81. Mutanen M. Bioavailability of selenium. *Annals of Clinical Research*, 1986, 18:48–54.

82. Levander OA et al. Bioavailability of selenium to Finnish men as assessed by platelet glutathione peroxidase activity and other blood parameters. *American Journal of Clinical Nutrition*, 1983, 37:887–897.

83. Levander OA. The global selenium agenda. In: Hurley LS et al., eds. *Trace elements in man and animals—6. Proceedings of the 6th International Symposium on Trace Elements in Man and Animals.* New York, NY, Plenum Press, 1988:1–5.

84. Gu Q-P et al. Distribution of selenium between plasma fractions in guinea pigs and humans with various intakes of selenium. *Journal of Trace Elements in Medicine and Biology*, 1998, 12:8–15.

85. *Trace elements in human nutrition and health.* Geneva, World Health Organization, 1996.

86. Subcommittee on the Tenth Edition of the Recommended Dietary Allowances, Food and Nutrition Board. *Recommended dietary allowances,* 10th ed. Washington, DC, National Academy Press, 1989.

87. Lombeck I et al. The selenium status of healthy children. I. Serum selenium concentration at different ages; activity of glutathione peroxidase of erythrocytes at different ages; selenium content of food of infants. *European Journal of Paediatrics*, 1977, 125:81–88.

88. Levander OA. Upper limit of selenium in infant formulas. *Journal of Nutrition*, 1989, 119:1869–1871.

89. *Nutrient and energy intakes for the European Community: a report of the*

Scientific Committee for Food. Brussels, Commission of the European Communities, 1993.

90. *Dietary reference values for food energy and nutrients for the United Kingdom.* London, Her Majesty's Stationery Office, 1991 (Report on Health and Social Subjects, No. 41).

91. *Recommended dietary allowances 1989 in the Netherlands.* The Hague, Netherlands Food and Nutrition Council, 1989.

92. Smith MI, Franke KW, Westfall BB. The selenium problem in relation to public health. *United States Public Health Report*, 1936, 51:1496–1505.

93. Smith MI, Westfall BB. Further field studies on the selenium problem in relation to public health. *United States Public Health Report*, 1937, 52:1375–1384.

94. Yang G et al. Endemic selenium intoxication of humans in China. *American Journal of Clinical Nutrition*, 1983, 37:872–881.

95. Hadjimarkos DM. Selenium in relation to dental caries. *Food and Cosmetic Toxicology*, 1973, 11:1083–1095.

96. Hadjimarkos DM, Storveik CA, Renmert LT. Selenium and dental caries. An investigation among school children of Oregon. *Journal of Paediatrics*, 1952, 40:451–455.

97. Commission on Natural Resources. *Mineral tolerance of domestic animals.* Washington, DC, National Academy of Sciences, 1980.

11. Magnesium

11.1 Tissue distribution and biological role of magnesium

The human body contains about 760 mg of magnesium at birth, approximately 5 g at age 4–5 months, and 25 g when adult (*1–3*). Of the body's magnesium, 30–40% is found in muscles and soft tissues, 1% is found in extracellular fluid, and the remainder is in the skeleton, where it accounts for up to 1% of bone ash (*4, 5*).

Soft tissue magnesium functions as a cofactor of many enzymes involved in energy metabolism, protein synthesis, RNA and DNA synthesis, and maintenance of the electrical potential of nervous tissues and cell membranes. Of particular importance with respect to the pathological effects of magnesium depletion is the role of this element in regulating potassium fluxes and its involvement in the metabolism of calcium (*6–8*). Magnesium depletion depresses both cellular and extracellular potassium and exacerbates the effects of low-potassium diets on cellular potassium content. Muscle potassium becomes depleted as magnesium deficiency develops, and tissue repletion of potassium is virtually impossible unless magnesium status is restored to normal. In addition, low plasma calcium often develops as magnesium status declines. It is not clear whether this occurs because parathyroid hormone release is inhibited or, more probably, because of a reduced sensitivity of bone to parathyroid hormone, thus restricting withdrawal of calcium from the skeletal matrix.

Between 50% and 60% of body magnesium is located within bone, where it is thought to form a surface constituent of the hydroxyapatite (calcium phosphate) mineral component. Initially much of this magnesium is readily exchangeable with serum and therefore represents a moderately accessible magnesium store which can be drawn on in times of deficiency. However, the proportion of bone magnesium in this exchangeable form declines significantly with increasing age (*9*).

Significant increases in bone mineral density of the femur have been associated positively with rises in erythrocyte magnesium when the diets of subjects with gluten-sensitive enteropathy were fortified with magnesium (*10*). Little is known of other roles for magnesium in skeletal tissues.

11.2 Populations at risk for, and consequences of, magnesium deficiency

Pathological effects of primary nutritional deficiency of magnesium occur infrequently in infants (*11*) but are even less common in adults unless a relatively low magnesium intake is accompanied by prolonged diarrhoea or excessive urinary magnesium losses (*12*). Susceptibility to the effects of magnesium deficiency rises when demands for magnesium increase markedly with the resumption of tissue growth during rehabilitation from general malnutrition (*6, 13*). Studies have shown that a decline in urinary magnesium excretion during protein–energy malnutrition (PEM) is accompanied by a reduced intestinal absorption of magnesium. The catch-up growth associated with recovery from PEM is achieved only if magnesium supply is increased substantially (*6, 14*).

Most of the early pathological consequences of depletion are neurologic or neuromuscular defects (*12, 15*), some of which probably reflect the influence of magnesium on potassium flux within tissues. Thus, a decline in magnesium status produces anorexia, nausea, muscular weakness, lethargy, staggering, and, if deficiency is prolonged, weight loss. Progressively increasing with the severity and duration of depletion are manifestations of hyperirritability, hyperexcitability, muscular spasms, and tetany, leading ultimately to convulsions. An increased susceptibility to audiogenic shock is common in experimental animals. Cardiac arrhythmia and pulmonary oedema frequently have fatal consequences (*12*). It has been suggested that a suboptimal magnesium status may be a factor in the etiology of coronary heart disease and hypertension but additional evidence is needed (*16*).

11.3 Dietary sources, absorption, and excretion of magnesium

Dietary deficiency of magnesium of a severity sufficient to provoke pathological changes is rare. Magnesium is widely distributed in plant and animal foods, and geochemical and other environmental variables rarely have a major influence on its content in foods. Most green vegetables, legume seeds, beans, and nuts are rich in magnesium, as are some shellfish, spices, and soya flour, all of which usually contain more than 500 mg/kg fresh weight. Although most unrefined cereal grains are reasonable sources, many highly-refined flours, tubers, fruits, fungi, and most oils and fats contribute little dietary magnesium (<100 mg/kg fresh weight) (*17–19*). Corn flour, cassava and sago flour, and polished rice flour have extremely low magnesium contents. Table 11.1 presents representative data for the dietary magnesium intakes of infants and adults.

TABLE 11.1
Typical daily intakes of magnesium by infants (6 kg) and adults (65 kg), in selected countries

Group and source of intake	Magnesium intake (mg/day)[a]	Reference(s)
Infants[b]		
Human-milk fed		
Finland	24 (23–25)	17
India	24 ± 0.9	20
United Kingdom	21 (20–23)	21,22
United States	23 (18–30)	11,23
Formula-fed		
United Kingdom (soya-based)	38–60	24
United Kingdom (whey-based)	30–52	24
United States	30–52	11,23
Adults: conventional diets		
China, Changle county	232 ± 62	25
China, Tuoli county	190 ± 59	25
China, females	333 ± 103	25
France, females	280 ± 84	26
France, males	369 ± 106	26
India	300–680	27
United Kingdom, females	237	28
United Kingdom, males	323	28
United States, females	207	29,30
United States, males	329	29,30

[a] Mean ± SD or mean (range).
[b] 750 ml liquid milk or formula as sole food source.

Stable isotope studies with ^{25}Mg and ^{26}Mg indicate that between 50% and 90% of the labelled magnesium from maternal milk and infant formula can be absorbed by infants (*11*, *23*). Studies with adults consuming conventional diets show that the efficiency of magnesium absorption can vary greatly depending on magnesium intake (*31*, *32*). One study showed that 25% of magnesium was absorbed when magnesium intake was high compared with 75% when intake was low (*33*). During a 14-day balance study a net absorption of 52 ± 8% was recorded for 26 adolescent females consuming 176 mg magnesium daily (*34*). Although this intake is far below the United States recommended dietary allowance (RDA) for this age group (280 mg/day), magnesium balance was still positive and averaged 21 mg/day. This study provided one of several sets of data that illustrate the homeostatic capacity of the body to adapt to a wide range of magnesium intakes (*35*, *36*). Magnesium absorption appears to be greatest within the duodenum and ileum and occurs by both passive and active processes (*37*).

High intakes of dietary fibre (40–50 g/day) lower magnesium absorption. This is probably attributable to the magnesium-binding action of phytate phosphorus associated with the fibre (*38–40*). However, consumption of phytate- and cellulose-rich products increases magnesium intake (as they usually contain high concentrations of magnesium) which often compensates for the decrease in absorption. The effects of dietary components such as phytate on magnesium absorption are probably critically important only when magnesium intake is low. There is no consistent evidence that modest increases in the intake of calcium (*34–36*), iron, or manganese (*22*) affect magnesium balance. In contrast, high intakes of zinc (142 mg/day) decrease magnesium absorption and contribute to a shift towards negative balance in adult males (*41*).

The kidney has a very significant role in magnesium homeostasis. Active reabsorption of magnesium takes place in the loop of Henle in the proximal convoluted tubule and is influenced by both the urinary concentration of sodium and probably by acid–base balance (*42*). The latter relationship may well account for the observation drawn from Chinese studies that dietary changes which result in increased urinary pH and decreased titratable acidity also reduce urinary magnesium output by 35% despite marked increases in magnesium input from vegetable protein diets (*25*). Several studies have now shown that dietary calcium intakes in excess of 2600 mg/day (*37*), particularly if associated with high sodium intakes, contribute to a shift towards negative magnesium balance or enhance its urinary output (*42, 43*).

11.4 Criteria for assessing magnesium requirements and allowances

In 1996, Shils and Rude (*44*) published a constructive review of past procedures used to derive estimates of magnesium requirements. They questioned the view of many authors that metabolic balance studies are probably the only practicable, non-invasive techniques for assessing the relationship of magnesium intake to magnesium status. At the same time, they emphasized the great scarcity of data on variations in urinary magnesium output and on magnesium levels in serum, erythrocytes, lymphocytes, bone, and soft tissues. Such data are needed to verify current assumptions that pathological responses to a decline in magnesium supply are not likely to occur if magnesium balance remains relatively constant.

In view of Shils and Rude's conclusion that many estimates of dietary requirements for magnesium were "based upon questionable and insufficient data" (*44*), a closer examination is needed of the value of biochemical criteria for defining the adequacy of magnesium status (*13*). Possible candidates for further investigation include the effects of changes in magnesium intake on urinary magnesium–creatinine ratios (*45*), the relationships between serum magnesium–calcium and magnesium–potassium concentrations (7, 8), and various other functional indicators of magnesium status.

The scarcity of studies from which to derive estimates of dietary allowances for magnesium has been emphasized by virtually all the agencies faced with this task. One United Kingdom agency commented particularly on the scarcity of studies with young subjects, and circumvented the problem of discordant data from work with adolescents and adults by restricting the range of studies considered (21). Using experimental data virtually identical to those used for a detailed critique of the basis for United States estimates (44), the Scientific Committee for Food of the European Communities (46) proposed an acceptable range of intakes for adults of 150–500 mg/day and described a series of quasi-population reference intakes for specific age groups, which included an increment of 30% to allow for individual variations in growth. Statements of acceptable intakes such as these leave uncertainty as to the extent of overestimation of derived recommended intakes.

It is questionable whether more reliable estimates of magnesium requirements can be made until data from balance studies are supported by the use of biochemical indexes of adequacy that could reveal the development of manifestations of suboptimal status. Such indexes have been examined, for example, by Nichols et al. (14) in their studies of the metabolic significance of magnesium depletion during PEM. A loss of muscle and serum magnesium resulted if total body magnesium retention fell below 2 mg/kg/day and was followed by a fall in the myofibrillar nitrogen–collagen ratio of muscle and a fall in muscle potassium content. Repletion of tissue magnesium status preceded a three-fold increase in muscle potassium content. Furthermore, it accelerated, by 7–10 days, the rate of recovery of muscle mass and composition initiated by restitution of nitrogen and energy supplies to infants previously deficient.

Neurologic signs such as hyperirritability, apathy, tremors, and occasional ataxia accompanied by low concentrations of potassium and magnesium in skeletal muscle and strongly negative magnesium balances were reported by many other studies of protein calorie deficiency in infants (47–49). Particularly noteworthy is evidence that all these effects are ameliorated or eliminated by increased oral magnesium, as were specific anomalies in the electrocardiographic T-wave profiles of such malnourished subjects (49). Evidence that the initial rate of growth at rehabilitation is influenced by dietary magnesium intake indicates the significance of this element for the etiology of the PEM syndromes (31, 50).

Regrettably, detailed studies have yet to be carried out to define the nature of changes resulting from a primary deficiency of dietary magnesium. Definition of magnesium requirements must therefore continue to be based on the limited information provided by balance techniques, which give little or no indication of responses by the body to inadequacy in magnesium supply that may induce covert pathological changes, and reassurance must be sought from the application of dietary standards for magnesium in communities consuming diets differing widely in magnesium content (27). The inadequate definition of lower acceptable limits of magnesium intake raises concern in communities or individuals suffering from malnutrition or a wider variety of nutritional or other diseases which influence magnesium metabolism adversely (12, 51, 52).

11.5 Recommended intakes for magnesium

The infrequency with which magnesium deficiency develops in human-milk-fed infants implies that the content and physiological availability of magnesium in human milk meets the infants' requirements. The intake of maternal milk from exclusively human-milk-fed infants 1–10 months of age ranges from 700 to 900 ml/day in both industrialized and developing countries (53). If the magnesium content of milk is assumed to be 29 mg/l (11, 54, 55), the intake from milk is 20–26 mg/day, or approximately 0.04 mg/kcal.

The magnesium in human milk is absorbed with substantially greater efficiency (about 80–90%) than that of formula milks (about 55–75%) or solid foods (about 50%) (56), and such differences must be taken into account when comparing differing dietary sources. For example, a daily intake of 23 mg from maternal milk probably yields 18 mg available magnesium, a quantity similar to that of the 36 mg or more suggested as meeting the requirements of young infants given formula or other foods (see below).

An indication of a likely requirement for magnesium at other ages can be derived from studies of magnesium–potassium relationships in muscle (57) and the clinical recovery of young children rehabilitated from malnutrition with or without magnesium fortification of therapeutic diets. Nichols et al. (14) showed that 12 mg magnesium/day was not sufficient to restore positive magnesium balance, serum magnesium content, or the magnesium and potassium contents of muscle of children undergoing PEM rehabilitation. Muscle potassium was restored to normal by 42 mg magnesium/day but higher intakes of dietary magnesium, up to 160 mg/day, were needed to restore muscle magnesium to normal. Although these studies show clearly that magnesium synergized growth responses resulting from nutritional rehabilitation, they also indicated that rectification of earlier deficits of protein and energy was a prerequisite to initiation of this effect of magnesium.

Similar studies by Caddell et al. (*49, 50*) also illustrate the secondary significance of magnesium accelerating clinical recovery from PEM. They indicate that prolonged consumption of diets low in protein and energy and with a low ratio (<0.02) of magnesium (in milligrams) to energy (in kilocalories) can induce pathological changes which respond to increases in dietary magnesium supply. It is noteworthy that of the balance trials intended to investigate magnesium requirements, none has yet included treatments with magnesium–energy ratios of <0.04 or induced pathological responses.

The relationship Mg = (kcal × 0.0099) – 0.0117 (SE ± 0.0029) holds for many conventional diets (*58*). Some staple foods in common use have very low magnesium contents; cassava, sago, corn flour or cornstarch, and polished rice all have low magnesium–energy ratios (0.003–0.02) (*18*). Their widespread use merits appraisal of total dietary magnesium content.

It has been reported with increasing frequency that a high percentage (e.g. <70%) (*26*) of individuals from some communities in Europe have magnesium intakes substantially lower than estimates of magnesium requirements derived principally from United States and United Kingdom sources (*21, 29*). Such reports emphasize the need for reappraisal of estimates for reasons previously discussed (*44*).

Recommended magnesium intakes proposed by the present Consultation are presented in Table 11.2 together with indications of the relationships of each recommendation to relevant estimates of the average requirements for dietary protein and energy (*19*). These recommended intakes must be regarded as provisional. Until additional data become available, these estimates reflect consideration of anxieties that previous recommendations for magnesium are overestimates. The estimates provided by the Consultation make greater allowance for developmental changes in growth rate and in protein and energy requirements. In reconsidering data on which estimates were based cited in previous reports (*21, 29, 46*), particular attention has been paid to balance data suggesting that the experimental conditions established have provided reasonable opportunity for the development of equilibrium during the investigation (*34, 60–62*).

The detailed studies of magnesium economy during malnutrition and subsequent therapy, with or without magnesium supplementation, provide reasonable grounds that the dietary magnesium recommendations derived herein for young children are realistic. Data for other ages are more scarce and are confined to magnesium balance studies. Some studies have paid little attention to the influence of variations in dietary magnesium content and of the effects of growth rate before and after puberty on the normality of magnesium-dependent functions.

TABLE 11.2
Recommended nutrient intakes (RNIs) for magnesium, by group

Group[a]	Assumed body weight (kg)[b]	RNI (mg/day)	Relative intake ratios		
			(mg/kg)	(mg/g protein[c])	(mg/kcal/day[d])
Infants and children					
0–6 months					
Human-milk-fed	6	26	4.3	2.5	0.05
Formula-fed	6	36	6.0	2.9	0.06
7–12 months	9	54	6.0	3.9	0.06
1–3 years	12	60	5.5	4.0	0.05
4–6 years	19	76	4.0	3.9	0.04
7–9 years	25	100	4.0	3.7	0.05
Adolescents					
Females, 10–18 years	49	220	4.5	5.2	0.10
Males, 10–18 years	51	230	3.5	5.2	0.09
Adults					
Females					
19–65 years	55	220	4.0	4.8	0.10
65+ years	54	190	3.5	4.1	0.10
Males					
19–65 years	65	260	4.0	4.6	0.10
65+ years	64	224	3.5	4.1	0.09

[a] No increment for pregnancy; 50 mg/day increment for lactation.
[b] Assumed body weights of age groups are derived by interpolation (59).
[c] Intake per gram of recommended protein intake for age of subject (21).
[d] Intake per kilocalorie estimated average requirement (21).

It is assumed that during pregnancy, the fetus accumulates 8 mg magnesium and fetal adnexa accumulate 5 mg magnesium. If it is assumed that this magnesium is absorbed with 50% efficiency, the 26 mg required over a pregnancy of 40 weeks (0.09 mg/day) can probably be accommodated by adaptation. A lactation allowance of 50–55 mg/day for dietary magnesium is made for the secretion of milk containing 25–28 mg magnesium (*21, 63*).

It is appreciated that magnesium demand probably declines in late adulthood as requirements for growth diminish. However, it is reasonable to expect that the efficiency with which magnesium is absorbed declines in elderly subjects. It may well be that the recommendations are overgenerous for elderly subjects, but data are not sufficient to support a more extensive reduction than that indicated. An absorption efficiency of 50% is assumed for all solid diets; data are not sufficient to allow for the adverse influence of phytic acid on magnesium absorption from high-fibre diets or from diets with a high content of pulses.

Not surprisingly, few of the representative dietary analyses presented in Table 11.1 fail to meet these recommended allowances. The few exceptions, deliberately selected for inclusion, are the marginal intakes (232 ± 62 mg) of the 168 women of Changle County, People's Republic of China, and the low intake (190 ± 59 mg) of 147 women surveyed from Tuoli County, People's Republic of China (25).

11.6 Upper limits

Magnesium from dietary sources is relatively innocuous. Contamination of food or water supplies with magnesium salt has been known to cause hypermagnesaemia, nausea, hypotension, and diarrhoea. Intakes of 380 mg magnesium as magnesium chloride have produced such signs in women. Upper limits of 65 mg for children aged 1–3 years, 110 mg for children aged 4–10 years, and 350 mg for adolescents and adults are suggested as tolerable limits for the daily intake of magnesium from foods and drinking water (64).

11.7 Comparison with other estimates

The recommended intakes for infants aged 0–6 months take account of differences in the physiological availability of magnesium from maternal milk as compared with infant formulas or solid foods. With the exception of the Canadian recommended nutrient intakes (RNIs), which are 20 mg/day for infants aged 0–4 months and 32 mg/day for those aged 5–12 months (63), other countries recommend intakes (as RDAs or RNIs) which substantially exceed the capacity of the lactating mother to supply magnesium for her offspring.

Recommendations for other ages are based subjectively on the absence of any evidence that magnesium deficiency of nutritional origin has occurred after consumption of a range of diets sometimes supplying considerably less than the United States RDA or the United Kingdom RNI recommendations, which are based on estimates of average magnesium requirements of 3.4–7 mg/kg body weight. The recommendations submitted herein assume that demands for magnesium, plus a margin of approximately 20% (to allow for methodological variability), are probably met by allowing approximately 3.5–5 mg/kg body weight from pre-adolescence to maturity. This assumption yields estimates virtually identical to those for Canada. Expressed as magnesium allowance (in milligrams) divided by energy allowance (in kilocalories) — the latter based upon energy recommendations from United Kingdom estimates (21) — all of the recommendations of Table 11.2 exceed the provisionally estimated critical minimum magnesium–energy ratio of 0.02.

11.8 Recommendations for future research

There is need for closer investigation of the biochemical changes that develop as magnesium status declines. The responses to magnesium intake, which influence the pathological effects resulting from disturbances in potassium utilization caused by low magnesium, should be studied. They may well provide an understanding of the influence of magnesium status on growth rate and neurologic integrity.

Closer investigation of the influence of magnesium status on the effectiveness of therapeutic measures during rehabilitation from PEM is also needed. The significance of magnesium in the etiology and consequences of PEM in children needs to be clarified. Claims that restoration of protein and energy supply aggravates the neurologic features of PEM if magnesium status is not improved merit priority of investigation. Failure to clarify these aspects may continue to obscure some of the most important pathological features of a nutritional disorder in which evidence already exists for the involvement of a magnesium deficit.

References

1. Widdowson EM, McCance RA, Spray CM. The chemical composition of the human body. *Clinical Science*, 1951, 10:113–125.
2. Forbes GB. *Human body composition: growth, aging, nutrition and activity.* New York, NY, Springer-Verlag, 1987.
3. Schroeder HA, Nason AP, Tipton IH. Essential metals in man: magnesium. *Journal of Chronic Diseases*, 1969, 21:815–841.
4. Heaton FW. Magnesium in intermediary metabolism. In: Canatin M, Seelig M, eds. *Magnesium in health and disease.* New York, NY, SP Medical and Scientific Books, 1976:43–55.
5. Webster PO. Magnesium. *American Journal of Clinical Nutrition*, 1987, 45:1305–1312.
6. Waterlow JC. *Protein-energy malnutrition.* London, Edwin Arnold, 1992.
7. Classen HG. Magnesium and potassium deprivation and supplementation in animals and man: aspects in view of intestinal absorption. *Magnesium*, 1984, 3:257–264.
8. Al-Ghamdi SM, Cameron EC, Sutton RA. Magnesium deficiency: pathophysiologic and clinical overview. *American Journal of Kidney Diseases*, 1994, 24:737–754.
9. Breibart S et al. Relation of age to radiomagnesium in bone. *Proceedings of the Society of Experimental Biology and Medicine*, 1960, 105:361–363.
10. Rude RK, Olerich M. Magnesium deficiency: possible role in osteoporosis associated with gluten-sensitive enteropathy. *Osteoporosis International*, 1996, 6:453–461.
11. Lönnerdal B. Magnesium nutrition of infants. *Magnesium Research*, 1995, 8:99–105.
12. Shils ME. Magnesium in health and disease. *Annual Review of Nutrition*, 1988, 8:429–460.
13. Gibson RS. *Principles of nutritional assessment.* New York, NY, Oxford University Press, 1990.
14. Nichols BL et al. Magnesium supplement in protein-calorie malnutrition. *American Journal of Clinical Nutrition*, 1978, 31:176–188.

15. Shils ME. Experimental human magnesium depletion. *Medicine*, 1969, 48: 61–85.
16. Elwood PC. Iron, magnesium and ischaemic heart disease. *Proceedings of the Nutrition Society*, 1994, 53:599–603.
17. Koivistoinen P. Mineral element composition of Finnish foods. *Acta Agricultura Scandinavica*, 1980, 22(Suppl.):S7–S171.
18. Paul AA, Southgate DAT. *The composition of foods.* London, Her Majesty's Stationery Office, 1978.
19. Tan SP, Wenlock RW, Buss DH. *Immigrant foods. Second supplement to the composition of foods.* London, Her Majesty's Stationery Office, 1985.
20. Belavady B. Lipid and trace element content of human milk. *Acta Pediatrica Scandinavica*, 1978, 67:566–569.
21. Department of Health. *Dietary reference values for food energy and nutrients for the United Kingdom.* London, Her Majesty's Stationery Office, 1991 (Report on Health and Social Subjects, No. 41).
22. Wisker E et al. Calcium, magnesium, zinc and iron balances in young women. *American Journal of Clinical Nutrition*, 1991, 54:533–559.
23. Lönnerdal B. Effects of milk and milk components on calcium, magnesium and trace element absorption during infancy. *Physiological Reviews*, 1997, 77:643–669.
24. Holland B, Unwin ID, Buss DH. *Milk products and eggs. Fourth supplement to the composition of foods.* Royal Society of Chemistry, Cambridge, 1989.
25. Hu J-F et al. Dietary intakes and urinary excretion of calcium and acids: a cross-sectional study of women in China. *American Journal of Clinical Nutrition*, 1993, 58:398–406.
26. Galan P et al. Dietary magnesium intake in a French adult population. *Magnesium Research*, 1997, 10:321–328.
27. Parr RM et al. *Human dietary intakes of trace elements: a global literature survey mainly for the period 1970–1991.* Vienna, International Atomic Energy Agency, 1992 (NAHRES 12).
28. Gregory J et al. *The Dietary and Nutritional Survey of British Adults.* London, Her Majesty's Stationery Office, 1990.
29. Subcommittee on the Tenth Edition of the Recommended Dietary Allowances, Food and Nutrition Board. *Recommended dietary allowances*, 10th ed. Washington, DC, National Academy Press, 1989.
30. Anonymous. Calcium and related nutrients: overview and methods. *Nutrition Reviews*, 1997, 55:335–341.
31. Spencer H et al. Magnesium absorption and metabolism in patients with chronic renal failure and in patients with normal renal function. *Gastroenterology*, 1980, 79:26–34.
32. Seelig MS. Magnesium requirements in human nutrition. *Journal of the Medical Society of New Jersey*, 1982, 70:849–854.
33. Schwartz R, Spencer H, Welsh JH. Magnesium absorption in human subjects. *American Journal of Clinical Nutrition*, 1984, 39:571–576.
34. Andon MB et al. Magnesium balance in adolescent females consuming a low- or high-calcium diet. *American Journal of Clinical Nutrition*, 1996, 63:950–953.
35. Abrams SA et al. Calcium and magnesium balance in 9–14 year old children. *American Journal of Clinical Nutrition*, 1997, 66:1172–1177.

36. Sojka J et al. Magnesium kinetics in adolescent girls determined using stable isotopes: effects of high and low calcium intakes. *American Journal of Physiology*, 1997, 273: R710–R715.
37. Greger JL, Smith SA, Snedeker SM. Effect of dietary calcium and phosphorus levels on the utilization of calcium, magnesium, manganese, and selenium by adult males. *Nutrition Research*, 1981, 1:315–325.
38. McCance RA, Widdowson EM. Mineral metabolism on dephytinised bread. *Journal of Physiology*, 1942, 101:304–313.
39. McCance RA, Widdowson EM. Mineral metabolism in healthy adults on white and brown bread dietaries. *Journal of Physiology*, 1942, 101:44–85.
40. Kelsay JL, Bahall KM, Prather ES. Effect of fiber from fruit and vegetables on the metabolic responses of human subjects. *American Journal of Clinical Nutrition*, 1979, 32:1876–1880.
41. Spencer H, Norris C, Williams D. Inhibitory effect of zinc on magnesium balance and absorption in man. *Journal of the American College of Nutrition*, 1994, 13:479–484.
42. Quarme GA, Disks JH. The physiology of renal magnesium handling. *Renal Physiology*, 1986, 9:257–269.
43. Kesteloot H, Joosens JV. The relationship between dietary intake and urinary excretion of sodium, potassium, calcium and magnesium. *Journal of Human Hypertension*, 1990, 4:527–533.
44. Shils ME, Rude RK. Deliberations and evaluations of the approaches, end-points and paradigms for magnesium dietary recommendations. *Journal of Nutrition*, 1996, 126(Suppl.):S2398–S2403.
45. Matos V et al. Urinary phosphate creatinine, calcium/creatinine and magnesium/creatinine ratios in a healthy pediatric population. *Journal of Pediatrics*, 1997, 131:252–257.
46. *Reference nutrient intakes for the European Community: a report of the Scientific Committee for Food.* Brussels, Commission of the European Communities, 1993.
47. Montgomery RD. Magnesium metabolism in infantile protein malnutrition. *Lancet*, 1960, 2:74–75.
48. Linder GC, Hansen DL, Karabus CD. The metabolism of magnesium and other inorganic cations and of nitrogen in acute kwashiorkor. *Pediatrics*, 1963, 31:552–568.
49. Caddell JL. Magnesium deficiency in protein-calorie malnutrition: a follow-up study. *Annals of the New York Academy of Sciences*, 1969, 162:874–890.
50. Caddell JL, Goodard DR. Studies in protein-calorie malnutrition. I. Chemical evidence for magnesium deficiency. *New England Journal of Medicine*, 1967, 276:533–535.
51. Brautbar N, Roy A, Hom P. Hypomagnesaemia and hypermagnesaemia. In: Sigel H, Sigel A, eds. *Metals in biological systems. 26. Magnesium and its role in biology, nutrition and physiology.* New York, NY, Marcel Dekker, 1990:215–320.
52. Elin RJ. The assessment of magnesium status in humans. In: Sigel H, Sigel A, eds. *Metals in biological systems. 26. Magnesium and its role in biology, nutrition and physiology.* New York, NY, Marcel Dekker, 1990:579–596.
53. *Complementary feeding of young children in developing countries: a review of current scientific knowledge.* Geneva, World Health Organization, 1998 (WHO/NUT/98.1).

54. Iyengar GV. *Elemental composition of human and animal milk.* Vienna, International Atomic Energy Agency, 1982 (IAEA-TECDOC-296).

55. Liu YMP et al. Absorption of calcium and magnesium from fortified human milk by very low birth weight infants. *Pediatric Research*, 1989, 25:496–502.

56. Lönnerdal B. Effects of milk and milk components on calcium, magnesium, and trace element absorption during infancy. *Physiological Reviews*, 1997, 77:643–669.

57. Dorup I. *Magnesium and potassium deficiency: its diagnosis, occurrence and treatment.* Aarhus, University of Aarhus Institute of Physiology, 1994.

58. Manalo E, Flora RE, Duel SE. A simple method for estimating dietary magnesium. *American Journal of Clinical Nutrition*, 1967, 20:627–631.

59. *Requirements of vitamin A, iron, folate and vitamin B_{12}.* Rome, Food and Agriculture Organization of the United Nations, 1988 (FAO Nutrition Series, No. 23).

60. Mahalko JR et al. Effect of a moderate increase in dietary protein on the retention and excretion of Ca, Cu, Fe, Mg, P, and Zn by adult males. *American Journal of Clinical Nutrition*, 1983, 37:8–14.

61. Hunt SM, Schofield FA. Magnesium balance and protein intake in the adult human female. *American Journal of Clinical Nutrition*, 1969, 22:367–373.

62. Marshall DH, Nordin BEC, Speed R. Calcium, phosphorus and magnesium requirement. *Proceedings of the Nutrition Society*, 1976, 35:163–173.

63. Scientific Review Committee. *Nutrition recommendations: Health and Welfare, Canada. Report of the Scientific Review Committee.* Ottawa, Supply and Services, 1992.

64. Food and Nutrition Board. *Dietary reference intakes for calcium, phosphorus, magnesium, vitamin D, and fluoride.* Washington, DC, National Academy Press, 1997.

12. Zinc

12.1 Role of zinc in human metabolic processes

Zinc is present in all body tissues and fluids. The total body zinc content has been estimated to be 30 mmol (2 g). Skeletal muscle accounts for approximately 60% of the total body content and bone mass, with a zinc concentration of 1.5–3 µmol/g (100–200 µg/g), for approximately 30%. The concentration of zinc in lean body mass is approximately 0.46 µmol/g (30 µg/g). Plasma zinc has a rapid turnover rate and it represents only about 0.1% of total body zinc content. This level appears to be under close homeostatic control. High concentrations of zinc are found in the choroid of the eye (4.2 µmol/g or 274 µg/g) and in prostatic fluids (4.6–7.7 mmol/l or 300–500 mg/l) (1).

Zinc is an essential component of a large number (>300) of enzymes participating in the synthesis and degradation of carbohydrates, lipids, proteins, and nucleic acids as well as in the metabolism of other micronutrients. Zinc stabilizes the molecular structure of cellular components and membranes and in this way contributes to the maintenance of cell and organ integrity. Furthermore, zinc has an essential role in polynucleotide transcription and thus in the process of genetic expression. Its involvement in such fundamental activities probably accounts for the essentiality of zinc for all life forms.

Zinc plays a central role in the immune system, affecting a number of aspects of cellular and humoral immunity (2). Shankar and Prasad have reviewed the role of zinc in immunity extensively (2).

The clinical features of severe zinc deficiency in humans are growth retardation, delayed sexual and bone maturation, skin lesions, diarrhoea, alopecia, impaired appetite, increased susceptibility to infections mediated via defects in the immune system, and the appearance of behavioural changes (1). The effects of marginal or mild zinc deficiency are less clear. A reduced growth rate and impairments of immune defence are so far the only clearly demonstrated signs of mild zinc deficiency in humans. Other effects, such as impaired taste and wound healing, which have been claimed to result from a low zinc intake, are less consistently observed.

12.2 Zinc metabolism and homeostasis

Zinc absorption is concentration dependent and occurs throughout the small intestine. Under normal physiological conditions, transport processes of uptake are not saturated. Zinc administered in aqueous solutions to fasting subjects is absorbed efficiently (60–70%), whereas absorption from solid diets is less efficient and varies depending on zinc content and diet composition (3).

The major losses of zinc from the body are through the intestine and urine, by desquamation of epithelial cells, and in sweat. Endogenous intestinal losses can vary from 7 μmol/day (0.5 mg/day) to more than 45 μmol/day (3 mg/day), depending on zinc intake—the higher the intake, the greater the losses (4). Urinary and integumental losses are of the order of 7–10 μmol/day (0.5–0.7 mg/day) each and depend less on normal variations in zinc intake (4). Starvation and muscle catabolism increase zinc losses in urine. Strenuous exercise and elevated ambient temperatures can lead to high losses through perspiration.

The body has no zinc stores in the conventional sense. In conditions of bone resorption and tissue catabolism, zinc is released and may be reutilized to some extent. Human experimental studies with low zinc diets containing 2.6–3.6 mg/day (40–55 μmol/day) have shown that circulating zinc levels and activities of zinc-containing enzymes can be maintained within a normal range over several months (5, 6), a finding which highlights the efficiency of the zinc homeostasis mechanism. Controlled depletion–repletion studies in humans have shown that changes in the endogenous excretion of intestinal, urinary, and integumental zinc as well as changes in absorptive efficiency are how body zinc content is maintained (7–10). However, the underlying mechanisms are poorly understood.

Sensitive indexes for assessing zinc status are unknown at present. Static indexes, such as zinc concentration in plasma, blood cells, and hair, and urinary zinc excretion are decreased in severe zinc deficiency. A number of conditions that are unrelated to zinc status can affect all these indexes, especially zinc plasma levels. Food intake, stress situations such as fever, infection, and pregnancy lower plasma zinc concentrations whereas, for example, long-term fasting increases it (11). However, on a population basis, reduced plasma zinc concentrations seem to be a marker for zinc-responsive growth reductions (12, 13). Experimental zinc depletion studies suggest that changes in immune response occur before reductions in plasma zinc concentrations are apparent (14). To date, it has not been possible to identify zinc-dependent enzymes which could serve as early markers for zinc status.

A number of functional indexes of zinc status have been suggested, for example, wound healing, taste acuity, and visual adaptation to the dark (11).

Changes in these functions are, however, not specific to zinc and these indexes have not been proven useful for identifying marginal zinc deficiency in humans thus far.

The introduction of stable isotope techniques in zinc research (15) has created possibilities for evaluating the relationship between diet and zinc status and is likely to lead to a better understanding of the mechanisms underlying the homeostatic regulation of zinc. Estimations of the turnover rates of administered isotopes in plasma or urine have revealed the existence of a relatively small but rapidly exchangeable body pool of zinc of about 1.5–3.0 mmol (100–200 mg) (16–19). The size of the pool seems to be correlated to habitual dietary intake and it is reduced in controlled depletion studies (18). The zinc pool was also found to be correlated to endogenous intestinal excretion of zinc (19) and to total daily absorption of zinc. These data suggest that the size of the pool depends on recently absorbed zinc and that a larger exchangeable pool results in larger endogenous excretion. Changes in endogenous intestinal excretion of zinc seem to be more important than changes in absorptive efficiency for maintenance of zinc homeostasis (19).

12.3 Dietary sources and bioavailability of zinc

Lean red meat, whole-grain cereals, pulses, and legumes provide the highest concentrations of zinc: concentrations in such foods are generally in the range of 25–50 mg/kg (380–760 μmol/kg) raw weight. Processed cereals with low extraction rates, polished rice, and chicken, pork or meat with high fat content have a moderate zinc content, typically between 10 and 25 mg/kg (150–380 μmol/kg). Fish, roots and tubers, green leafy vegetables, and fruits are only modest sources of zinc, having concentrations <10 mg/kg (<150 μmol/kg) (20). Saturated fats and oils, sugar, and alcohol have very low zinc contents.

The utilization of zinc depends on the overall composition of the diet. Experimental studies have identified a number of dietary factors as potential promoters or antagonists of zinc absorption (21). Soluble organic substances of low relative molecular mass, such as amino and hydroxy acids, facilitate zinc absorption. In contrast, organic compounds forming stable and poorly soluble complexes with zinc can impair absorption. In addition, competitive interactions between zinc and other ions with similar physicochemical properties can affect the uptake and intestinal absorption of zinc. The risk of competitive interactions with zinc seems to be mainly related to the consumption of high doses of these other ions, in the form of supplements or in aqueous solutions. However, at levels present in food and at realistic fortification levels, zinc absorption appears not to be affected, for example, by iron or copper (21).

Isotope studies with human subjects have identified two factors that, together with the total zinc content of the diet, are major determinants of absorption and utilization of dietary zinc. The first is the content of inositol hexaphosphate (phytate) in the diet and the second is the level and source of dietary protein. Phytates are present in whole-grain cereals and legumes and in smaller amounts in other vegetables. They have a strong potential for binding divalent cations and their depressive effect on zinc absorption has been demonstrated in humans (21). The molar ratio between phytates and zinc in meals or diets is a useful indicator of the effect of phytates in depressing zinc absorption. At molar ratios above the range of 6–10, zinc absorption starts to decline; at ratios above 15, absorption is typically less than 15% (20). The effect of phytate is, however, modified by the source and amount of dietary proteins consumed. Animal proteins improve zinc absorption from a phytate-containing diet (22). Zinc absorption from some legume-based diets (e.g. white beans and lupin protein) is comparable with that from animal-protein-based diets despite a higher phytate content in the former (22, 23). High dietary calcium potentiated the antagonistic effects of phytates on zinc absorption in experimental studies. The results from human studies are less consistent and any effects seem to depend on the source of calcium and the composition of the diet (21, 23).

Several recently published absorption studies illustrate the effect of zinc content and diet composition on fractional zinc absorption (19, 24–26). The results from the total diet studies, where all main meals of a day's intake were extrinsically labelled, show a remarkable consistency in fractional absorption despite relatively large variations in meal composition and zinc content (see Table 12.1). Thus, approximately twice as much zinc is absorbed from a non-vegetarian or high-meat diet (25, 26) than from a diet based on rice and wheat flour (19). Data are lacking on zinc absorption from typical diets of developing countries, which usually have high phytate contents.

The availability of zinc from the diet can be improved by reducing the phytate content and including sources of animal protein. Lower extraction rates of cereal grains will result in lower phytate content but at the same time the zinc content is reduced, so that the net effect on zinc supply is limited. The phytate content can be reduced by activating the phytase present in most phytate-containing foods or through the addition of microbial or fungal phytases. Phytases hydrolyse the phytate to lower inositol phosphates, resulting in improved zinc absorption (27, 28). The activity of phytases in tropical cereals such as maize and sorghum is lower than that in wheat and rye (29). Germination of cereals and legumes increases phytase activity and addition of some germinated flour to ungerminated maize or sorghum followed by

TABLE 12.1
Examples of fractional zinc absorption from total diets measured by isotope techniques

Subject characteristics (reference)	Diet characteristics	Isotope technique	Zinc content (μmol)	Zinc content (mg)	Phytate– zinc molar ratio	Zinc absorption, % (± SD)
Young adults (n = 8) (24)	High-fibre	Radioisotope	163	10.7	7	27 ± 6
Young women (n = 10) (19)	Self-selected rice- and wheat-based	Stable isotope	80	8.1	11	31 ± 9
Women (20–42 years) (n = 21) (25)	Lacto-ovo vegetarian	Radioisotope	139	9.1	14	26[a]
Women (20–42 years) (n = 21) (25)	Non-vegetarian	Radioisotope	169	11.1	5	33[a]
Postmenopausal women (n = 14) (26)	Low meat	Radioisotope	102	6.7	—	30[b]
Postmenopausal women (n = 14) (26)	High meat	Radioisotope	198	13.0	—	28[b]

SD, standard deviation.
[a] Pooled SD = 5.
[b] Pooled SD = 4.6.

soaking at ambient temperature for 12–24 hours can reduce the phytate content substantially (29). Additional reduction can be achieved by the fermentation of porridge for weaning foods or dough for bread making. Commercially available phytase preparations could also be used but may not be economically accessible in many populations.

12.4 Populations at risk for zinc deficiency

The central role of zinc in cell division, protein synthesis, and growth is especially important for infants, children, adolescents, and pregnant women; these groups suffer most from an inadequate zinc intake. Zinc-responsive stunting has been identified in several studies; for example, a more rapid body weight gain in malnourished children from Bangladash supplemented with zinc was reported (30). However, other studies have failed to show a growth-promoting effect of zinc supplementation. A recent meta-analysis of 25 intervention trials comprising 1834 children under 13 years of age, with a mean duration of approximately 7 months and a mean dose of zinc of 14 mg/day (214 μmol/day), showed a small but significant positive effect of zinc supplementation on height and weight increases (13). Zinc supplementation had a positive effect when stunting was initially present; a more pronounced effect on weight gain was associated with initial low plasma zinc concentrations.

Results from zinc supplementation studies suggest that a low zinc status in children not only affects growth but is also associated with an increased risk of severe infectious diseases (*31*). Episodes of acute diarrhoea were characterized by shorter duration and less severity in zinc-supplemented groups; reductions in incidence of diarrhoea were also reported. Other studies indicate that the incidence of acute lower respiratory tract infections and malaria may also be reduced by zinc supplementation. Prevention of suboptimal zinc status and zinc deficiency in children by an increased intake and availability of zinc could consequently have a significant effect on child health in developing countries.

The role of maternal zinc status on pregnancy outcome is still unclear. Positive as well as negative associations between plasma zinc concentration and fetal growth or labour and delivery complications have been reported (*32*). Results of zinc supplementation studies also remain inconclusive (*32*). Interpretation of plasma zinc concentrations in pregnancy is complicated by the effect of haemodilution, and the fact that low plasma zinc levels may reflect other metabolic disturbances (*11*). Zinc supplementation studies of pregnant women have been performed mainly in relatively well-nourished populations, which may be one of the reasons for the mixed results (*32*). A recent study among low-income American women with plasma zinc concentrations below the mean at enrolment in prenatal care showed that a zinc intake of 25 mg/day resulted in greater infant birth weights and head circumferences as well as a reduced frequency of very low-birth-weight infants among non-obese women compared with the placebo group (*12*).

12.5 Evidence used to estimate zinc requirements

The lack of specific and sensitive indexes for zinc status limits the possibilities for evaluating zinc requirements from epidemiological observations. Previous estimates, including those published in 1996 as a result of a collaborative effort by WHO, the Food and Agriculture Organization of the United Nations (FAO) and the International Atomic Energy Agency (IAEA) (*33*) have relied on the factorial technique, which involves totalling the requirements for tissue growth, maintenance, metabolism, and endogenous losses. Experimental zinc repletion studies with low zinc intakes have clearly shown that the body has a pronounced ability to adapt to different levels of zinc intakes by changing the endogenous intestinal, urinary and integumental zinc losses (*5–9, 34*). The normative requirement for absorbed zinc was thus defined as the obligatory loss during the early phase of zinc depletion before adaptive reductions in excretion take place and was set at 1.4 mg/day for men and 1.0 mg/day for women. To estimate the normative maintenance requirements for other age groups, the respective basal metabolic rates were used for extrapolation. In growing individuals the rate of accretion and zinc content of newly-formed tissues were used to derive estimates of requirements for tissue growth. Similarly, the retention of zinc during pregnancy (35) and the zinc concentration in milk at different stages of lactation (36) were used to estimate the physiological requirements in pregnancy and lactation.

The translation of these estimates of absorbed zinc into requirements for dietary zinc involves several considerations. First, the nature of the diet (i.e. its content of promoters and inhibitors of zinc absorption) determines the fraction of the dietary zinc that is potentially absorbable. Second, the efficiency of absorption of potentially available zinc is inversely related to the content of zinc in the diet. The review of available data from experimental zinc absorption studies of single meals or total diets resulted in a division of diets into three categories—high, moderate, and low zinc bioavailability—as detailed in Table 12.2 (33). To take account of the fact that the relationship between efficiency of absorption and zinc content differs for these diets, algorithms were developed (33) and applied to the estimates of requirements for absorbed zinc to achieve a set of figures for the average individual dietary zinc requirements (Table 12.3). The fractional absorption figures applied for the three diet categories at intakes adequate to meet the normative requirements for absorbed zinc were 50%, 30%, and 15%, respectively. From these estimates and from the evaluation of data from dietary intake studies, mean population intakes were identified which were deemed sufficient to ensure a low prevalence of individuals at risk of inadequate zinc intake (33). Assumptions made in deriving zinc requirements for specific population groups are summarized below.

12.5.1 Infants, children, and adolescents

Endogenous losses of zinc in human-milk-fed infants were assumed to be 20 µg/kg/day (0.31 µmol/kg/day) whereas 40 µg/kg/day (0.6 µmol/kg/day) was assumed for infants fed formula or weaning foods (33). For other age groups an average loss of 0.002 µmol/basal kJ (0.57 µg/basal kcal) was derived from the estimates in adults. Estimated zinc increases for infant growth were set at 120 and 140 µg/kg/day (1.83–2.14 µmol/kg/day) for female and male infants, respectively, for the first 3 months (33). These values decrease to 33 µg/kg/day (0.50 µmol/kg/day) for ages 6–12 months. For ages 1–10 years, the requirements for growth were based on the assumption that new tissue contains 30 µg/g (0.46 µmol zinc/g) (33). For adolescent growth, a tissue-zinc

TABLE 12.2
Criteria for categorizing diets according to the potential bioavailability of their zinc

Nominal category[a]	Principal dietary characteristics
High availability	Refined diets low in cereal fibre, low in phytic acid content, and with phytate–zinc molar ratio <5; adequate protein content principally from non-vegetable sources, such as meats and fish. Includes semi-synthetic formula diets based on animal protein.
Moderate availability	Mixed diets containing animal or fish protein. Lacto-ovo, ovo-vegetarian, or vegan diets not based primarily on unrefined cereal grains or high-extraction-rate flours. Phytate–zinc molar ratio of total diet within the range 5–15, or not exceeding 10 if more than 50% of the energy intake is accounted for by unfermented, unrefined cereal grains and flours and the diet is fortified with inorganic calcium salts (>1 g Ca^{2+}/day). Availability of zinc improves when the diet includes animal protein or milks, or other protein sources or milks.
Low availability	Diets high in unrefined, unfermented, and ungerminated cereal grain[b], especially when fortified with inorganic calcium salts and when intake of animal protein is negligible. Phytate–zinc molar ratio of total diet exceeds 15[c], High-phytate, soya-protein products constitute the primary protein source. Diets in which, singly or collectively, approximately 50% of the energy intake is accounted for by the following high-phytate foods: high-extraction-rate (≥90%) wheat, rice, maize, grains and flours, oatmeal, and millet; chapatti flours and *tanok*; and sorghum, cowpeas, pigeon peas, grams, kidney beans, black-eyed beans, and groundnut flours. High intakes of inorganic calcium salts (>1 g Ca^{2+}/day), either as supplements or as adventitious contaminants (e.g. from calcareous geophagia), potentiate the inhibitory effects and low intakes of animal protein exacerbates these effects.

[a] At intakes adequate to meet the average normative requirements for absorbed zinc (Table 12.3) the three availability levels correspond to 50%, 30% and 15% absorption. With higher zinc intakes, the fractional absorption is lower.
[b] Germination of cereal grains or fermentation (e.g. leavening) of many flours can reduce antagonistic potency of phytates; if done, the diet should then be classified as having moderate zinc availability.
[c] Vegetable diets with phytate–zinc ratios exceeding 30 are not unknown; for such diets, an assumption of 10% availability of zinc or less may be justified, especially if the intake of protein is low, that of inorganic calcium salts is excessive (e.g. calcium salts providing >1.5 g Ca^{2+}/day), or both.
Source: adapted from reference (33).

content of 23 µg/g (0.35 µmol/g) was assumed. Pubertal growth spurts increase physiological zinc requirements substantially. Growth of adolescent males corresponds to an increase in body zinc requirement of about 0.5 mg/day (7.6 µmol/day) (33).

TABLE 12.3
Average individual normative requirements for zinc (µg/kg body weight/day) from diets differing in zinc bioavailability[a]

Group	High bioavailability[b]	Moderate bioavailability[c]	Low bioavailability[d]
Infants and children			
Females, 0–3 months	175[e]	457[f]	1067[g]
Males, 0–3 months	200[e]	514[f]	1200[g]
3–6 months	79[e]	204[f]	477[g]
6–12 months	66[e], 186	311	621
1–3 years	138	230	459
3–6 years	114	190	380
6–10 years	90	149	299
Adolescents			
Females, 10–12 years	68	113	227
Males, 10–12 years	80	133	267
Females, 12–15 years	64	107	215
Males, 12–15 years	76	126	253
Females, 15–18 years	56	93	187
Males, 15–18 years	61	102	205
Adults			
Females, 18–60+ years	36	59	119
Males, 18–60+ years	43	72	144

[a] For information on diets, see Table 12.2.
[b] Assumed bioavailability of dietary zinc, 50%.
[c] Assumed bioavailability of dietary zinc, 30%.
[d] Assumed bioavailability of dietary zinc, 15%.
[e] Applicable to infants fed maternal milk alone for which the bioavailability of zinc is assumed to be 80% and infant endogenous losses to be 20 µg/kg (0.31 µmol/kg). Corresponds to basal requirements with no allowance for storage.
[f] Applicable to infants partly human-milk-fed or fed whey-adjusted cow milk formula or milk plus low-phytate solids. Corresponds to basal requirements with no allowance for storage.
[g] Applicable to infants receiving phytate-rich vegetable protein-based infant formula with or without whole-grain cereals. Corresponds to basal requirements with no allowance for storage.
Source: adapted from reference (33).

12.5.2 Pregnant women

The total amount of zinc retained during pregnancy has been estimated to be 1.5 mmol (100 mg) (35). During the third trimester, the physiological requirement of zinc is approximately twice as high as that in women who are not pregnant (33).

12.5.3 Lactating women

Zinc concentrations in human milk are high in early lactation, i.e. 2–3 mg/l (31–46 µmol/l) in the first month, and fall to 0.9 mg/l (14 µmol/l) after 3 months (36). From data on maternal milk volume and zinc content, it was estimated that the daily output of zinc in milk during the first 3 months of lactation could amount to 1.4 mg/day (21.4 µmol/l), which would theoretically triple the physiological zinc requirements in lactating women compared with non-lactating, non-pregnant women. In setting the estimated requirements for early lactation, it was assumed that part of this requirement is covered by postnatal involution of the uterus and from skeletal resorption (*33*).

12.5.4 Elderly

A lower absorptive efficiency has been reported in the elderly, which could justify a dietary requirement higher than that for other adults. On the other hand, endogenous losses seem to be lower in the elderly. Because of the suggested role of zinc in infectious diseases, an optimal zinc status in the elderly could have a significant public health effect and is an area of zinc metabolism requiring further research. Currently however, requirements for the elderly are estimated to be the same as those for other adults.

12.6 Interindividual variations in zinc requirements and recommended nutrient intakes

The studies (*6–10*) used to estimate the average physiological zinc requirements with the factorial technique are based on a relatively small number of subjects and do not make any allowance for interindividual variations in obligatory losses at different intakes. Because zinc requirements are related to tissue turnover rate and growth, it is reasonable to assume that variations in physiological zinc requirements are of the same magnitude as variations in protein requirements (*37*) and that the same figure (12.5%) for the interindividual coefficient of variation (CV) could be adopted. However, unlike protein requirements, the derivation of dietary zinc requirements involves estimating absorption efficiences. Consequently, variations in absorptive efficiency, not relevant in relation to estimates of protein requirements, may have to be taken into account in the estimates of the total interindividual variation in zinc requirements. Systematic studies of the interindividual variations in zinc absorption under different conditions are few. In small groups of healthy well-nourished subjects, the reported variations in zinc absorption from a defined meal or diet are of the order of 20–40% and seem to be largely independent of age, sex, or diet characteristics (see Table 12.1). How much these variations, besides being attributable to methodological imprecision, reflect variations in physiological requirement, effects of preceding zinc intake, etc. is not known. Based on the available data from zinc absorption studies (*19, 20, 23–28*), it is tentatively suggested that the interindividual variation in dietary zinc requirements, which includes variation in requirement for absorbed zinc (i.e. variations in metabolism and turnover rate of zinc) and variation in absorptive efficiency, corresponds to a CV of 25%. The recom-

TABLE 12.4
Recommended nutrient intakes (RNIs) for dietary zinc (mg/day) to meet the normative storage requirements from diets differing in zinc bioavailability[a]

Group	Assumed body weight (kg)	High bioavailability	Moderate bioavailability	Low bioavailability
Infants and children				
0–6 months	6	1.1[b]	2.8[c]	6.6[d]
7–12 months	9	0.8[b], 2.5[e]	4.1	8.4
1–3 years	12	2.4	4.1	8.3
4–6 years	17	2.9	4.8	9.6
7–9 years	25	3.3	5.6	11.2
Adolescents				
Females, 10–18 years	47	4.3	7.2	14.4
Males, 10–18 years	49	5.1	8.6	17.1
Adults				
Females, 19–65 years	55	3.0	4.9	9.8
Males, 19–65 years	65	4.2	7.0	14.0
Females, 65+ years	55	3.0	4.9	9.8
Males, 65+ years	65	4.2	7.0	14.0
Pregnant women				
First trimester	—	3.4	5.5	11.0
Second trimester	—	4.2	7.0	14.0
Third trimester	—	6.0	10.0	20.0
Lactating women				
0–3 months	—	5.8	9.5	19.0
3–6 months	—	5.3	8.8	17.5
6–12 months	—	4.3	7.2	14.4

[a] For information on diets, see Table 12.2. Unless otherwise specified, the interindividual variation of zinc requirements is assumed to be 25%. Weight data interpolated from reference (*38*).
[b] Exclusively human-milk-fed infants. The bioavailability of zinc from human milk is assumed to be 80%; assumed coefficient of variation, 12.5%.
[c] Formula-fed infants. Applies to infants fed whey-adjusted milk formula and to infants partly human-milk-fed or given low-phytate feeds supplemented with other liquid milks; assumed coefficient of variation, 12.5%.
[d] Formula-fed infants. Applicable to infants fed a phytate-rich vegetable protein-based formula with or without whole-grain cereals; assumed coefficient of variation, 12.5%.
[e] Not applicable to infants consuming human milk only.

mended nutrient intakes (RNIs) derived from the estimates of average individual dietary requirements (Table 12.3) with the addition of 50% (2 standard deviations) are given in Table 12.4.

12.7 Upper limits

Only a few occurrences of acute zinc poisoning have been reported. The toxicity signs are nausea, vomiting, diarrhoea, fever, and lethargy and have been observed after ingestion of 4–8 g (60–120 mmol) of zinc. Long-term zinc intakes higher than requirements could, however, interact with the metabolism of other trace elements. Copper seems to be especially sensitive to high zinc doses. A zinc intake of 50 mg/day (760 μmol) affects copper status indexes, such as CuZn-superoxide dismutase in erythrocytes (*39, 40*). Low copper and ceruloplasmin levels and anaemia have been observed after zinc intakes of 450–660 mg/day (6.9–10 mmol/day) (*41, 42*). Changes in serum lipid pattern and in immune response have also been observed in zinc supplementation studies (*43, 44*). Because copper also has a central role in immune defence, these observations should be studied further before large-scale zinc supplementation programmes are undertaken. Any positive effects of zinc supplementation on growth or infectious diseases could be offset by associated negative effects on copper-related functions.

The upper level of zinc intake for an adult man is set at 45 mg/day (690 μmol/day) and extrapolated to other groups in relation to basal metabolic rate. For children this extrapolation means an upper limit of intake of 23–28 mg/day (350–430 μmol/day), which is close to what has been used in some of the zinc supplementation studies. Except for excessive intakes of some types of seafood, such intakes are unlikely to be attained with most diets. Adventitious zinc in water from contaminated wells and from galvanized cooking utensils could also lead to high zinc intakes.

12.8 Adequacy of zinc intakes in relation to requirement estimates

The risk of inadequate zinc intakes in children has been evaluated by comparing the suggested estimates of zinc requirements (*33*) with available data on food composition and dietary intake in different parts of the world (*45*). For this assessment, it was assumed that zinc requirements follow a Gaussian distribution with a CV of 15% and that the correlation between intake and requirement is very low. Zinc absorption from diets in Kenya, Malawi, and Mexico was estimated to be 15%, based on the high phytate–zinc molar ratio (> 25) of these diets, whereas an absorption of 30% was assumed for diets in Egypt, Ghana, Guatemala, and Papua New Guinea. Diets of fermented maize and cassava products (*kenkey, banku,* and *gari*) in Ghana, yeast leavened wheat-based bread in Egypt, and the use of sago with a low phytate content as the staple in Papua New Guinea were assumed to result in a lower phytate–zinc molar ratio and a better zinc availability. However, on these diets, 68–94% of children were estimated to be at risk for zinc deficiency in these populations, with the exception of those in Egypt where the estimate was 36% (*45*). The average daily zinc intakes of the children in the high-risk countries were between 3.7 and 6.6 mg (56–100 μmol), and in Egypt, 5.2 mg (80 μmol) illustrating the impact of a low availability.

Most of the zinc supplementation studies have not provided dietary intake data, which could be used to identify the zinc intake critical for beneficial growth effects. In a recent study in Chile, positive effects on height gain in boys after 14 months of zinc supplementation were noted (*46*). The intake in the placebo group at the start of the study was 6.3 ± 1.3 mg/day (96 ± 20 µmol/day) (n = 49). Because only 15% of the zinc intake of the Chilean children was derived from flesh foods, availability was assumed to be relatively low.

Krebs et al. (*47*) observed no effect of zinc supplementation on human-milk zinc content or on maternal zinc status of a group of lactating women and judged their intake sufficient to maintain adequate zinc status through 7 months or more of lactation. The mean zinc intake of the non-supplemented women was 13.0 ± 3.4 mg/day (199 ± 52 µmol/day).

The efficiency of the homeostatic mechanisms for maintaining body zinc content at low intakes, which formed the basis for the estimates of physiological requirements in the WHO/FAO/IAEA report (*33*), as well as the presumed negative impact of a high-phytate diet on zinc status, has been confirmed in several experimental studies (*10*, *46*, *48*, *49*). Reductions in urinary and intestinal losses maintained normal plasma zinc concentrations over a 5-week period in 11 men with zinc intakes of 2.45 mg/day (37 µmol/day) (*10*). In a similar repletion–depletion study with 15 men, an intake of 4 mg/day (61 µmol/day) from a diet with a molar phytate–zinc ratio of 58 for 7 weeks resulted in a reduction of urinary zinc excretion from 0.52 ± 0.18 to 0.28 ± 0.15 mg/day (7.9 ± 2.8 µmol/day to 4.3 ± 2.3 µmol/day) (*48*). A significant reduction of plasma zinc concentrations and changes in cellular immune response were observed. Effects on immunity were also observed when five young male volunteers consumed a zinc-restricted diet with a high-phytate content (molar ratio approximately 20) for 20–24 weeks (*14*). Suboptimal zinc status has also been documented in pregnant women consuming diets with high phytate–zinc ratios (>17) (*49*). Frequent reproductive cycling and high malaria prevalence also seemed to contribute to the impairment of zinc status in this population group.

In conclusion, the approach used for derivation of average individual requirements of zinc used in the 1996 WHO/FAO/IAEA report (*33*) and the resulting estimates still seem valid and useful for assessment of the adequacy of zinc intakes in population groups and for planning diets for defined population groups.

12.9 Recommendations for future research

As already indicated in the 1996 WHO/FAO/IAEA report (*33*), there is still an urgent need to characterize the early functional effects of zinc deficiency and to define their relation to pathologic changes. This knowledge is vital to the understanding of the role of zinc deficiency in the etiology of stunting and impaired immunocompetence.

For a better understanding of the relationship between diet and zinc supply, there is a need for further research which evaluates the availability of zinc from diets typical of developing countries. The research should include an assessment of the feasibility of adopting realistic and culturally-accepted food preparation practices, such as fermentation, germination, and soaking, and of including available and inexpensive animal protein sources in plant-food-based diets.

References

1. Hambridge KM, Casey CE, Krebs NF. Zinc. In: Mertz W, ed. *Trace elements in human and animal nutrition*, 5th ed. *Volume 2*. Orlando, FL, Academic Press, 1987:1–137.
2. Shankar AH, Prasad AS. Zinc and immune function: the biological basis of altered resistance to infection. *American Journal of Clinical Nutrition*, 1998, 68(Suppl.):S447–S463.
3. Sandström B. Bioavailability of zinc. *European Journal of Clinical Nutrition*, 1997, 51(Suppl. 1):S17–S19.
4. King JC, Turnlund JR. Human zinc requirements. In: Mills CF, ed. *Zinc in human biology*. New York, NY, Springer-Verlag, 1989:335–350.
5. Lukaski HC et al. Changes in plasma zinc content after exercise in men fed a low-zinc diet. *American Journal of Physiology*, 1984, 247:E88–E93.
6. Milne DB et al. Ethanol metabolism in postmenopausal women fed a diet marginal in zinc. *American Journal of Clinical Nutrition*, 1987, 46:688–693.
7. Baer MJ, King JC. Tissue zinc levels and zinc excretion during experimental zinc depletion in young men. *American Journal of Clinical Nutrition*, 1984, 39:556–570.
8. Hess FM, King JC, Margen S. Zinc excretion in young women on low zinc intakes and oral contraceptive agents. *Journal of Nutrition*, 1977, 107:1610–1620.
9. Milne DB et al. Effect of dietary zinc on whole body surface loss of zinc: impact on estimation of zinc retention by balance method. *American Journal of Clinical Nutrition*, 1983, 38:181–186.
10. Johnson PE et al. Homeostatic control of zinc metabolism in men: zinc excretion and balance in men fed diets low in zinc. *American Journal of Clinical Nutrition*, 1993, 57:557–565.
11. Agett PJ, Favier A. Zinc. *International Journal for Vitamin and Nutrition Research*, 1993, 63:247–316.
12. Goldenberg RL et al. The effect of zinc supplementation on pregnancy outcome. *Journal of the American Medical Association*, 1995, 274:463–468.
13. Brown KH, Peerson JM, Allen LH. Effect of zinc supplementation on children's growth: a meta-analysis of intervention trials. Bibliotheca Nutritio et Dieta, 1998, 54:76–83.
14. Beck FWJ et al. Changes in cytokine production and T cell subpopulations in experimentally induced zinc-deficient humans. *American Journal of Physiology*, 1997, 272:E1002–E1007.
15. Sandström B et al. Methods for studying mineral and trace element absorp-

tion in humans using stable isotopes. *Nutrition Research Reviews*, 1993, 6:71–95.

16. Wastney ME et al. Kinetic analysis of zinc metabolism in humans after simultaneous administration of [65]Zn and [70]Zn. *American Journal of Physiology*, 1991, 260:R134–R141.

17. Fairweather-Tait SJ et al. The measurement of exchangeable pools of zinc using the stable isotope [70]Zn. *British Journal of Nutrition*, 1993, 70:221–234.

18. Miller LV et al. Size of the zinc pools that exchange rapidly with plasma zinc in humans: alternative techniques for measuring and relation to dietary zinc intake. *Journal of Nutrition*, 1994, 124:268–276.

19. Sian L et al. Zinc absorption and intestinal losses of endogenous zinc in young Chinese women with marginal zinc intakes. *American Journal of Clinical Nutrition*, 1996, 63:348–353.

20. Sandström B. Dietary pattern and zinc supply. In: Mills CF, ed. *Zinc in human biology*. New York, NY, Springer-Verlag, 1989:350–363.

21. Sandström B, Lönnerdal B. Promoters and antagonists of zinc absorption. In: Mills CF, ed. *Zinc in human biology*. New York, NY, Springer-Verlag, 1989:57–78.

22. Sandström B et al. Effect of protein level and protein source on zinc absorption in humans. *Journal of Nutrition*, 1998, 119:48–53.

23. Petterson D, Sandström B, Cederblad Å. Absorption of zinc from lupin (*Lupinus angustifolius*)-based foods. *British Journal of Nutrition*, 1994, 72:865–871.

24. Knudsen E et al. Zinc absorption estimated by fecal monitoring of zinc stable isotopes validated by comparison with whole-body retention of zinc radioisotopes in humans. *Journal of Nutrition*, 1995, 125:1274–1282.

25. Hunt JR, Matthys LA, Johnson LK. Zinc absorption, mineral balance, and blood lipids in women consuming controlled lactoovovegetarian and omnivorous diets for 8 weeks. *American Journal of Clinical Nutrition*, 1998, 67:421–430.

26. Hunt JR et al. High- versus low-meat diets: effects on zinc absorption, iron status, and calcium, copper, iron, magnesium, manganese, nitrogen, phosphorus, and zinc balance in postmenopausal women. *American Journal of Clinical Nutrition*, 1995, 62:621–632.

27. Nävert B, Sandström B, Cederblad Å. Reduction of the phytate content of bran by leavening in bread and its effect on absorption of zinc in man. *British Journal of Nutrition*, 1985, 53:47–53.

28. Sandström B, Sandberg AS. Inhibitory effects of isolated inositol phosphates on zinc absorption in humans. *Journal of Trace Elements and Electrolytes in Health and Disease*, 1992, 6:99–103.

29. Gibson RS et al. Dietary interventions to prevent zinc deficiency. *American Journal of Clinical Nutrition*, 1998, 68(Suppl.):S484–S487.

30. Simmer K et al. Nutritional rehabilitation in Bangladesh—the importance of zinc. *American Journal of Clinical Nutrition*, 1988, 47:1036–1040.

31. Black MM. Zinc deficiency and child development. *American Journal of Clinical Nutrition*, 1998, 68(Suppl.):S464–S469.

32. Caulfield LE et al. Potential contribution of maternal zinc supplementation during pregnancy to maternal and child survival. *American Journal of Clinical Nutrition*, 1998, 68(Suppl.):S499–S508.

33. *Trace elements in human nutrition and health*. Geneva, World Health Organization, 1996.

34. Taylor CM et al. Homeostatic regulation of zinc absorption and endogenous losses in zinc-deprived men. *American Journal of Clinical Nutrition*, 1991, 53:755–763.

35. Swanson CA, King JC. Zinc and pregnancy outcome. *American Journal of Clinical Nutrition*, 1987, 46:763–771.

36. *Complementary feeding of young children in developing countries: a review of current scientific knowledge.* Geneva, World Health Organization, 1998 (WHO/NUT/98.1).

37. *Energy and protein requirements. Report of a Joint FAO/WHO/UNU Expert Consultation.* Geneva, World Health Organization, 1985 (WHO Technical Report Series, No. 724).

38. *Requirements of vitamin A, iron, folate, and vitamin B_{12}. Report of a Joint FAO/WHO Expert Consultation.* Rome, Food and Agriculture Organization of the United Nations, 1988 (FAO Food and Nutrition Series, No. 23).

39. Fischer PWF, Giroux A, L'Abbé MR. Effect of zinc supplementation on copper status in adult man. *American Journal of Clinical Nutrition*, 1984, 40:743–746.

40. Yadrick MK, Kenney MA, Winterfeldt EA. Iron, copper, and zinc status: response to supplementation with zinc or zinc and iron in adult females. *American Journal of Clinical Nutrition*, 1989, 49:145–150.

41. Patterson WP, Winkelmann M, Perry MC. Zinc-induced copper deficiency: megamineral sideroblastic anemia. *Annals of Internal Medicine*, 1985, 103:385–386.

42. Porter KG et al. Anaemia and low serum-copper during zinc therapy. *Lancet*, 1977, 2:774.

43. Hooper PL et al. Zinc lowers high-density lipoprotein-cholesterol levels. *Journal of the American Medical Association*, 1980, 244:1960–1962.

44. Chandra RK. Excessive intake of zinc impairs immune responses. *Journal of the American Medical Association*, 1984, 252:1443–1446.

45. Gibson RS, Ferguson EL. Assessment of dietary zinc in a population. *American Journal of Clinical Nutrition*, 1998, 68(Suppl.):S430–S434.

46. Ruz M et al. A 14-month zinc-supplementation trial in apparently healthy Chilean preschool children. *American Journal of Clinical Nutrition*, 1997, 66:1406–1413.

47. Krebs NF et al. Zinc supplementation during lactation: effects on maternal status and milk zinc concentrations. *American Journal of Clinical Nutrition*, 1995, 61:1030–1036.

48. Ruz M et al. Erythrocytes, erythrocyte membranes, neutrophils and platelets as biopsy materials for the assessment of zinc status in humans. *British Journal of Nutrition*, 1992, 68:515–527.

49. Gibson RS, Huddle J-M. Suboptimal zinc status in pregnant Malawian women: its association with low intakes of poorly available zinc, frequent reproductive cycling, and malaria. *American Journal of Clinical Nutrition*, 1998, 67:702–709.

13. Iron

13.1 Role of iron in human metabolic processes

Iron has several vital functions in the body. It serves as a carrier of oxygen to the tissues from the lungs by red blood cell haemoglobin, as a transport medium for electrons within cells, and as an integrated part of important enzyme systems in various tissues. The physiology of iron has been extensively reviewed (1–6).

Most of the iron in the body is present in the erythrocytes as haemoglobin, a molecule composed of four units, each containing one haem group and one protein chain. The structure of haemoglobin allows it to be fully loaded with oxygen in the lungs and partially unloaded in the tissues (e.g. in the muscles). The iron-containing oxygen storage protein in the muscles, myoglobin, is similar in structure to haemoglobin but has only one haem unit and one globin chain. Several iron-containing enzymes, the cytochromes, also have one haem group and one globin protein chain. These enzymes act as electron carriers within the cell and their structures do not permit reversible loading and unloading of oxygen. Their role in the oxidative metabolism is to transfer energy within the cell and specifically in the mitochondria. Other key functions for the iron-containing enzymes (e.g. cytochrome P450) include the synthesis of steroid hormones and bile acids; detoxification of foreign substances in the liver; and signal controlling in some neurotransmitters, such as the dopamine and serotonin systems in the brain. Iron is reversibly stored within the liver as ferritin and haemosiderin whereas it is transported between different compartments in the body by the protein transferrin.

13.2 Iron metabolism and absorption

13.2.1 Basal iron losses

Iron is not actively excreted from the body in urine or in the intestines. Iron is only lost with cells from the skin and the interior surfaces of the body— intestines, urinary tract, and airways. The total amount lost is estimated at 14 µg/kg body weight/day (7). In children, it is probably more correct to relate these losses to body surface. A non-menstruating 55-kg woman loses about

0.8 mg Fe/day and a 70-kg man loses about 1 mg/day. The range of individual variation has been estimated to be ±15% (8).

Earlier studies suggested that sweat iron losses could be considerable, especially in a hot, humid climate. However, new studies which took extensive precautions to avoid the interference of contamination of iron from the skin during the collection of total body sweat have shown that sweat iron losses are negligible (9).

13.2.2 Requirements for growth

The newborn term infant has an iron content of about 250–300 mg (75 mg/kg body weight). During the first 2 months of life, haemoglobin concentration falls because of the improved oxygen situation in the newborn infant compared with the intrauterine fetus. This leads to a considerable redistribution of iron from catabolized erythrocytes to iron stores. This iron will cover the needs of the term infant during the first 4–6 months of life and is why iron requirements during this period can be provided by human milk, which contains very little iron. Because of the marked supply of iron to the fetus during the last trimester of pregnancy, the iron situation is much less favourable in the premature and low-birth-weight infant than in the healthy term infant. An extra supply of iron is therefore needed in these infants during the first 6 months of life.

In the term infant, iron requirements rise markedly after age 4–6 months and amount to about 0.7–0.9 mg/day during the remaining part of the first year. These requirements are very high, especially in relation to body size and energy intake (Table 13.1) (10).

In the first year of life, the term infant almost doubles its total iron stores and triples its body weight. The increase in body iron during this period occurs mainly during the latter 6 months. Between 1 and 6 years of age, the body iron content is again doubled. The requirements for absorbed iron in infants and children are very high in relation to their energy requirements. For example, in infants 6–12 months of age, about 1.5 mg of iron need to be absorbed per 4.184 MJ and about half of this amount is required up to age 4 years.

In the weaning period, the iron requirements in relation to energy intake are at the highest level of the lifespan except for the last trimester of pregnancy, when iron requirements to a large extent have to be covered from the iron stores of the mother (see section 13.4 on iron and pregnancy). Infants have no iron stores and have to rely on dietary iron alone. It is possible to meet these high requirements if the diet has a consistently high content of meat and foods rich in ascorbic acid. In most developed countries today, infant

TABLE 13.1

Iron intakes required for growth under the age of 18 years, median basal iron losses, menstrual losses in women, and total absolute iron requirements

Group	Age (years)	Mean body weight (kg)	Required iron intakes for growth (mg/day)	Median basal iron losses (mg/day)	Menstrual losses		Total absolute requirements[a]	
					Median (mg/day)	95th percentile (mg/day)	Median (mg/day)	95th percentile (mg/day)
Infants and children	0.5–1	9	0.55	0.17			0.72	0.93
	1–3	13	0.27	0.19			0.46	0.58
	4–6	19	0.23	0.27			0.50	0.63
	7–10	28	0.32	0.39			0.71	0.89
Males	11–14	45	0.55	0.62			1.17	1.46
	15–17	64	0.60	0.90			1.50	1.88
	18+	75		1.05			1.05	1.37
Females	11–14[b]	46	0.55	0.65			1.20	1.40
	11–14	46	0.55	0.65	0.48[c]	1.90[c]	1.68	3.27
	15–17	56	0.35	0.79	0.48[c]	1.90[c]	1.62	3.10
	18+	62		0.87	0.48[c]	1.90[c]	1.46	2.94
Postmenopausal		62		0.87			0.87	1.13
Lactating		62		1.15			1.15	1.50

[a] Total absolute requirements = Requirement for growth + basal losses + menstrual losses.
[b] Pre-menarche.
[c] Effect of the normal variation in haemoglobin concentration not included in this figure.
Source: adapted, in part, from reference (8) and in part on new calculations of the distribution of iron requirements in menstruating women.

cereal products are the staple foods for that period of life. Commercial products are regularly fortified with iron and ascorbic acid, and they are usually given together with fruit juices and solid foods containing meat, fish, and vegetables. The fortification of cereal products with iron and ascorbic acid is important in meeting the high dietary needs, especially considering the importance of an optimal iron nutrititure during this phase of brain development.

Iron requirements are also very high in adolescents, particularly during the period of rapid growth (*11*). There is a marked individual variation in growth rate, and the requirements of adolescents may be considerably higher than the calculated mean values given in Table 13.1. Girls usually have their growth spurt before menarche, but growth is not finished at that time. Their total iron requirements are therefore considerable. In boys during puberty there is a marked increase in haemoglobin mass and concentration, further increasing iron requirements to a level above the average iron requirements in menstruating women (Figure 13.1).

13.2.3 Menstrual iron losses

Menstrual blood losses are very constant from month to month for an individual woman but vary markedly from one woman to another (*16*). The main part of this variation is genetically controlled by the fibrinolytic activators in

FIGURE 13.1
Iron requirements of boys and girls at different ages

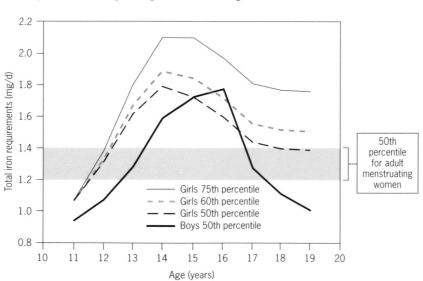

Sources: based on data from references (*8* and *12–16*).

the uterine mucosa—even in populations which are geographically widely separated (Burma, Canada, China, Egypt, England, and Sweden) (*17, 18*). These findings strongly suggest that the main source of variation in iron status in different populations is not related to a variation in iron requirements but to a variation in the absorption of iron from the diets. (This statement disregards infestations with hookworms and other parasites.) The mean menstrual iron loss, averaged over the entire menstrual cycle of 28 days, is about 0.56 mg/day. The frequency distribution of physiological menstrual blood losses is highly skewed. Adding the average basal iron loss (0.8 mg/day) and its variation allows the distribution of the total iron requirements in adult women to be calculated as the convolution of the distributions of menstrual and basal iron losses (Figure 13.2). The mean daily total iron requirement is 1.36 mg. In 10% of women, it exceeds 2.27 mg and in 5% it exceeds 2.84 mg (*19*). In 10% of menstruating (still-growing) teenagers, the corresponding daily total iron requirement exceeds 2.65 mg, and in 5% of girls, it exceeds 3.2 mg. The marked skewness of menstrual losses is a great nutritional problem because assessment of an individual's iron losses is unreliable. This means that women with physiological but heavy losses cannot be identified and reached by iron supplementation. The choice of contraceptive method also greatly influences menstrual losses.

In postmenopausal women and in physically active elderly people, the iron requirements per unit of body weight are the same as in men. When physical activity decreases as a result of ageing, blood volume decreases and haemoglobin mass diminishes, leading to a shift of iron usage from haemoglobin and muscle to iron stores. This implies a reduction of the daily iron requirements. Iron deficiency in the elderly is therefore seldom of nutritional origin but is usually caused by pathologic iron losses.

The absorbed iron requirements in different groups are summarized in Table 13.1. The iron requirements during pregnancy and lactation are dealt with separately (see section 13.4).

13.2.4 Iron absorption

With respect to the mechanism of absorption, there are two kinds of dietary iron: haem iron and non-haem iron (*20*). In the human diet, the primary sources of haem iron are the haemoglobin and myoglobin from consumption of meat, poultry, and fish whereas non-haem iron is obtained from cereals, pulses, legumes, fruits, and vegetables. The average absorption of haem iron from meat-containing meals is about 25% (*21*). The absorption of haem iron can vary from about 40% during iron deficiency to about 10% during iron repletion (*22*). Haem iron can be degraded and converted to non-haem

FIGURE 13.2
Distribution of daily iron requirements in menstruating adult women and teenagers: the probability of adequacy at different amounts of iron absorbed

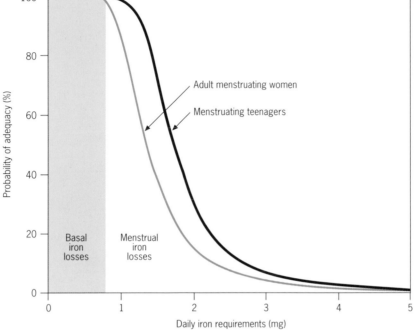

The left-hand side of the graph shows the basal obligatory losses that amount to 0.8 mg/day. The right-hand side shows the variation in menstrual iron losses. This graph illustrates that growth requirements in teenagers vary considerably at different ages and between individuals.

iron if foods are cooked at a high temperature for too long. Calcium (discussed below) is the only dietary factor that negatively influences the absorption of haem iron and does so to the same extent that it influences non-haem iron (23).

Non-haem iron is the main form of dietary iron. The absorption of non-haem iron is influenced by individual iron status and by several factors in the diet. Dietary factors influencing iron absorption are outlined in Box 13.1. Iron compounds used for the fortification of foods will only be partially available for absorption. Once dissolved, however, the absorption of iron from fortificants (and food contaminants) is influenced by the same factors as the iron native to the food substance (24, 25). Iron from the soil (e.g. from various forms of clay) is sometimes present on the surface of foods as a contaminant, having originated from dust on air-dried foods or from the residue of the water used in irrigation. Even if the fraction of iron that is available is often

BOX 13.1 FACTORS INFLUENCING DIETARY IRON ABSORPTION

Haem iron absorption

Factors determining iron status of subject:

Amount of dietary haem iron, especially from meat

Content of calcium in meal (e.g. from milk, cheese)

Food preparation (i.e. time, temperature)

Non-haem iron absorption

Factors determining iron status of subject:

Amount of potentially available non-haem iron (includes adjustment for fortification iron and contamination iron)

Balance between the following enhancing and inhibiting factors:

Enhancing factors

Ascorbic acid (e.g. certain fruit juices, fruits, potatoes, and certain vegetables)

Meat, fish and other seafood

Fermented vegetables (e.g. sauerkraut), fermented soy sauces, etc.

Inhibiting factors

Phytate and other lower inositol phosphates (e.g. bran products, bread made from high-extraction flour, breakfast cereals, oats, rice – especially unpolished rice – pasta products, cocoa, nuts, soya beans, and peas)

Iron-binding phenolic compounds (e.g. tea, coffee, cocoa, certain spices, certain vegetables, and most red wines)

Calcium (e.g. from milk, cheese)

Soya

Source: reference (*23*).

small, contamination iron may still be nutritionally significant because of its addition to the overall dietary intake of iron (*26, 27*).

Reducing substances (i.e. substances that keep iron in the ferrous form) must be present for iron to be absorbed (*28*). The presence of meat, poultry, and fish in the diet enhance iron absorption. Other foods contain chemical entities (ligands) that strongly bind ferrous ions, and thus inhibit absorption. Examples are phytates and certain iron-binding polyphenols (see Box 13.1).

13.2.5 Inhibition of iron absorption

Phytates are found in all kinds of grains, seeds, nuts, vegetables, roots (e.g. potatoes), and fruits. Chemically, phytates are inositol hexaphosphate salts and are a storage form of phosphates and minerals. Other phosphates have not been shown to inhibit non-haem iron absorption. In North American and European diets, about 90% of phytates originate from cereals. Phytates strongly inhibit iron absorption in a dose-dependent fashion and even small amounts of phytates have a marked effect (29, 30).

Bran has a high content of phytate and strongly inhibits iron absorption. Wholewheat flour, therefore, has a much higher phytate content than does white-wheat flour (31). In bread, some of the phytates in bran are degraded during the fermentation of the dough. Fermentation for a couple of days (sourdough fermentation) can almost completely degrade the phytate and increase the bioavailability of iron in bread made from wholewheat flour (32). Oats strongly inhibit iron absorption because of their high phytate content that results from native phytase in oats being destroyed by the normal heat process used to avoid rancidity (33). Sufficient amounts of ascorbic acid can counteract this inhibition (34). In contrast, non-phytate-containing dietary fibre components have almost no influence on iron absorption.

Almost all plants contain phenolic compounds as part of their defence system against insects and animals. Only some of the phenolic compounds (mainly those containing galloyl groups) seem to be responsible for the inhibition of iron absorption (35). Tea, coffee, and cocoa are common plant products that contain iron-binding polyphenols (36–39). Many vegetables, especially green leafy vegetables (e.g. spinach), and herbs and spices (e.g. oregano) contain appreciable amounts of galloyl groups, which strongly inhibit iron absorption as well. Consumption of betel leaves, common in areas of Asia, also has a marked negative effect on iron absorption.

Calcium, consumed as a salt or in dairy products interferes significantly with the absorption of both haem and non-haem iron (40–42). However, because calcium is an essential nutrient, it cannot be considered to be an inhibitor of iron absorption in the same way as phytates or phenolic compounds. In order to lessen this interference, practical solutions include increasing iron intake, increasing its bioavailability, or avoiding the intake of foods rich in calcium and foods rich in iron at the same meal (43).

The mechanism of action for absorption inhibition is unknown, but the balance of evidence strongly suggests that the inhibitory effect takes place within the mucosal cell itself at the common final transfer step for haem and non-haem iron. Recent analyses of the dose–effect relationship show that the first 40 mg of calcium in a meal does not inhibit absorption of haem and non-haem iron. Above this level of calcium intake, a sigmoid relationship develops, and at levels of 300–600 mg calcium, reaches a 60% maximal inhibition of iron absorption. The form of this curve suggests a one-site competitive

FIGURE 13.3
Effect of different amounts of calcium on iron absorption

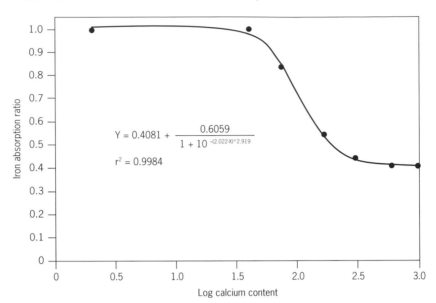

$$Y = 0.4081 + \frac{0.6059}{1 + 10^{-(2.022-X)^{2.919}}}$$

$$r^2 = 0.9984$$

binding of iron and calcium (Figure 13.3). This relationship explains some of the seemingly conflicting results obtained in studies on the interaction between calcium and iron (*44*).

For unknown reasons, the addition of soya to a meal reduces the fraction of iron absorbed (*45–48*). This inhibition is not solely explained by the high phytate content of soya. However, because of the high iron content of soya, the net effect on iron absorption with an addition of soya products to a meal is usually positive. In infant foods containing soya, the inhibiting effect can be overcome by the addition of sufficient amounts of ascorbic acid. Conversely, some fermented soy sauces have been found to enhance iron absorption (*49, 50*).

13.2.6 Enhancement of iron absorption

Ascorbic acid is the most potent enhancer of non-haem iron absorption (*34, 51–53*). Synthetic vitamin C increases the absorption of iron to the same extent as the native ascorbic acid in fruits, vegetables, and juices. The effect of ascorbic acid on iron absorption is so marked and essential that this effect could be considered as one of vitamin C's physiological roles (*54*). Each meal should preferably contain at least 25 mg of ascorbic acid and possibly more if the meal contains many inhibitors of iron absorption. Therefore, ascorbic acid's role in iron absorption should be taken into account when establishing the requirements for vitamin C, which currently are set only to prevent vitamin C deficiency (especially scurvy). (See Chapter 7.)

Meat, fish, and seafood all promote the absorption of non-haem iron (55–58). The mechanism for this effect has not been determined. It should be pointed out that meat also enhances the absorption of haem iron to about the same extent (21). Meat thus promotes iron nutrition in two ways: it stimulates the absorption of both haem and non-haem iron and it provides the well-absorbed haem iron. Epidemiologically, the intake of meat has been found to be associated with a lower prevalence of iron deficiency.

Organic acids, such as citric acid, have been found to enhance the absorption of non-haem iron in some studies (29). This effect is not observed as consistently as is that of ascorbic acid (47, 52). Sauerkraut (59) and other fermented vegetables and even some fermented soy sauces (49, 50) enhance iron absorption. However, the nature of this enhancement has not yet been determined.

13.2.7 Iron absorption from meals

The pool concept in iron absorption implies that there are two main pools in the gastrointestinal lumen—one pool of haem iron and another pool of non-haem iron—and that iron absorption takes place independently from each pool (24). The pool concept also implies that the absorption of iron from the non-haem iron pool is a function of all the ligands present in the mixture of foods included in a meal. The absorption of non-haem iron from a certain meal not only depends on its iron content but also, and to a marked degree, on the composition of the meal (i.e. the balance among all factors enhancing and inhibiting the absorption of iron). The bioavailability can vary more than 10-fold in meals with similar contents of iron, energy, protein, and fat (20). The simple addition of certain spices (e.g. oregano) to a meal or the intake of a cup of tea with a meal may reduce the bioavailability by one half or more. Conversely, the addition of certain vegetables or fruits containing ascorbic acid may double or even triple iron absorption, depending on the other properties of the meal and the amounts of ascorbic acid present.

13.2.8 Iron absorption from the whole diet

There is limited information about the total amount of iron absorbed from the diet because no simple method for measuring iron absorption from the whole diet has been available. Traditionally, it has been measured by chemical balance methods using long balance periods or by determining the haemoglobin regeneration rate in subjects with induced iron deficiency anaemia and a well-controlled diet over a long period of time.

More recently, however, new techniques, based on radioiron tracers, have been developed to measure iron absorption from the whole diet. In the first studies of this type to be conducted, all non-haem iron in all meals over periods of 5–10 days was homogeneously labelled to the same specific activity with an extrinsic inorganic radioiron tracer (43, 60). Haem iron absorption was then estimated. In a further study, haem and non-haem iron were separately labelled with two radioiron tracers as biosynthetically labelled haemoglobin and as an inorganic iron salt (22). These studies showed that new information could be obtained, for example, about the average bioavailability of dietary iron in different types of diets, the overall effects of certain factors (e.g. calcium) on iron nutrition, and the regulation of iron absorption in relation to iron status. Iron absorption from the whole diet has been extrapolated from the sum of the absorption of iron from the single meals included in the diet. However, it has been suggested that the iron absorption of single meals may exaggerate the absorption of iron from the whole diet (61, 62), as there is a large variation of absorption between meals. Despite this, studies where all meals in a diet are labelled to the same specific activity (the same amount of radioactivity in each meal per unit iron) show that the sum of iron absorption from a great number of single meals agrees with the total absorption from the diet. One study showed that iron absorption from a single meal was the same when the meal was served in the morning after an overnight fast or at lunch or supper (63). The same observation was made in another study when a hamburger meal was served in the morning or 2–4 hours after a breakfast (42).

Because the sum of energy expenditure and intake set the limit for the amount of food eaten and for meal size, it is practical to relate the bioavailability of iron in different meals to energy content (i.e. the bioavailable nutrient density). The use of the concept of bioavailable nutrient density is a feasible way to compare bioavailability of iron in different meals, construct menus, and calculate recommended intakes of iron (64).

Intake of energy and essential nutrients such as iron was probably considerably higher for early humans than it is today (65–67). The fact that low iron intake is associated with a low-energy lifestyle implies that the interaction between different factors influencing iron absorption, will be more critical. For example, the interaction between calcium and iron absorption probably had no importance in the nutrition of early humans, who had a diet with ample amounts of both iron and calcium.

13.2.9 Iron balance and regulation of iron absorption

The body has three unique mechanisms for maintaining iron balance. The first is the continuous reutilization of iron from catabolized erythrocytes in the body. When an erythrocyte dies after about 120 days, it is usually degraded by the macrophages of the reticular endothelium. The iron is released and delivered to transferrin in the plasma, which brings the iron back to red blood cell precursors in the bone marrow or to other cells in different tissues. Uptake and distribution of iron in the body is regulated by the synthesis of transferrin receptors on the cell surface. This system for internal iron transport not only controls the rate of flow of iron to different tissues according to their needs, but also effectively prevents the appearance of free iron and the formation of free radicals in the circulation.

The second mechanism involves access to the specific storage protein, ferritin. This protein stores iron in periods of relatively low need and releases it to meet excessive iron demands. This iron reservoir is especially important in the third trimester of pregnancy.

The third mechanism involves the regulation of absorption of iron from the intestines; decreasing body iron stores trigger increased iron absorption and increasing iron stores trigger decreased iron absorption. Iron absorption decreases until equilibrium is established between absorption and requirement. For a given diet this regulation of iron absorption, however, can only balance losses up to a certain critical point beyond which iron deficiency will develop (68). About half of the basal iron losses are from blood and occur primarily in the gastrointestinal tract. Both these losses and the menstrual iron losses are influenced by the haemoglobin level; during the development of an iron deficiency, menstrual and basal iron losses will successively decrease when the haemoglobin level decreases. In a state of more severe iron deficiency, skin iron losses may also decrease. Iron balance (absorption equals losses) may be present not only in normal subjects but also during iron deficiency and iron overload.

The three main factors that affect iron balance are absorption (intake and bioavailability of iron), losses, and stored amount. The interrelationship among these factors has recently been described in mathematical terms, making it possible to predict, for example, the amount of stored iron when iron losses and bioavailability of dietary iron are known (69). In states of increased iron requirement or decreased bioavailability, the regulatory capacity to prevent iron deficiency is limited (68). However, the regulatory capacity seems to be extremely good in preventing iron overload in a state of increased dietary iron intake or bioavailability (69).

13.3 Iron deficiency
13.3.1 Populations at risk for iron deficiency

Populations most at risk for iron deficiency are infants, children, adolescents, and women of childbearing age, especially pregnant women. The weaning period in infants is especially critical because of the very high iron requirement needed in relation to energy requirement (see section 13.2.2). Thanks to better information about iron deficiency and the addition of fortified cereals to the diets of infants and children, the iron situation has markedly improved in these groups in most developed countries, such that the groups currently considered to be most at risk are menstruating and pregnant women, and adolescents of both sexes. In developing countries, however, the iron situation is still very critical in many groups—especially in infants in the weaning period. During this period, iron nutrition is of great importance for the adequate development of the brain and other tissues such as muscles, which are differentiated early in life.

Iron deficiency and iron deficiency anaemia are often incorrectly used as synonyms. A definition of these terms may clarify some of the confusion about different prevalence figures given in the literature (70). Iron deficiency is defined as a haemoglobin concentration below the optimum value in an *individual*, whereas iron deficiency anaemia implies that the haemoglobin concentration is below the 95th percentile of the distribution of haemoglobin concentration in a *population* (disregarding effects of altitude, age and sex, etc. on haemoglobin concentration). The confusion arises due to the very wide distribution of the haemoglobin concentration in healthy, fully iron-replete subjects (in women, 120–160 g/l; in men, 140–180 g/l) (71). During the development of a negative iron balance in subjects with no mobilizable iron from iron stores (i.e. no visible iron in technically perfect bone marrow smears or a serum ferritin concentration <15 μg/l), there will be an immediate impairment in the production of haemoglobin with a resulting decrease in haemoglobin and different erythrocyte indexes (e.g. mean corpuscular haemoglobin and mean corpuscular volume). In turn, this will lead to an overlap in the distributions of haemoglobin in iron-deficient and iron-replete women (Figure 13.4). The extent of overlap depends on the prevalence and severity of iron deficiency. In populations with more severe iron deficiency, for example, the overlap is much less marked.

In women, anaemia is defined as a haemoglobin level <120 g/l. For a woman who has her normal homeostatic value set at 150 g/l, her haemoglobin level must decrease by 26% to 119 g/l before she is considered to be anaemic, whereas for a woman who has her normal haemoglobin set at 121 g/l, her haemoglobin level must only decrease by 1.5% to 119 g/l. Iron

FIGURE 13.4

Distribution of haemoglobin concentration in a sample of 38-year-old women with and without stainable bone marrow iron

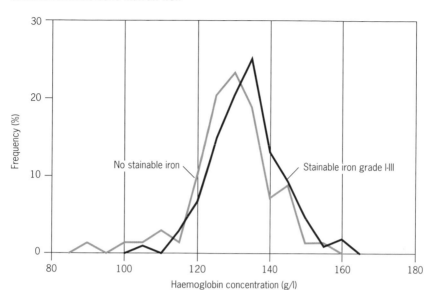

The main fraction (91%) of the iron-deficient women in this sample had haemoglobin levels above the lowest normal level for the population: 120 g/l (mean ± 2 SD). The degree of overlap of the two distributions depends on the severity of anaemia in a population.
Source: reference (*68*).

deficiency anaemia is a rather imprecise concept for evaluating the single subject and has no immediate physiological meaning. By definition, this implies that the prevalence of iron deficiency anaemia is less frequent than iron deficiency and that the presence of anaemia in a subject is a statistical rather than a functional concept. The main use of the cut-off value in defining anaemia is in comparisons between population groups (*72*). In practical work, iron deficiency anaemia should be replaced by the functional concept of iron deficiency. Anaemia per se is mainly important when it becomes so severe that oxygen delivery to tissues is impaired. An iron deficiency anaemia which develops slowly in otherwise healthy subjects with moderately heavy work output will not give any symptoms until the haemoglobin level is about 80 g/l or lower (*71*). The reason for the continued use of the concept of iron deficiency anaemia is the ease of determining haemoglobin. Therefore, in clinical practice, knowledge of previous haemoglobin values in a subject is of great importance for evaluating the diagnosis.

Iron deficiency being defined as an absence of iron stores combined with signs of an iron-deficient erythropoiesis implies that in a state of iron deficiency there is an insufficient supply of iron to various tissues. This occurs at a serum ferritin level <15 µg/l. At this point, insufficient amounts of iron will be delivered to transferrin, the circulating transport protein for iron, and the binding sites for iron on transferrin will therefore contain less and less iron. This is usually described as a reduction in transferrin saturation. When transferrin saturation drops to a certain critical level, erythrocyte precursors, which continuously need iron for the formation of haemoglobin, will get an insufficient supply of iron. At the same time, the supply of iron by transferrin to other tissues will also be impaired. Liver cells will get less iron, more transferrin will be synthesized, and the concentration of transferrin in plasma will then suddenly increase. Cells with a high turnover rate are the first ones to be affected (e.g. intestinal mucosal cells with a short lifespan). The iron–transferrin complex binds to transferrin receptors on certain cell surfaces and is then taken up by invagination of the whole complex on the cell wall. The uptake of iron seems to be related both to transferrin saturation and the number of transferrin receptors on the cell surface (73, 74). There is a marked diurnal variation in the saturation of transferrin because the turnover rate of iron in plasma is very high. This fact makes it difficult to evaluate the iron status from single determinations of transferrin saturation.

13.3.2 Indicators of iron deficiency

The absence of iron stores (iron deficiency) can be diagnosed by showing that there is no stainable iron in the reticuloendothelial cells in bone marrow smears or, more easily, by a low concentration of ferritin in serum (<15 µg/l). Even if an absence of iron stores per se may not necessarily be associated with any immediate adverse effects, it is a reliable and good indirect indicator of iron-deficient erythropoiesis and of an increased risk of a compromised supply of iron to different tissues.

Even before iron stores are completely exhausted, the supply of iron to the erythrocyte precursors in the bone marrow is compromised, leading to iron-deficient erythropoiesis (70). A possible explanation is that the rate of release of iron from stores is influenced by the amount of iron remaining. As mentioned above, it can then be assumed that the supply of iron to other tissues needing iron is also insufficient because the identical transport system is used. During the development of iron deficiency haemoglobin concentration, transferrin concentration, transferrin saturation, transferrin receptors in plasma, erythrocyte protoporphyrin, and erythrocyte indexes are changed. All these indicators, however, show a marked overlap between normal and iron-deficient subjects, which makes it impossible to identify the single subject with mild iron deficiency by looking at any single one of these indicators.

Therefore, these tests are generally used in combination (e.g. for interpreting results from the second National Health and Nutrition Examination Survey in the United States [75, 76]). By increasing the number of tests used, the diagnostic specificity then increases but the sensitivity decreases, and thus the true prevalence of iron deficiency is markedly underestimated if multiple diagnostic criteria are used. Fortunately, a low serum ferritin (<15 µg/l) is always associated with an iron-deficient erythropoiesis. The use of serum ferritin alone as a measure will also underestimate the true prevalence of iron deficiency but to a lesser degree than when the combined criteria are used.

A diagnosis of iron deficiency anaemia can be suspected if anaemia is present in subjects who are iron-deficient as described above. Preferably, to fully establish the diagnosis, the subjects should respond adequately to iron treatment. The pitfalls with this method are the random variation in haemoglobin concentrations over time and the effect of the regression towards the mean when a new measurement is made.

The use of serum ferritin has improved the diagnostic accuracy of iron deficiency. It is the only simple method available to detect early iron deficiency. Its practical value is somewhat reduced, however, by the fact that serum ferritin is a very sensitive acute-phase reactant and may be increased for weeks after a simple infection with fever for a day or two (77). Several other conditions, such as use of alcohol (78, 79), liver disease, and collagen diseases, may also increase serum ferritin concentrations. Determination of transferrin receptors in plasma has also been recommended in the diagnosis of iron deficiency. The advantage of this procedure is that it is not influenced by infections. Its main use is in subjects who are already anaemic and it is not sensitive enough for the early diagnosis of iron deficiency. The use of a combination of determinations of serum ferritin and serum transferrin receptors has also been suggested (80).

13.3.3 Causes of iron deficiency

Nutritional iron deficiency implies that the diet cannot supply enough iron to cover the body's physiological requirements for this mineral. Worldwide this is the most common cause of iron deficiency. In many tropical countries, infestations with hookworms lead to intestinal blood losses that in some individuals can be considerable. The average blood loss can be reliably estimated by egg counts in stools. Usually the diet in these populations is also limited with respect to iron content and availability. The severity of the infestations varies markedly between subjects and regions.

In clinical practice, a diagnosis of iron deficiency must always lead to a search for pathologic causes of blood loss (e.g. tumours in the gastrointestinal tract or uterus, especially if uterine bleedings have increased or changed in regularity). Patients with achlorhydria absorb dietary iron less well (a reduction of about 50%) than healthy individuals, and patients who have undergone gastric surgery, especially if the surgery was extensive, may eventually develop iron deficiency because of impaired iron absorption. Gluten enteropathy is another possibility to consider, especially in young patients.

13.3.4 Prevalence of iron deficiency

Iron deficiency is probably the most common nutritional deficiency disorder in the world. A recent estimate based on WHO criteria indicated that around 600–700 million people worldwide have marked iron deficiency anaemia (*81*), and the bulk of these people live in developing countries. In developed countries, the prevalence of iron deficiency anaemia is much lower and usually varies between 2% and 8%. However, the prevalence of iron deficiency, including both anaemic and non-anaemic subjects (see definitions above), is much higher. In developed countries, for example, an absence of iron stores or subnormal serum ferritin values is found in about 20–30% of women of fertile age. In adolescent girls, the prevalence is even higher.

It is difficult to determine the prevalence of iron deficiency more exactly because representative populations for clinical investigation are hard to obtain. Laboratory methods and techniques for blood sampling need careful standardization. One often neglected source of error (e.g. when samples from different regions, or samples taken at different times, are compared) comes from the use of reagent kits for determining serum ferritin that are not adequately calibrated to international WHO standards. In addition, seasonal variations in infection rates influence the sensitivity and specificity of most methods used.

Worldwide, the highest prevalence figures for iron deficiency are found in infants, children, adolescents, and women of childbearing age. Both better information about iron deficiency prevention and increased consumption of fortified cereals by infants and children have markedly improved the iron situation in these groups in most developed countries, such that, the highest prevalence of iron deficiency today is observed in menstruating and pregnant women, and adolescents of both sexes.

In developing countries, where the prevalence of iron deficiency is very high and the severity of anaemia is marked, studies on the distribution of haemoglobin in different population groups can provide important information that can then be used as a basis for action programmes (*72*). A more detailed analysis of subsamples may then give excellent information for the planning of more extensive programmes.

13.3.5 Effects of iron deficiency

Studies in animals have clearly shown that iron deficiency has several negative effects on important functions in the body (3). The physical working capacity of rats is significantly reduced in states of iron deficiency, especially during endurance activities (82, 83). This negative effect seems to be less related to the degree of anaemia than to impaired oxidative metabolism in the muscles with an increased formation of lactic acid. Thus, the effect witnessed seems to be due to a lack of iron-containing enzymes which are rate limiting for oxidative metabolism (84). Further to this, several groups have observed a reduction in physical working capacity in human populations with long-standing iron deficiency, and demonstrated an improvement in working capacity in these populations after iron administration (84).

The relationship between iron deficiency and brain function and development is very important to consider when choosing a strategy to combat iron deficiency (85–88). Several structures in the brain have a high iron content; levels are of the same order of magnitude as those observed in the liver. The observation that the lower iron content of the brain in iron-deficient growing rats cannot be increased by giving iron at a later date strongly suggests that the supply of iron to brain cells takes place during an early phase of brain development and that, as such, early iron deficiency may lead to irreparable damage to brain cells. In humans about 10% of brain-iron is present at birth; at the age of 10 years the brain has only reached half its normal iron content, and optimal amounts are first reached between the ages of 20 and 30 years.

Iron deficiency also negatively influences the normal defence systems against infections. In animal studies, the cell-mediated immunologic response by the action of T-lymphocytes is impaired as a result of a reduced formation of these cells. This in turn is due to a reduced DNA synthesis dependent on the function of ribonucleotide reductase, which requires a continuous supply of iron for its function. In addition, the phagocytosis and killing of bacteria by the neutrophil leukocytes is an important component of the defence mechanism against infections. These functions are impaired in iron deficiency as well. The killing function is based on the formation of free hydroxyl radicals within the leukocytes, the respiratory burst, and results from the activation of the iron-sulfur enzyme NADPH oxidase and probably also cytochrome b (a haem enzyme) (89).

The impairment of the immunologic defence against infections that was found in animals is also regularly found in humans. Administration of iron normalizes these changes within 4–7 days. It has been difficult to demonstrate, however, that the prevalence of infections is higher or that their severity is more marked in iron-deficient subjects than in control subjects. This may well be ascribed to the difficulty in studying this problem with an adequate experimental design.

Several groups have demonstrated a relationship between iron deficiency and attention, memory, and learning in infants and small children. In the most recent well-controlled studies, no effect was noted from the administration of iron. This finding is consistent with the observations in animals. Therapy-resistant behavioural impairment and the fact that there is an accumulation of iron during the whole period of brain growth should be considered strong arguments for the early detection and treatment of iron deficiency. This is valid for women, especially during pregnancy, and for infants and children, up through the period of adolescence to adulthood. In a recent well-controlled study, administration of iron to non-anaemic but iron-deficient adolescent girls improved verbal learning and memory (90).

Well-controlled studies in adolescent girls show that iron-deficiency without anaemia is associated with reduced physical endurance (91) and changes in mood and ability to concentrate (92). Another recent study showed that there was a reduction in maximum oxygen consumption in non-anaemic women with iron deficiency that was unrelated to a decreased oxygen-transport capacity of the blood (93).

13.4 Iron requirements during pregnancy and lactation

Iron requirements during pregnancy are well established (Table 13.2). Most of the iron required during pregnancy is used to increase the haemoglobin mass of the mother; this increase occurs in all healthy pregnant women who

TABLE 13.2
Iron requirements during pregnancy

	Iron requirements (mg)
Iron requirements during pregnancy	
Fetus	300
Placenta	50
Expansion of maternal erythrocyte mass	450
Basal iron losses	240
Total iron requirement	**1040**
Net iron balance after delivery	
Contraction of maternal erythrocyte mass	+450
Maternal blood loss	−250
Net iron balance	**+200**
Net iron requirements for pregnancy[a]	**840**

[a] Assuming sufficient material iron stores are present.

have sufficiently large iron stores or who are adequately supplemented with iron. The increased haemoglobin mass is directly proportional to the increased need for oxygen transport during pregnancy and is one of the important physiological adaptations that occurs in pregnancy (94, 95). A major problem in maintaining iron balance in pregnancy is that iron requirements are not equally distributed over its duration. The exponential growth of the fetus in the last trimester of pregnancy means that more than 80% of fetal iron needs relate to this period. The total daily iron requirements, including the basal iron losses (0.8 mg), increase during pregnancy from 0.8 mg to about 10 mg during the last 6 weeks of pregnancy.

In lactating women, the daily iron loss in milk is about 0.3 mg. Together with the basal iron losses of 0.8 mg, the total iron requirements during the lactation period amount to 1.1 mg/day.

Iron absorption during pregnancy is determined by the amount of iron in the diet, its bioavailability (meal composition), and the changes in iron absorption that occur during pregnancy. There are marked changes in the fraction of iron absorbed during pregnancy. In the first trimester, there is a marked, somewhat paradoxical, decrease in the absorption of iron, which is closely related to the reduction in iron requirements during this period as compared with the non-pregnant state (see below). In the second trimester, iron absorption is increased by about 50%, and in the last trimester it may increase by up to about four times the norm. Even considering the marked increase in iron absorption, it is impossible for the mother to cover her iron requirements from diet alone, even if her diet's iron content and bioavailability are very high. In diets prevailing in most developed countries, there will be a deficit of about 400–500 mg in the amount of iron absorbed versus required during pregnancy (Figure 13.5).

An adequate iron balance can be achieved if iron stores of 500 mg are available during the second and third trimesters. However, it is uncommon for women today to have iron stores of this size. It is therefore recommended that iron supplements in tablet form, preferably together with folic acid, be given to all pregnant women because of the difficulties in correctly evaluating iron status in pregnancy with routine laboratory methods. In the non-anaemic pregnant woman, daily supplements of 100 mg of iron (e.g. as ferrous sulphate) given during the second half of pregnancy are adequate. In anaemic women, higher doses are usually required.

During the birth process, the average blood loss corresponds to about 250 mg iron. At the same time, however, the haemoglobin mass of the mother gradually normalizes, which implies that about 200 mg iron from the expanded haemoglobin mass (150–250 mg) is returned to the mother. To cover

FIGURE 13.5
Daily iron requirements and daily dietary iron absorption in pregnancy

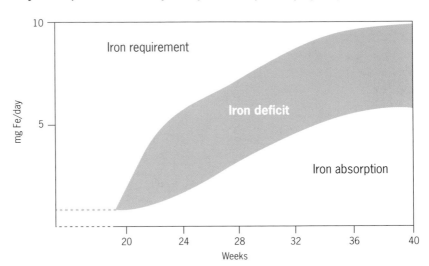

The shaded area represents the deficit of iron that has to be covered by iron from stores or iron supplementation.

the needs of a woman after pregnancy, a further 300 mg of iron must be accumulated in the iron stores in order for the woman to start her next pregnancy with about 500 mg of stored iron; such restitution is not possible with present types of diets.

There is an association between low haemoglobin values and premature birth. An extensive study (96) showed that a woman with a haematocrit of 37% had twice the risk of having a premature birth, as did a woman with a haematocrit between 41% and 44% ($P \leq 0.01$). A similar observation was reported in another extensive study in the United States (97). The subjects were examined retrospectively and the cause of the lower haematocrit was not investigated.

Early in pregnancy there are marked hormonal, haemodynamic, and haematologic changes. There is, for example, a very early increase in the plasma volume, which has been used to explain the physiological anaemia of pregnancy observed in iron-replete women. The primary cause of this phenomenon, however, is more probably an increased ability of the haemoglobin to deliver oxygen to the tissues (fetus). This change is induced early in pregnancy by increasing the content of 2,3-diphospho-D-glycerate in the erythrocytes, which shifts the haemoglobin–oxygen dissociation curve to the right. The anaemia is a consequence of this important adaptation and it is not primarily a desirable change, for example, to improve placental blood flow by reducing blood viscosity.

Another observation has similarly caused some confusion about the rationale of giving extra iron routinely in pregnancy. In extensive studies of pregnant women, a U-shaped relationship between various pregnancy complications and the haemoglobin level has been noted (i.e. there are more complications at both low and high levels). There is nothing to indicate, however, that high haemoglobin levels (within the normal non-pregnant range) per se have any negative effects. The haemoglobin increase is caused by pathologic hormonal and haemodynamic changes induced by an increased sensitivity to angiotensin II, which occurs in some pregnant women, leading to a reduction in plasma volume, hypertension, and toxaemia of pregnancy.

Pregnancy in adolescents presents a special problem because iron is needed to cover the requirements of growth for the mother and the fetus. In countries with very early marriage, a girl may get pregnant before menstruating. The combined iron requirements for growth and pregnancy are very high and the iron situation is very serious for these adolescents.

In summary, the physiological adjustments occurring in pregnancy are not sufficient to balance its very marked iron requirements, and the pregnant woman has to rely on her iron stores. In developed countries, the composition of the diet has not been adjusted to the present low-energy-demanding lifestyles found there. As a result, women in these countries have insufficient or empty iron stores during pregnancy. This is probably the main cause of the critical iron-balance situation in pregnant women in these countries today. The unnatural necessity to give extra nutrients such as iron and folate to otherwise healthy pregnant women should be considered in this perspective.

13.5 Iron supplementation and fortification

The prevention of iron deficiency has become more urgent in recent years with the accumulation of evidence strongly suggesting a relationship between even mild iron deficiency and impaired brain development, and especially so in view of the observation that functional defects affecting learning and behaviour cannot be reversed by giving iron at a later date. As mentioned, iron deficiency is common both in developed and in developing countries. Great efforts have been made by WHO to develop methods to combat iron deficiency.

Iron deficiency can generally be combated by one or more of the following three strategies: (1) iron supplementation (i.e. giving iron tablets to certain target groups such as pregnant women and preschool children); (2) iron fortification of certain foods, such as flour; and (3) food and nutrition education on improving the amount of iron absorbed from the diet by increasing the intake of iron and especially by improving the bioavailability of the dietary iron.

Several factors determine the feasibility and effectiveness of different strategies, such as the health infrastructure of a society, the economy, and access to suitable methods of iron fortification. The solutions are therefore often quite different in developing and developed countries. There is a need to obtain new knowledge about the feasibility of different methods to improve iron nutrition and to apply present knowledge in more effective ways. Further to this, initiation of local activities on the issue of iron nutrition should be stimulated while actions from governments are awaited.

13.6 Evidence used for estimating recommended nutrient intakes

To translate physiological iron requirements, given in Table 13.1, into dietary iron requirements, the bioavailability of iron in different diets must be calculated. It is also necessary to define an iron status where the supply of iron to the erythrocyte precursors and other tissues begins to be compromised. A state of iron-deficient erythropoiesis occurs when iron can no longer be mobilized from iron stores; iron can no longer be mobilized when stores are almost completely empty. A reduction then occurs, for example, in the concentration of haemoglobin and in the average content of haemoglobin in the erythrocytes (i.e. a reduction in mean corpuscular haemoglobin). At the same time the concentration of transferrin in the plasma increases because of an insufficient supply of iron to liver cells. These changes were recently shown to occur rather suddenly at a level of serum ferritin <15 μg/l (68, 70). A continued negative iron balance will further reduce the level of haemoglobin. Symptoms related to iron deficiency are less related to the haemoglobin level and more to the fact that there is a compromised supply of iron to tissues.

The bioavailability of iron in meals consumed in countries with a Western-type diet has been measured by using different methods. Numerous single-meal studies have shown absorption of non-haem iron ranging from 5% to 40% (59, 98, 99). Attempts have also been made to estimate the bioavailability of dietary iron in populations consuming Western-type diets by using indirect methods (e.g. calculation of the coverage of iron requirements in groups of subjects with known dietary intake). Such studies suggest that in borderline iron-deficient subjects, the bioavailability from healthy diets may reach a level of around 14–16% (15% relates to subjects who have a serum ferritin value of <15 μg/l or a reference dose absorption of 56.5%) (19).

New radioiron tracer techniques have enabled direct measurements of the average bioavailability of iron in different Western-type diets to be made (22, 43, 60). Expressed as total amounts of iron absorbed from the whole diet, it was found that 53.2 µg/kg/day could be absorbed daily from each of the two main meals of an experimental diet which included ample amounts of meat or fish. For a body weight of 55 kg and an iron intake of 14 mg/day, this corresponds to a bioavailability of 21% in subjects with no iron stores and an iron-deficient erythropoiesis. A diet common among women in Sweden containing smaller portions of meat and fish, higher amounts of phytate-containing foods, and some vegetarian meals each week was found to have a bioavailability of 12%. Reducing the intake of meat and fish further reduced the bioavailability to about 10% (25 µg Fe/kg/day).

In vegetarians, the bioavailability of iron is usually low because of the absence of meat and fish and a high intake of foods containing phytates and polyphenols. A Western-type diet that includes servings of fruits and vegetables, along with meat and fish has a bioavailability of about 15%, but for the typical Western-type diet—especially among women—the bioavailability is around 12% or even 10%. In countries or for certain groups in a population with a very high meat intake, the bioavailability may be around 18%. In the more developed countries, a high bioavailability of iron from the diet is mainly associated with a high meat intake, a high intake of ascorbic acid with meals, a low intake of phytate-rich cereals, and no coffee or tea within 2 hours of the main meals (38). Table 13.3 shows examples of diets with different iron bioavailability. Table 13.4 shows the bioavailability of iron for two levels of iron intake in a 55-kg woman with no iron stores.

Iron absorption data are also available from several population groups in Africa (100), South America (101), India (102), and south-east (103–107) Asia. The bioavailability of different Indian diets, after an adjustment to a reference dose absorption of 56.5%, was 1.7–1.8% for millet-based diets, 3.5–4.0% for

TABLE 13.3
Examples of diets with different iron bioavailability

Type of diet	Bioavailability (µg/kg/day)
Very high meat in two main meals daily and high ascorbic acid (theoretical)	75.0
High meat/fish in two main meals daily	66.7
Moderate meat/fish in two main meals daily	53.2
Moderate meat/fish in two main meals daily; low phytate and calcium	42.3
Meat/fish in 60% of two main meals daily; high phytate and calcium	31.4
Low meat intake; high phytate; often one main meal	25.0
Meat/fish negligible; high phytate; high tannin and low ascorbic acid	15.0
Pre-agricultural ancestors	
Plant/animal subsistence: 65/35; *very high meat and ascorbic acid intake*	150

TABLE 13.4

Translation of bioavailability (expressed as amount of iron absorbed) into percentage absorbed for two levels of iron intake (15 and 17 mg/day)

Bioavailability (µg/kg/day)	Absorption in a 55-kg woman with no iron stores (mg/day)	Bioavailability (%)	
		15 mg/day	17 mg/day
150	8.25	55.0	48.8
75.0	4.13	27.5	24.4
66.7	3.67	24.5	21.8
53.2	2.93	19.5	17.0
42.3	2.32	15.5	13.5
31.4	1.73	11.5	10.0
25.0	1.38	9.2	8.2
15.0	0.83	5.5	4.7

wheat-based diets, and 8.3–10.3% for rice-based diets (*102*). In south-east Asia, iron absorption data has been reported from Burma and Thailand. In Burma, iron absorption from a basal rice-based meal was 1.7%; when the meal contained 15 g of fish the bioavailability of iron was 5.5%, and with 40 g of fish, it was 10.1% (*103*). In Thailand, iron absorption from a basal rice-based meal was 1.9%; adding 100 g of fresh fruit increased absorption to 4.8% and adding 80 g of lean meat increased non-haem iron absorption to 5.4% (*104*, *105*). In three other studies where basal meals included servings of vegetables rich in ascorbic acid, the absorption figures were 5.9%, 10.0%, and 10.8%, respectively (*106*). In a further study in Thailand, 60 g of fish were added to the same basal meal, which increased absorption to 21.6% (*106*). Another such study in central Thailand examined the reproducibility of dietary iron absorption measurements under optimal field conditions for 20 farmers and labourers (16 men, 4 women). The subjects had a free choice of foods (i.e. rice, vegetables, soup, a curry, and a fish dish). All foods consumed were weighed and the rice was labelled with an extrinsic radioiron tracer. The mean absorption of iron was 20.3% (adjusted to reference dose absorption of 56.5%) (*107*).

It is obvious that absorbed iron requirements need to be adjusted to different types of diets, especially in vulnerable groups. In setting recommended intakes in the 1980s FAO and WHO proposed, for didactic reasons, the use of three bioavailability levels, 5%, 10%, and 15% (*8*). In light of more recent studies discussed herein, for developing countries, it may be more realistic to use the figures of 5% and 10%. In populations consuming more Western-type diets, two levels would be appropriate—12% and 15%—depending mainly on meat intake.

The amount of dietary iron absorbed is mainly determined by the amount of body stores of iron and by the properties of the diet (iron content and bioavailability). (In anaemic subjects, the rate of erythrocyte production also influences iron absorption.) For example, in a 55-kg woman with average iron losses who consumes a diet with an iron bioavailability of 15%, the mean iron stores would be about 120 mg. Furthermore, approximately 10–15% of women consuming this diet would have no iron stores. In a 55-kg woman who consumes a diet with an iron bioavailability of 12%, iron stores would be approximately 75 mg and about 25–30% of women consuming this diet would have no iron stores. When the bioavailability of iron decreases to 10%, mean iron stores are reduced to about 25 mg, and about 40–50% of women consuming this diet would have no iron stores. Women consuming diets with an iron bioavailability of 5% have no iron stores and they are iron deficient.

13.7 Recommendations for iron intakes

The recommended nutrient intakes (RNIs) for varying dietary iron bioavailabilities are shown in Table 13.5. The RNIs are based on the 95th percentile of the absorbed iron requirements (Table 13.1). No figures are given for dietary iron requirements in pregnant women because the iron balance in pregnancy depends not only on the properties of the diet but also and especially on the amounts of stored iron.

TABLE 13.5
The recommended nutrient intakes (RNIs) for iron for different dietary iron bioavailabilities (mg/day)

Group	Age (years)	Mean body weight (kg)	Recommended nutrient intake (mg/day) for a dietary iron bioavailability of			
			15%	12%	10%	5%
Infants and	0.5–1	9	6.2[a]	7.7[a]	9.3[a]	18.6[a]
children	1–3	13	3.9	4.8	5.8	11.6
	4–6	19	4.2	5.3	6.3	12.6
	7–10	28	5.9	7.4	8.9	17.8
Males	11–14	45	9.7	12.2	14.6	29.2
	15–17	64	12.5	15.7	18.8	37.6
	18+	75	9.1	11.4	13.7	27.4
Females	11–14[b]	46	9.3	11.7	14.0	28.0
	11–14	46	21.8	27.7	32.7	65.4
	15–17	56	20.7	25.8	31.0	62.0
	18+	62	19.6	24.5	29.4	58.8
Postmenopausal		62	7.5	9.4	11.3	22.6
Lactating		62	10.0	12.5	15.0	30.0

[a] Bioavailability of dietary iron during this period varies greatly.
[b] Pre-menarche.
Source: adapted, in part, from reference (8) and in part on new calculations of the distribution of iron requirements in menstruating women. Because of the very skewed distribution of iron requirements in these women, dietary iron requirements are calculated for four levels of dietary iron bioavailability.

13.8 Recommendations for future research

The following were identified as priority areas for future research efforts:

- Acquire knowledge of the content of phytate and iron-binding polyphenols in food, condiments, and spices and produce new food tables which include such data.

- Acquire knowledge about detailed composition of common meals in different regions of the world and their usual variation in composition to examine the feasibility of making realistic recommendations about changes in meal composition, taking into consideration the effect of such changes on other nutrients (e.g. vitamin A).

- Give high priority to systematic research in the area of iron requirements. The very high iron requirements, especially in relation to energy requirements, in the weaning period make it difficult to develop appropriate diets based on recommendations that are effective and realistic. Alternatives such as home fortification of weaning foods should also be considered.

- Critically analyse the effectiveness of iron compounds used for fortification.

- Study models for improving iron supplementation—from the distribution of iron tablets to increasing the motivation of individuals to take iron supplements, especially during pregnancy.

References

1. Bothwell TH et al. *Iron metabolism in man.* London, Blackwell Scientific Publications, 1979.
2. Hallberg L. Iron absorption and iron deficiency. *Human Nutrition: Clinical Nutrition,* 1982, 36:259–278.
3. Dallman PR. Biochemical basis for the manifestations of iron deficiency. *Annual Review of Nutrition,* 1986, 6:13–40.
4. Brock JH, Halliday JW, Powell LW. *Iron metabolism in health and disease.* London, WB Saunders, 1994.
5. Kühn LC. Control of cellular iron transport and storage at the molecular level. In: Hallberg L, Asp N-G, eds. *Iron nutrition in health and disease.* London, John Libbey, 1996:17–29.
6. Mascotti DP, Rup D, Thach RE. Regulation of iron metabolism: translational effects mediated by iron, heme and cytokines. *Annual Review of Nutrition,* 1995, 15:239–261.
7. Green R et al. Body iron excretion in man. A collaborative study. *American Journal of Medicine,* 1968, 45:336–353.
8. *Requirements of vitamin A, iron, folate and vitamin B_{12}. Report of a Joint FAO/WHO Expert Consultation.* Rome, Food and Agriculture Organization of the United Nations, 1988 (FAO Food and Nutrition Series, No. 23).
9. Brune M et al. Iron losses in sweat. *American Journal of Clinical Nutrition,* 1986, 43:438–443.

10. *Nutrient and energy intakes for the European Community: a report of the Scientific Committee for Food.* Brussels, Commission of the European Communities, 1993.

11. Rossander-Hulthén L, Hallberg L. Prevalence of iron deficiency in adolescents. In: Hallberg L, Asp N-G, eds. *Iron nutrition in health and disease.* London, John Libby, 1996:149–156.

12. Dallman PR, Siimes M. Percentile curves for hemoglobin and red cell volume in infancy and childhood. *Journal of Pediatrics*, 1979, 94:26–31.

13. Tanner JM, Whitehouse RH, Takaishi M. Standards from birth to maturity for height, eight, height velocity, and weight velocity in British children, 1965, Part I. *Archives of Diseases in Childhood*, 1966, 41:454–471.

14. Tanner JM, Whitehouse RH, Takaishi M. Standards from birth to maturity for height, weight, height velocity, and weight velocity in British children, 1965, Part II. *Archives of Diseases in Childhood*, 1966, 41: 613–632.

15. Karlberg P et al. The somatic development of children in a Swedish urban community. *Acta Paediatrica Scandinavica*, 1976, 258(Suppl.):S5–S147.

16. Hallberg L et al. Menstrual blood loss—a population study. Variation at different ages and attempts to define normality. *Acta Obstetricia Gynecologica Scandinavica*, 1966, 45:320–351.

17. Rybo G-M, Hallberg L. Influence of heredity and environment on normal menstrual blood loss. A study of twins. *Acta Obstetricia Gynecologica Scandinavica*, 1966, 45:389–410.

18. Rybo G-M. Plasminogen activators in the endometrium. I. Methodological aspects. II. Clinical aspects. *Acta Obstetricia Gynecologica Scandinavica*, 1966, 45:411–450.

19. Hallberg L, Rossander-Hulthén L. Iron requirements in menstruating women. *American Journal of Clinical Nutrition*, 1991, 54:1047–1058.

20. Hallberg L. Bioavailability of dietary iron in man. *Annual Review of Nutrition*, 1981, 1:123–147.

21. Hallberg L et al. Dietary heme iron absorption. A discussion of possible mechanisms for the absorption-promoting effect of meat and for the regulation of iron absorption. *Scandinavian Journal of Gastroenterology*, 1979, 14:769–779.

22. Hallberg L, Hulthén L, Gramatkovski E. Iron absorption from the whole diet in men: how effective is the regulation of iron absorption? *American Journal of Clinical Nutrition*, 1997, 66:347–356.

23. Hallberg L et al. Inhibition of haem-iron absorption in man by calcium. *British Journal of Nutrition*, 1993, 69:533–540.

24. Hallberg L. The pool concept in food iron absorption and some of its implications. *Proceedings of the Nutrition Society*, 1974, 33:285–291.

25. Hallberg L. Factors influencing the efficacy of iron fortification and the selection of fortification vehicles. In: Clydesdale FM, Wiemer KL, eds. *Iron fortification of foods.* New York, NY, Academic Press, 1985:17–28.

26. Hallberg L, Björn-Rasmussen E. Measurement of iron absorption from meals contaminated with iron. *American Journal of Clinical Nutrition*, 1981, 34: 2808–2815.

27. Hallberg L et al. Iron absorption from some Asian meals containing contamination iron. *American Journal of Clinical Nutrition*, 1983, 37: 272–277.

28. Wollenberg P, Rummel W. Dependence of intestinal iron absorption on the

valency state of iron. *Naunyn-Schmiedeberg's Archives of Pharmacology*, 1987, 36:578–582.

29. Gillooly M et al. The effect of organic acids, phytates and polyphenols on absorption of iron from vegetables. *British Journal of Nutrition*, 1983, 49:331–342.

30. Hallberg L, Brune M, Rossander L. Iron absorption in man: ascorbic acid and dose-dependent inhibition by phytate. *American Journal of Clinical Nutrition*, 1989, 49:140–144.

31. Hallberg L, Rossander L, Skånberg A-B. Phytates and the inhibitory effect of bran on iron absorption in man. *American Journal of Clinical Nutrition*, 1987, 45:988–996.

32. Brune M et al. Iron absorption from bread in humans: inhibiting effects of cereal fiber, phytate and inositol phosphates with different numbers of phosphate groups. *Journal of Nutrition*, 1992, 122:442–449.

33. Rossander-Hulthén L, Gleerup A, Hallberg L. Inhibitory effect of oat products on non-haem iron absorption in man. *European Journal of Clinical Nutrition*, 1990, 44:783–791.

34. Siegenberg D et al. Ascorbic acid prevents the dose-dependent inhibitory effects of polyphenols and phytates on non-heme iron absorption. *American Journal of Clinical Nutrition*, 1991, 53:537–541.

35. Brune M, Rossander L, Hallberg L. Iron absorption and phenolic compounds: importance of different phenolic structures. *European Journal of Clinical Nutrition*, 1989, 43:547–558.

36. Disler PB et al. The effect of tea on iron absorption. *Gut*, 1975, 16:193–200.

37. Derman D et al. Iron absorption from a cereal-based meal containing cane sugar fortified with ascorbic acid. *British Journal of Nutrition*, 1977, 38: 261–269.

38. Morck TA, Lynch SE, Cook JD. Inhibition of food iron absorption by coffee. *American Journal of Clinical Nutrition*, 1983, 37:416–420.

39. Hallberg L, Rossander L. Effect of different drinks on the absorption of non-heme iron from composite meals. *Human Nutrition: Applied Nutrition*, 1982, 36:116–123.

40. Hallberg L et al. Calcium: effect of different amounts on nonheme- and heme-iron absorption in humans. *American Journal of Clinical Nutrition*, 1991, 53:112–119.

41. Hallberg L et al. Calcium and iron absorption: mechanism of action and nutritional importance. *European Journal of Clinical Nutrition*, 1992, 46: 317–327.

42. Gleerup A, Rossander-Hulthén L, Hallberg L. Duration of the inhibitory effect of calcium on non-haem iron absorption in man. *European Journal of Clinical Nutrition*, 1993, 47:875–879.

43. Gleerup A et al. Iron absorption from the whole diet: comparison of the effect of two different distributions of daily calcium intake. *American Journal of Clinical Nutrition*, 1995, 61:97–104.

44. Hallberg L. Does calcium interfere with iron absorption? *American Journal of Clinical Nutrition*, 1998, 68:3–4.

45. Cook JD, Morck TA, Lynch SR. The inhibitory effects of soy products on nonheme iron absorption in man. *American Journal of Clinical Nutrition*, 1981, 34:2622–2629.

46. Hallberg L, Hulthén L. Effect of soy protein on nonheme iron absorption in man. *American Journal of Clinical Nutrition*, 1982, 36:514–520.

47. Hallberg L, Rossander L. Improvement of iron nutrition in developing countries: comparison of adding meat, soy protein, ascorbic acid, citric acid, and ferrous sulphate on iron absorption from a simple Latin American-type of meal. *American Journal of Clinical Nutrition*, 1984, 39:577–583.

48. Hurrell RF et al. Soy protein, phytate, and iron absorption in humans. *American Journal of Clinical Nutrition*, 1992, 56:573–578.

49. Baynes RD et al. The promotive effect of soy sauce on iron absorption in human subjects. *European Journal of Clinical Nutrition*, 1990, 44:419–424.

50. Macfarlane BJ et al. The effect of traditional oriental soy products on iron absorption. *American Journal of Clinical Nutrition*, 1990, 51:873–880.

51. Cook JD, Monsen ER. Vitamin C, the common cold and iron absorption. *American Journal of Clinical Nutrition*, 1977, 30:235–241.

52. Hallberg L, Brune M, Rossander L. Effect of ascorbic acid on iron absorption from different types of meals. Studies with ascorbic-acid-rich foods and synthetic ascorbic acid given in different amounts with different meals. *Human Nutrition: Applied Nutrition*, 1986, 40:97–113.

53. Derman DP et al. Importance of ascorbic acid in the absorption of iron from infant foods. *Scandinavian Journal of Haematology*, 1980, 25:193–201.

54. Hallberg L, Brune M, Rossander-Hulthén L. Is there a physiological role of vitamin C in iron absorption? *Annals of the New York Academy of Sciences*, 1987, 498:324–332.

55. Layrisse M, Martinez-Torres C, Roch M. The effect of interaction of various foods on iron absorption. *American Journal of Clinical Nutrition*, 1968, 21:1175–1183.

56. Layrisse M et al. Food iron absorption: a comparison of vegetable and animal foods. *Blood*, 1969, 33:430–443.

57. Cook JD, Monson RR. Food iron absorption in human subjects. III. Comparison of the effect of animal proteins on nonheme iron absorption. *American Journal of Clinical Nutrition*, 1976, 29:859–867.

58. Björn-Rasmussen E, Hallberg L. Effect of animal proteins on the absorption of food iron in man. *Nutrition and Metabolism*, 1979, 23:192–202.

59. Hallberg L, Rossander L. Absorption of iron from Western-type lunch and dinner meals. *American Journal of Clinical Nutrition*, 1982, 35:502–509.

60. Hulthén L et al. Iron absorption from the whole diet. Relation to meal composition, iron requirements and iron stores. *European Journal of Clinical Nutrition*, 1995, 49:794–808.

61. Hallberg L, Hulthén L. Methods to study dietary iron absorption in man — an overview. In: Hallberg L, Asp N-G, eds. *Iron nutrition in health and disease*. London, John Libbey, 1996:81–95.

62. Cook JD, Dassenko SA, Lynch SR. Assessment of the role of nonheme iron availability in iron balance. *American Journal of Clinical Nutrition*, 1991, 54:717–722.

63. Taylor PG et al. Iron bioavailability from diets consumed by different socio-economic strata of the Venezuelan population. *Journal of Nutrition*, 1995, 25:1860–1868.

64. Hallberg L. Bioavailable nutrient density: a new concept applied in the interpretation of food iron absorption data. *American Journal of Clinical Nutrition*, 1981, 34:2242–2247.

65. Eaton SB, Konner M. Paleolithic nutrition: a consideration of its nature and current implications. *New England Journal of Medicine*, 1985, 312:283–289.
66. Eaton SB, Nelson DA. Calcium in evolutionary perspective. *American Journal of Clinical Nutrition*, 1991, 54(Suppl.):S281–S287.
67. Eaton SB, Eaton III SB, Konner M. Paleolithic nutrition revisited: a twelve year retrospective on its nature and implications. *European Journal of Clinical Nutrition*, 1997, 51:207–216.
68. Hallberg L et al. Iron balance in menstruating women. *European Journal of Clinical Nutrition*, 1995, 49:200–207.
69. Hallberg L, Hulthén L, Garby L. Iron stores in man in relation to diet and iron requirements. *European Journal of Clinical Nutrition*, 1998, 52:623–631.
70. Hallberg L et al. Screening for iron deficiency: an analysis based on bone-marrow examinations and serum ferritin determinations in a population sample of women. *British Journal of Haematology*, 1993, 85:787–798.
71. Wintrobe MM. *Clinical hematology*, 8th ed. Philadelphia, PA, Lea & Febiger, 1981.
72. Yip R, Stoltzfus RJ. Assessment of the prevalence and the nature of iron deficiency for populations: the utility of comparing haemoglobin distributions. In: Hallberg L, Asp N-G, eds. *Iron nutrition in health and disease*. London, John Libby, 1996, 31–38.
73. Harford JB, Röuault TA, Klausner RD. The control of cellular iron homeostasis. In: Brock JH et al., eds. *Iron metabolism in health and disease*. London, WB Saunders, 1994:123–149.
74. Baker E, Morgan EH. Iron transport. In: Brock JH et al., eds. *Iron metabolism in health and disease*. London, WB Saunders, 1994:63–95.
75. Pilch SM, Senti FRE. *Assessment of the iron nutritional status of the US population based on data collected in the second National Health and Nutrition Examination Survey, 1976–1980*. Bethesda, MD, Life Sciences Research Office, Federation of American Societies for Experimental Biology, 1984.
76. Group ESW. Summary of a report on assessment of the iron nutritional status of the United States population. *American Journal of Clinical Nutrition*, 1985, 2:1318–1330.
77. Hulthén L et al. Effect of a mild infection on serum ferritin concentration — clinical and epidemiological implications. *European Journal of Clinical Nutrition*, 1998, 52:1–4.
78. Osler M, Minman N, Heitman BL. Dietary and non-dietary factors associated with iron status in a cohort of Danish adults followed for six years. *European Journal of Clinical Nutrition*, 1998, 52:459–463.
79. Leggett BA et al. Factors affecting the concentrations of ferritin in serum in a healthy Australian population. *Clinical Chemistry*, 1990, 36:1350–1355.
80. Cook JD, Skikne B, Baynes R. The use of transferrin receptor for the assessment of iron status. In: Hallberg L, Asp N-G, eds. *Iron nutrition in health and disease*. London, John Libbey, 1996, 49–58.
81. DeMaeyer E, Adiels-Tegman M, Raystone E. The prevalence of anemia in the world. *World Health Statistics Quarterly*, 1985, 38:302–316.
82. Edgerton VR et al. Iron deficiency anemia and physical performance and activity of rats. *Journal of Nutrition*, 1972, 102:381–399.
83. Finch CA et al. Iron deficiency in the rat. Physiological and biochemical studies of muscle dysfunction. *Journal of Clinical Investigation*, 1976, 58:447–453.

84. Scrimshaw NS. Functional consequences of iron deficiency in human populations. *Journal of Nutrition Science and Vitaminology*, 1984, 30:47–63.
85. Lozoff B, Jimenez E, Wolf A. Long-term developmental outcome of infants with iron deficiency. *New England Journal of Medicine*, 1991, 325:687–694.
86. Youdim MBH. *Brain iron: neurochemical and behavioural aspects.* New York, NY, Taylor & Francis, 1988.
87. Beard JL, Connor JR, Jones BC. Iron in the brain. *Nutrition Reviews*, 1993, 1:157–170.
88. Pollitt E. Iron deficiency and cognitive function. *Annual Review of Nutrition*, 1993, 13:521–537.
89. Brock JH. Iron in infection, immunity, inflammation and neoplasia. In: Brock JH et al., eds. *Iron metabolism in health and disease.* London, WB Saunders, 1994:353–389.
90. Bruner AB et al. Randomised study of cognitive effects of iron supplementation in non-anaemic iron-deficient adolescent girls. *Lancet*, 1996, 348:992–996.
91. Rowland TW et al. The effect of iron therapy on the exercise capacity of non-anemic iron-deficient adolescent runners. *American Journal of Diseases of Children*, 1988, 142:165–169.
92. Ballin A et al. Iron state in female adolescents. *American Journal of Diseases of Children*, 1992, 146:803–805.
93. Zhu YI, Haas JD. Iron depletion without anemia and physical performance in young women. *American Journal of Clinical Nutrition*, 1997, 66:334–341.
94. Hallberg L. Iron balance in pregnancy. In: Berger H, ed. *Vitamins and minerals in pregnancy and lactation.* New York, NY, Raven Press, 1988:115–127 (Nestlé Nutrition Workshop Series, Vol. 16).
95. Hallberg L. Iron balance in pregnancy and lactation. In: Fomon SJ, Zlotkin S, eds. *Nutritional anemias.* New York, NY, Raven Press, 1992:13–25 (Nestlé Nutrition Workshop Series, Vol. 30).
96. Lieberman E et al. Association of maternal hematocrit with premature labor. *American Journal of Obstetrics and Gynecology*, 1988, 159:107–114.
97. Garn SM et al. Maternal hematological levels and pregnancy outcome. *Seminars in Perinatology*, 1981, 5:155–162.
98. Rossander L, Hallberg L, Björn-Rasmussen E. Absorption of iron from breakfast meals. *American Journal of Clinical Nutrition*, 1979, 32:2484–2489.
99. Hallberg L, Rossander L. Bioavailability of iron from Western-type whole meals. *Scandinavian Journal of Gastroenterology*, 1982, 17:151–160.
100. Galan P et al. Iron absorption from typical West African meals containing contaminating Fe. *British Journal of Nutrition*, 1990, 64:541–546.
101. Acosta A et al. Iron absorption from typical Latin American meals. *American Journal of Clinical Nutrition*, 1984, 39:953–962.
102. Rao BSN, Vijayasarathy C, Prabhavathi T. Iron absorption from habitual diets of Indians studied by the extrinsic tag technique. *Indian Journal of Medicine*, 1983, 77:648–657.
103. Aung-Than-Batu, Thein-Than, Thane-Toe. Iron absorption from Southeast Asian rice-based meals. *American Journal of Clinical Nutrition*, 1976, 29:219–225.
104. Hallberg L et al. Iron absorption from Southeast Asian diets. *American Journal of Clinical Nutrition*, 1974, 27:826–836.
105. Hallberg L et al. Iron absorption from Southeast Asian diets. II. Role of

various factors that might explain low absorption. *American Journal of Clinical Nutrition*, 1977, 30:539–548.

106. Hallberg L et al. Iron absorption from Southeast Asian diets and the effect of iron fortification. *American Journal of Clinical Nutrition*, 1978, 31:1403–1408.

107. Hallberg L, Björn-Rasmussen E, Rossander L. The measurement of food iron absorption in man. A methodological study on the measurement of dietary non-haem-Fe absorption when the subjects have a free choice of food items. *British Journal of Nutrition*, 1979, 41:283–289.

14. Vitamin B$_{12}$

14.1 Role of vitamin B$_{12}$ in human metabolic processes

Although the nutritional literature still uses the term vitamin B$_{12}$, a more specific name for vitamin B$_{12}$ is cobalamin. Vitamin B$_{12}$ is the largest of the B complex vitamins, with a relative molecular mass of over 1000. It consists of a corrin ring made up of four pyrroles with cobalt at the centre of the ring (*1, 2*).

There are several vitamin B$_{12}$-dependent enzymes in bacteria and algae, but no species of plants have the enzymes necessary for vitamin B$_{12}$ synthesis. This fact has significant implications for the dietary sources and availability of vitamin B$_{12}$. In mammalian cells, there are only two vitamin B$_{12}$-dependent enzymes (*3*). One of these enzymes, methionine synthase, uses the chemical form of the vitamin which has a methyl group attached to the cobalt and is called methylcobalamin (see Chapter 15, Figure 15.2). The other enzyme, methylmalonyl coenzyme (CoA) mutase, uses a form of vitamin B$_{12}$ that has a 5'-adeoxyadenosyl moiety attached to the cobalt and is called 5'-deoxyadenosylcobalamin, or coenzyme B$_{12}$. In nature, there are two other forms of vitamin B$_{12}$: hydroxycobalamin and aquacobalamin, where hydroxyl and water groups, respectively, are attached to the cobalt. The synthetic form of vitamin B$_{12}$ found in supplements and fortified foods is cyanocobalamin, which has cyanide attached to the cobalt. These three forms of vitamin B$_{12}$ are enzymatically activated to the methyl- or deoxyadenosylcobalamins in all mammalian cells.

14.2 Dietary sources and availability

Most microorganisms, including bacteria and algae, synthesize vitamin B$_{12}$, and they constitute the only source of the vitamin (*4*). The vitamin B$_{12}$ synthesized in microorganisms enters the human food chain through incorporation into food of animal origin. In many animals, gastrointestinal fermentation supports the growth of these vitamin B$_{12}$ synthesizing microorganisms, and subsequently the vitamin is absorbed and incorporated into the animal tissues. This is particularly true for the liver, where vitamin B$_{12}$ is stored in large concentrations. Products from herbivorous animals, such as milk, meat, and eggs, thus constitute important dietary sources of the vitamin, unless the animal is subsisting in one of the many regions known to be geochemically deficient in cobalt (5). Milk from cows and humans contains binders with very high affinity for vitamin B_{12}, though whether they hinder or promote intestinal absorption is not entirely clear. Omnivores and carnivores, including humans, derive dietary vitamin B_{12} almost exclusively from animal tissues or products (i.e. milk, butter, cheese, eggs, meat, poultry). It appears that the vitamin B_{12} required by humans is not derived from microflora in any appreciable quantities, although vegetable fermentation preparations have been reported as being possible sources of vitamin B_{12} (6).

14.3 Absorption

The absorption of vitamin B_{12} in humans is complex (1, 2). Vitamin B_{12} in food is bound to proteins and is only released by the action of a high concentration of hydrochloric acid present in the stomach. This process results in the free form of the vitamin, which is immediately bound to a mixture of glycoproteins secreted by the stomach and salivary glands. These glycoproteins, called R-binders (or haptocorrins), protect vitamin B_{12} from chemical denaturation in the stomach. The stomach's parietal cells, which secrete hydrochloric acid, also secrete a glycoprotein called intrinsic factor. Intrinsic factor binds vitamin B_{12} and ultimately enables its active absorption. Although the formation of the vitamin B_{12}–intrinsic factor complex was initially thought to happen in the stomach, it is now clear that this is not the case. At an acidic pH, the affinity of the intrinsic factor for vitamin B_{12} is low whereas its affinity for the R-binders is high. When the contents of the stomach enter the duodenum, the R-binders become partly digested by the pancreatic proteases, which in turn causes them to release their vitamin B_{12}. Because the pH in the duodenum is more neutral than that in the stomach, the intrinsic factor has a high binding affinity to vitamin B_{12}, and it quickly binds the vitamin as it is released from the R-binders. The vitamin B_{12}–intrinsic factor complex then proceeds to the lower end of the small intestine, where it is absorbed by phagocytosis by specific ileal receptors (1, 2).

14.4 Populations at risk for, and consequences of, vitamin B_{12} deficiency

14.4.1 Vegetarians

Because plants do not synthesize vitamin B_{12}, individuals who consume diets completely free of animal products (vegan diets) are at risk of vitamin B_{12} deficiency. This is not true of lacto-ovo vegetarians, who consume the vitamin in eggs, milk, and other dairy products.

14.4.2 Pernicious anaemia

Malabsorption of vitamin B$_{12}$ can occur at several points during digestion (*1*, *4*). By far the most important condition resulting in vitamin B$_{12}$ malabsorption is the autoimmune disease called pernicious anaemia (PA). In most cases of PA, antibodies are produced against the parietal cells causing them to atrophy, and lose their ability to produce intrinsic factor and secrete hydrochloric acid. In some forms of PA, the parietal cells remain intact but autoantibodies are produced against the intrinsic factor itself and attach to it, thus preventing it from binding vitamin B$_{12}$. In another less common form of PA, the antibodies allow vitamin B$_{12}$ to bind to the intrinsic factor but prevent the absorption of the intrinsic factor–vitamin B$_{12}$ complex by the ileal receptors. As is the case with most autoimmune diseases, the incidence of PA increases markedly with age. In most ethnic groups, it is virtually unknown to occur before the age of 50, with a progressive rise in incidence thereafter (*4*). However, African American populations are known to have an earlier age of presentation (*4*). In addition to causing malabsorption of dietary vitamin B$_{12}$, PA also results in an inability to reabsorb the vitamin B$_{12}$ which is secreted in the bile. Biliary secretion of vitamin B$_{12}$ is estimated to be between 0.3 and 0.5 µg/day. Interruption of this so-called enterohepatic circulation of vitamin B$_{12}$ causes the body to go into a significant negative balance for the vitamin. Although the body typically has sufficient vitamin B$_{12}$ stores to last 3–5 years, once PA has been established, the lack of absorption of new vitamin B$_{12}$ is compounded by the loss of the vitamin because of negative balance. When the stores have been depleted, the final stages of deficiency are often quite rapid, resulting in death in a period of months if left untreated.

14.4.3 Atrophic gastritis

Historically, PA was considered to be the major cause of vitamin B$_{12}$ deficiency, but it was a fairly rare condition, perhaps affecting between one and a few per cent of elderly populations. More recently, it has been suggested that a far more common problem is that of hypochlorhydria associated with atrophic gastritis, where there is a progressive reduction with age of the ability of the parietal cells to secrete hydrochloric acid (*7*). It is claimed that perhaps up to one quarter of elderly subjects could have various degrees of hypochlorhydria as a result of atrophic gastritis. It has also been suggested that bacterial overgrowth in the stomach and intestine in individuals suffering from atrophic gastritis may also reduce vitamin B$_{12}$ absorption. The absence of acid in the stomach is postulated to prevent the release of protein-bound vitamin B_{12} contained in food but not to interfere with the absorption of the free vitamin B_{12} found in fortified foods or supplements. Atrophic gastritis does not prevent the reabsorption of biliary vitamin B_{12} and therefore does not result in the negative balance seen in individuals with PA. Nonetheless, it is agreed that with time, a reduction in the amount of vitamin B_{12} absorbed from the diet will eventually deplete vitamin B_{12} stores, resulting in overt deficiency.

When considering recommended nutrient intakes (RNIs) for vitamin B_{12} for the elderly, it is important to take into account the absorption of vitamin B_{12} from sources such as fortified foods or supplements as compared with dietary vitamin B_{12}. In the latter instances, it is clear that absorption of intakes of less than 1.5–2.0 µg/day is complete—that is, for daily intakes of less than 1.5–2.0 µg of free vitamin B_{12}, the intrinsic factor-mediated system absorbs that entire amount. It is probable that this is also true of vitamin B_{12} in fortified foods, although this has not been specifically examined. However, absorption of food-bound vitamin B_{12} has been reported to vary from 9% to 60% depending on the study and the source of the vitamin, which is perhaps related to its incomplete release from food (8). This has led many to estimate absorption as being up to 50% to correct for the bioavailability of vitamin B_{12} from food.

14.5 Vitamin B_{12} interaction with folate or folic acid

One of the vitamin B_{12}-dependent enzymes, methionine synthase, functions in one of the two folate cycles, namely, the methylation cycle (see Chapter 15). This cycle is necessary to maintain availability of the methyl donor, S-adenosylmethionine. Interruption of the cycle reduces the level of S-adenosylmethionine. This occurs in PA and other causes of vitamin B_{12} deficiency, producing as a result demyelination of the peripheral nerves and the spinal column, giving rise to the clinical condition called subacute combined degeneration (1, 2). This neuropathy is one of the main presenting conditions in PA. The other principal presenting condition in PA is a megaloblastic anaemia morphologically identical to that seen in folate deficiency. Disruption of the methylation cycle also causes a lack of DNA biosynthesis and anaemia.

The methyl trap hypothesis is based on the fact that once the cofactor 5,10-methylenetetrahydrofolate is reduced by its reductase to form 5-methyltetrahydrofolate, the reverse reaction cannot occur. This suggests that the only way for the 5-methyltetrahydrofolate to be recycled to tetrahydrofolate, and thus to participate in DNA biosynthesis and cell division, is through the vitamin B_{12}-dependent enzyme methionine synthase. When the activity of this synthase is compromised, as it would be in PA, the cellular folate will become progressively trapped as 5-methyltetrahydrofolate (see Chapter 15, Figure 15.2). This will result in a cellular pseudo-folate deficiency where, despite adequate amounts of folate, anaemia will develop, which is identical to that seen in true folate deficiency. Clinical symptoms of PA, therefore, include neuropathy, anaemia, or both. Treatment with vitamin B$_{12}$, if given intramuscularly, will reactivate methionine synthase, allowing myelination to restart. The trapped folate will be released and DNA synthesis and generation of red cells will cure the anaemia. Treatment with high concentrations of folic acid will treat the anaemia but not the neuropathy of PA. It should be stressed that the so-called "masking" of the anaemia of PA is generally agreed not to occur at concentrations of folate found in food or at intakes of the synthetic form of folic acid at usual RNI levels of 200 or 400µg/day (1). However, there is some evidence that amounts less than 400µg may cause a haematologic response and thus potentially treat the anaemia (9). The masking of the anaemia definitely occurs at high concentrations of folic acid (>1000µg/day). This becomes a concern when considering fortification with synthetic folic acid of a dietary staple such as flour (see Chapter 15).

In humans, the vitamin B$_{12}$-dependent enzyme methylmalonyl CoA mutase functions both in the metabolism of propionate and certain amino acids—converting them into succinyl CoA—and in the subsequent metabolism of these amino acids via the citric acid cycle. It is clear that in vitamin B$_{12}$ deficiency the activity of the mutase is compromised, resulting in high plasma or urine concentrations of methylmalonic acid (MMA), a degradation product of methylmalonyl CoA mutase. In adults, this mutase does not appear to have any vital function, but it clearly has an important role during embryonic life and in early development. Children deficient in this enzyme, through rare genetic mutations, suffer from mental retardation and other developmental defects.

14.6 Criteria for assessing vitamin B$_{12}$ status

Traditionally it was thought that low vitamin B$_{12}$ status was accompanied by a low serum or plasma vitamin B$_{12}$ level (4). Recently, Lindenbaum et al. (10) challenged this assumption, by suggesting that a proportion of people with normal serum and plasma vitamin B$_{12}$ levels are in fact vitamin B$_{12}$ deficient. They also suggested that elevation of plasma homocysteine and plasma MMA are more sensitive indicators of vitamin B$_{12}$ status. Although plasma homocysteine can also be elevated because of folate or vitamin B$_6$ deficiency, elevation of MMA apparently always occurs with poor vitamin B$_{12}$ status. However, there may be other reasons why MMA is elevated, such as renal insufficiency, so the elevation of MMA, in itself, is not diagnostic. Thus, low serum or plasma levels of vitamin B_{12} should be the first indication of poor status and this could be confirmed by an elevated MMA if this assay was available.

14.7 Recommendations for vitamin B₁₂ intakes

The Food and Nutrition Board of the National Academy of Sciences (NAS) Institute of Medicine (8) has recently conducted an exhaustive review of the evidence regarding vitamin B_{12} intake, status, and health implications for all age groups, including the periods of pregnancy and lactation. This review has lead to calculations of what they have called an estimated average requirement (EAR), which is defined by NAS as "the daily intake value that is estimated to meet the requirement, as defined by the specific indicator of adequacy, in half of the individuals in a life-stage or gender group" (8). The NAS then estimated a recommended dietary allowance (RDA) for vitamin B_{12}, as this daily intake value plus 2 standard deviations (SDs).

Some members of the present FAO/WHO Consultation were involved in the preparation and review of the NAS recommendations and judge them to be the best estimates currently available. The FAO/WHO Consultation thus felt it appropriate to adopt the same approach used by the NAS in deriving the RNIs for vitamin B_{12}. Therefore, the EARs given in Table 14.1 are the same as those proposed by the NAS, and the RNIs (which are equivalent to

TABLE 14.1
Estimated average requirements (EARs) and recommended nutrient intakes (RNIs) for vitamin B₁₂, by group

Group	EAR (µg/day)	RNI (µg/day)
Infants and children		
0–6 months	0.3	0.4
7–12 months	0.6	0.7
1–3 years	0.7	0.9
4–6 years	1.0	1.2
7–9 years	1.5	1.8
Adolescents		
10–18 years	2.0	2.4
Adults		
19–65 years	2.0	2.4
65+ years	2.0	2.4
Pregnant women	2.2	2.6
Lactating women	2.4	2.8

Source: adapted from reference (8).

the RDAs used by the NAS) calculated as the EAR plus 2 SD. Supporting evidence for the recommendations for each age group is summarized below.

14.7.1 Infants

As with other nutrients, the principal way to determine requirements of infants is to examine the levels in milk from mothers on adequate diets. There is a wide difference in the vitamin B$_{12}$ values reported in human milk because of differences in methodology. The previous FAO/WHO Expert Consultation (11) based their recommendations on milk vitamin B$_{12}$ values of normal women of about 0.4μg/l. For an average milk production of 0.75l/day, the vitamin B$_{12}$ intake by infants would be 0.3μg/day (12). Other studies have reported concentrations of vitamin B$_{12}$ in human milk in the range 0.4–0.8μg/l (13–17). Although daily intakes ranging from 0.02 to 0.05μg/day have been found to prevent deficiency (18, 19), these intakes are totally inadequate for long-term health. Thus, based on the assumption that human milk contains enough vitamin B$_{12}$ for optimum health, an EAR between 0.3 and 0.6μg/day seems reasonable giving an RNI of between 0.4 and 0.7μg/day. It would seem appropriate to use the lower RNI figure of 0.4μg/day for infants aged 0–6 months and the higher RNI figure of 0.7μg/day for infants aged 7–12 months (Table 14.1).

14.7.2 Children

The Food and Nutrition Board of the NAS Institute of Medicine (8) suggested the same intakes for adolescents as those for adults (see section 14.7.3) with progressive reduction of intake for younger groups.

14.7.3 Adults

Several lines of evidence point to an adult average requirement of about 2.0μg/day. The amount of intramuscular vitamin B$_{12}$ needed to maintain remission in people with PA suggests a requirement of about 1.5μg/day (10), but they would also be losing 0.3–0.5μg/day through interruption of their enterohepatic circulation. This might suggest a requirement of 0.7–1.0μg/day for those without PA. Because vitamin B$_{12}$ is not completely absorbed from food, an adjustment of 50% has to be added, giving a range of 1.4–2.0μg/day (4). Therapeutic response to dietary vitamin B$_{12}$ suggests a minimum requirement of something less than 1.0μg/day (8), which again suggests a requirement of 2.0μg/day, allowing for the conservative correction that only half of dietary vitamin B$_{12}$ is absorbed (8). Diets containing 1.8μg/day seemed to maintain adequate status but intakes lower than this resulted in subjects showing some signs of deficiency (8). Furthermore, dietary intakes of less than 1.5 μg/day were reported to be inadequate in some subjects (20).

In summary, the average requirement could be said to be 2 μg/day (8). Assuming the variability of the requirements for vitamin B_{12} is accounted for by adding 2 SDs, the RNI for adults and the elderly becomes 2.4 μg/day.

14.7.4 Pregnant women

The previous FAO/WHO Expert Consultation (11) estimated that 0.1–0.2 μg/day of vitamin B_{12} is transferred to the fetus during the last two trimesters of pregnancy. On the basis of fetal liver content from postmortem samples (21–23), there is further evidence that the fetus accumulates, on average, 0.1–0.2 μg/day of vitamin B_{12} during pregnancies of women with diets which provide adequate levels of vitamin B_{12}. It has been reported that children born to vegetarians or other women with a low vitamin B_{12} intake subsequently develop signs of clinical vitamin B_{12} deficiency such as neuropathy (13). Therefore, in order to derive an EAR for pregnant women, 0.2 μg/day of vitamin B_{12} was added to the EAR for adults, to give an EAR of 2.2 μg/day and a RNI of 2.6 μg/day during pregnancy.

14.7.5 Lactating women

It is estimated that 0.4 μg/day of vitamin B_{12} is found in the human milk of women with adequate vitamin B_{12} status (8). Therefore, an extra 0.4 μg/day of vitamin B_{12} is needed during lactation in addition to the normal adult requirement of 2.0 μg/day, giving a total EAR of 2.4 μg/day and a RNI of 2.8 μg/day during lactation.

14.8 Upper limits

The absorption of vitamin B_{12} mediated by the glycoprotein, intrinsic factor, is limited to 1.5–2.0 μg per meal because of the limited capacity of the receptors. In addition, between 1% and 3% of any particular oral administration of vitamin B_{12} is absorbed by passive diffusion. Thus, if 1000 μg vitamin B_{12} (sometimes used to treat those with PA) is taken orally, the amount absorbed would be 2.0 μg by active absorption plus up to about 30 μg by passive diffusion. Intake of 1000 μg vitamin B_{12} has never been reported to have any side-effects (8). Similar large amounts have been used in some preparations of nutritional supplements without apparent ill effects. However, there are no established benefits for such amounts. Such high intakes thus represent no benefit in those without malabsorption and should probably be avoided.

14.9 Recommendations for future research

Because they do not consume any animal products, vegans are at risk of vitamin B$_{12}$ deficiency. It is generally agreed that in some communities the only source of vitamin B$_{12}$ is from contamination of food by microorganisms. When vegans move to countries where standards of hygiene are more stringent, there is good evidence that risk of vitamin B$_{12}$ deficiency increases in adults and, particularly, in children born to and breastfed by women who are strict vegans.

As standards of hygiene improve in developing countries, there is a concern that the prevalence of vitamin B$_{12}$ deficiency might increase. This should be ascertained by estimating plasma vitamin B$_{12}$ levels, preferably in conjunction with plasma MMA levels in representative adult populations and in infants.

Further research needs include the following:

- ascertaining the contribution that fermented vegetable foods make to the vitamin B$_{12}$ status of vegan communities;
- investigating the prevalence of atrophic gastritis in developing countries to determine its extent in exacerbating vitamin B$_{12}$ deficiency.

References

1. Weir DG, Scott JM. Cobalamins physiology, dietary sources and requirements. In: Sadler M, Strain JJ, Caballero B, eds. *Encyclopedia of human nutrition. Volume 1.* San Diego, CA, Academic Press, 1998:394–401.
2. Weir DG, Scott JM. Vitamin B12. In: Shils ME et al., eds. *Modern nutrition in health and disease.* Baltimore, MA, Williams & Wilkins, 1999:447–458.
3. Scott JM, Weir DG. Folate/vitamin B$_{12}$ interrelationships. *Essays in Biochemistry*, 1994, 28:63–72.
4. Chanarin I. *The megaloblastic anaemias*, 2nd ed. Oxford, Blackwell Scientific Publications, 1979.
5. Smith RM. Cobalt. In: Mertz W, ed. *Trace elements in human and animal nutrition*, 5th ed. San Diego, CA, Academic Press, 1987:143–184.
6. van den Berg H, Dagnelie PC, van Staveren WA. Vitamin B$_{12}$ and seaweed. *Lancet*, 1988, 1:242–243.
7. Carmel R. Prevalence of undiagnosed pernicious anaemia in the elderly. *Archives of Internal Medicine*, 1996, 156:1097–1100.
8. Food and Nutrition Board. *Dietary reference intakes for thiamin, riboflavin, niacin, vitamin B$_6$, folate, vitamin B$_{12}$, pantothenic acid, biotin, and choline.* Washington, DC, National Academy Press, 1998.
9. Savage DG, Lindenbaum J. Neurological complications of acquired cobalamin deficiency: clinical aspects. In: Wickramasinghe SM, ed. *Bailliere's clinical haematology: megaloblastic anaemia.* London, Bailliere Tindall, 1995, 8:657–678.
10. Lindenbaum J et al. Diagnosis of cobalamin deficiency. II. Relative sensitivities of serum cobalamin, methylmalonic acid, and total homocysteine concentrations. *American Journal of Hematology*, 1990, 34:99–107.
11. *Requirements of vitamin A, iron, folate and vitamin B$_{12}$. Report of a Joint*

FAO/WHO Expert Consultation. Rome, Food and Agriculture Organization of the United Nations, 1988 (FAO Food and Nutrition Series, No. 23).

12. Collins RA et al. The folic acid and vitamin B_{12} content of the milk of various species. *Journal of Nutrition*, 1951, 43:313–321.

13. Specker BL et al. Vitamin B-12: low milk concentrations are related to low serum concentrations in vegetarian women and to methylmalonic aciduria in their infants. *American Journal of Clinical Nutrition*, 1990, 52:1073–1076.

14. Donangelo CM et al. Iron, zinc, folate and vitamin B_{12} nutritional status and milk composition of low-income Brazilian mothers. *European Journal of Clinical Nutrition*, 1989, 43:253–266.

15. Dagnelie PC et al. Nutrients and contaminants in human milk from mothers on macrobiotic and omnivorous diets. *European Journal of Clinical Nutrition*, 1992, 46:355–366.

16. Trugo NM, Sardinha F. Cobalamin and cobalamin-binding capacity in human milk. *Nutrition Research*, 1994, 14:22–33.

17. Ford C et al. Vitamin B_{12} levels in human milk during the first nine months of lactation. *International Journal of Vitamin and Nutrition Research*, 1996, 66:329–331.

18. Srikantia SG, Reddy V. Megaloblastic anaemia of infancy and vitamin B_{12}. *British Journal of Haematology*, 1967, 13:949–953.

19. Roberts PD et al. Vitamin B_{12} status in pregnancy among immigrants to Britain. *British Medical Journal*, 1973, 3:67–72.

20. Narayanan MM, Dawson DW, Lewis MJ. Dietary deficiency of vitamin B_{12} in association with low serum cobalamin levels in non-vegetarians. *European Journal of Haematology*, 1991, 47:115–118.

21. Baker SJ et al. Vitamin B_{12} deficiency in pregnancy and the puerperium. *British Medical Journal*, 1962, 1:1658–1661.

22. Loria A et al. Nutritional anemia. VI. Fetal hepatic storage of metabolites in the second half of pregnancy. *Journal of Pediatrics*, 1977, 91:569–573.

23. Vaz Pinto A et al. Folic acid and vitamin B_{12} determination in fetal liver. *American Journal of Clinical Nutrition*, 1975, 28:1085–1086.

15. Folate and folic acid

15.1 Role of folate and folic acid in human metabolic processes

Folates accept one-carbon units from donor molecules and pass them on via various biosynthetic reactions (1). In their reduced form cellular folates function conjugated to a polyglutamate chain. These folates are a mixture of unsubstituted polyglutamyl tetrahydrofolates and various substituted one-carbon forms of tetrahydrofolate (e.g. 10-formyl-, 5,10-methylene-, and 5-methyl-tetrahydrofolate) (Figure 15.1). The reduced forms of the vitamin, particularly the unsubstituted dihydro and tetrahydro forms, are unstable chemically. They are easily split between the C-9 and N-10 bond to yield a substituted pteridine and p-aminobenzoylglutamate, which have no biologic activity (2). Substituting a carbon group at N-5 or N-10 decreases the tendency of the molecule to split; however, the substituted forms are also susceptible to oxidative chemical rearrangements and, consequently, loss of activity (2). The folates found in food consist of a mixture of reduced folate polyglutamates.

The chemical lability of all naturally-occurring folates results in a significant loss of biochemical activity during harvesting, storage, processing, and preparation. Half or even three quarters of initial folate activity may be lost during these processes. Although natural folates rapidly lose activity in foods over periods of days or weeks, the synthetic form of this vitamin, folic acid, (e.g. in fortified foods) is almost completely stable for months or even years (2). In this form, the pteridine (2-amino-4-hydroxypteridine) ring is not reduced (Figure 15.1), rendering it very resistant to chemical oxidation. However, folic acid is reduced in cells by the enzyme dihydrofolate reductase to the dihydro and tetrahydro forms (Figure 15.2). This takes place within the intestinal mucosal cells, and 5-methyltetrahydrofolate is released into the plasma.

Natural folates found in foods are all conjugated to a polyglutamyl chain containing different numbers of glutamic acids depending on the type of food. This polyglutamyl chain is removed in the brush border of the mucosal cells

FIGURE 15.1

The chemical formula of folic acid (synthetic form) and the most important natural folates (in cells and thus in food the latter are conjugated to a polyglutamate tail)

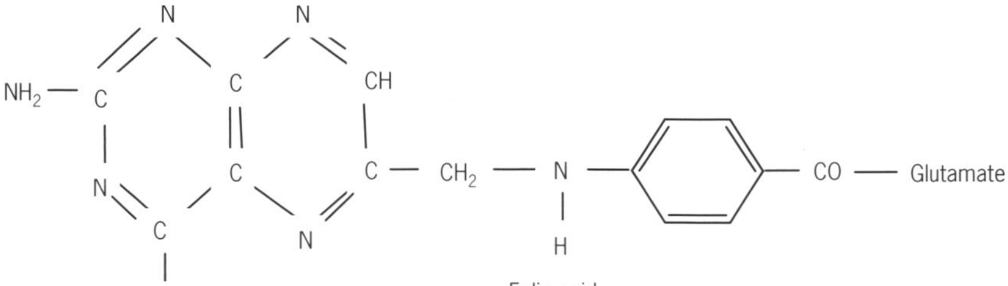

Folic acid

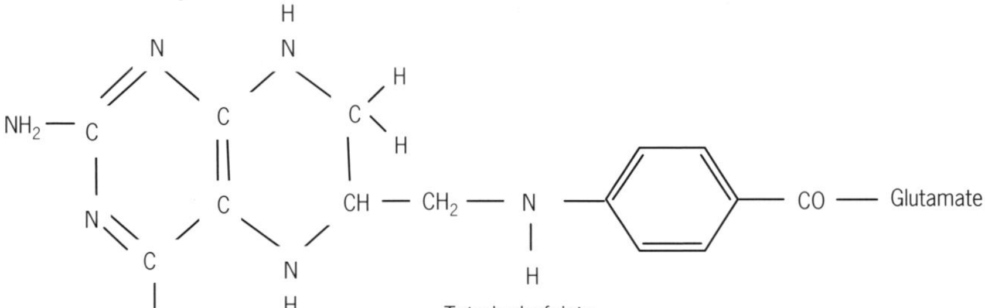

Tetrahydrofolate

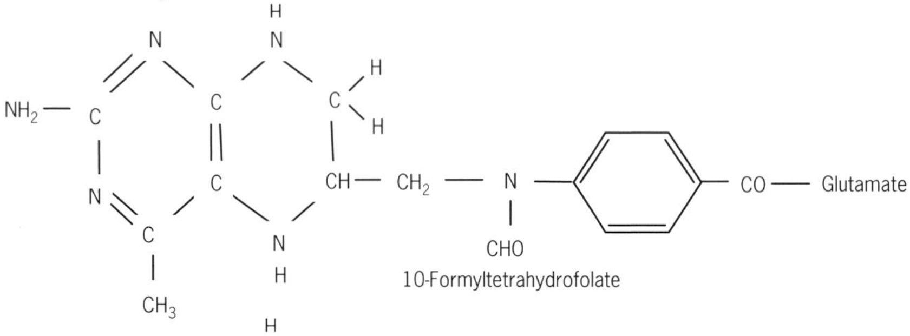

10-Formyltetrahydrofolate

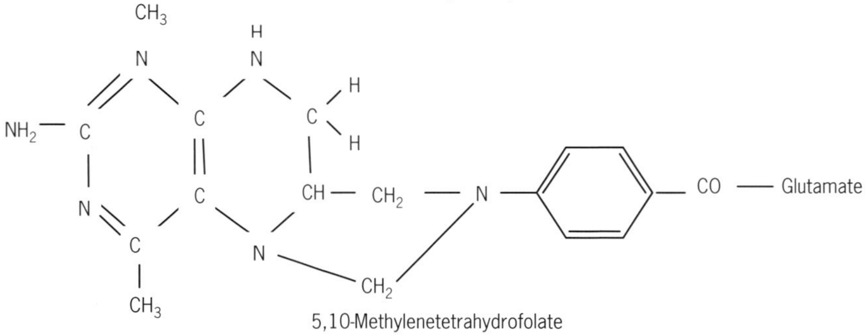

5,10-Methylenetetrahydrofolate

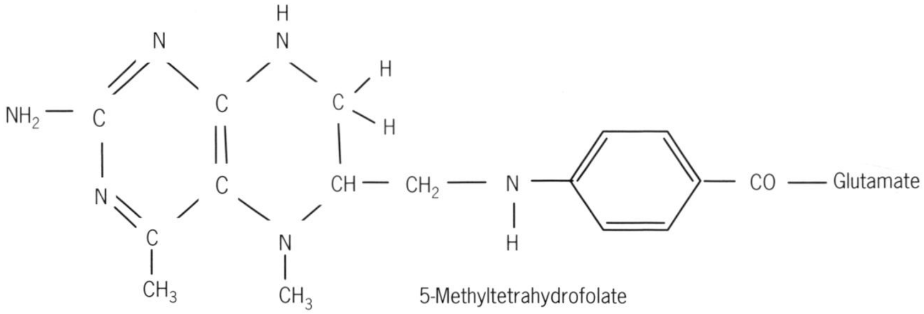

5-Methyltetrahydrofolate

FIGURE 15.2

The role of the folate cofactors in the DNA cycle and the methylation cycle (the enzyme methionine synthase requires vitamin B$_{12}$ as well as folate for activity)

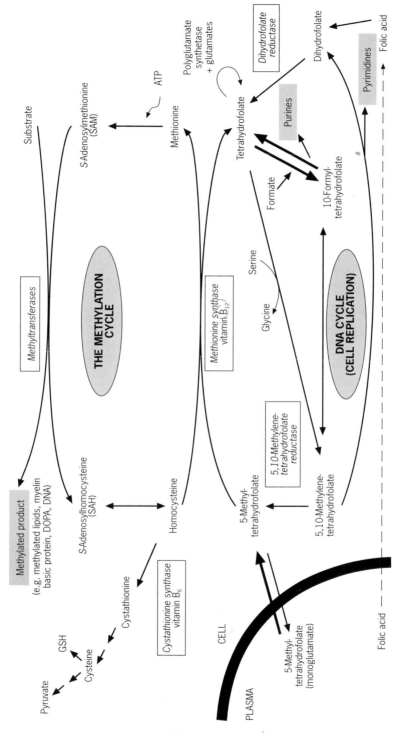

by the enzyme, folate conjugase, and folate monoglutamate is subsequently absorbed (1). The primary form of folate entering human circulation from the intestinal cells is 5-methyltetrahydrofolate monoglutamate. This process is, however, limited in capacity. If enough folic acid is given orally, unaltered folic acid appears in the circulation (3), is taken up by cells, and is reduced by dihydrofolate reductase to tetrahydrofolate.

The bioavailability of natural folates is affected by the removal of the polyglutamate chain by the intestinal conjugase. This process is apparently not complete (4), thereby reducing the bioavailability of natural folates by as much as 25–50%. In contrast, synthetic folic acid appears to be highly bioavailable—85% or greater (4, 5). The low bioavailability and, more importantly, the poor chemical stability of the natural folates have a profound influence on the development of nutrient recommendations. This is particularly true if some of the dietary intake is as the more stable and bioavailable synthetic form, folic acid. Fortification of foods such as breakfast cereals and flour can add significant amounts of folic acid to the diet.

Functional folates have one-carbon groups derived from several metabolic precursors (e.g. serine, N-formino-L-glutamate, and folate). With 10-formyltetrahydrofolate, the formyl group is incorporated sequentially into C-2 and C-8 of the purine ring during its biosynthesis. Similarly, the conversion of deoxyuridylate (a precursor to RNA) into thymidylate (a precursor to DNA) is catalysed by thymidylate synthase, which requires 5,10-methylenetetrahydrofolate. Thus, folate in its reduced and polyglutamylated forms is essential for the DNA biosynthesis cycle shown in Figure 15.2.

Alternatively, 5,10-methylenetetrahydrofolate can be channelled to the methylation cycle (Figure 15.2) (1). This cycle has two functions. It ensures that the cell always has an adequate supply of S-adenosylmethionine, an activated form of methionine which acts as a methyl donor to a wide range of methyltransferases. The methyltransferases methylate a wide range of substrates including lipids, hormones, DNA, and proteins. One particularly important methylation is that of myelin basic protein, which acts as insulation for nerve cells. When the methylation cycle is interrupted, as it is during vitamin B_{12} deficiency (see Chapter 14), one of the clinical consequences is the demyelination of nerve cells resulting in a neuropathy which leads to ataxia, paralysis, and, if untreated, ultimately death. Other important methyltransferase enzymes down-regulate DNA and suppress cell division (1).

In the liver, the methylation cycle also serves to degrade methionine. Methionine is an essential amino acid in humans and is present in the diet of people in developed countries at about 60% over that required for protein synthesis and other uses. The excess methionine is degraded via the methylation cycle to homocysteine, which can either be catabolized to sulfate and pyruvate (with the latter being used for energy) or remethylated to methionine. All cells including the liver metabolize methionine to homocysteine as part of the methylation cycle. This cycle results in converting methionine to S-adenosylmethionine, which is used as a methyl donor for the numerous methyltransferences that exist in all cells. This cycle effectively consumes methyl (-CH_3) groups and these must be replenished if the cycle is to maintain an adequate concentration of S-adenosylmethionine, and thus the methylation reactions necessary for cell metabolism and survival. These methyl groups are added to the cycle as 5-methyltetrahydrofolate, which the enzyme methionine synthase uses to remethylate homocysteine back to methionine and thus to S-adenosylmethionine (Figure 15.2).

The DNA and methylation cycles both regenerate tetrahydrofolate. However, there is a considerable amount of catabolism of folate (6) and a small loss of folate via excretion from the urine, skin, and bile. Thus, there is a need to replenish the body's folate content by uptake from the diet. If there is inadequate dietary folate, the activity of both the DNA and the methylation cycles will be reduced. A decrease in the former will reduce DNA biosynthesis and thereby reduce cell division. Although this will be seen in all dividing cells, the deficiency will be most obvious in cells that rapidly divide, including for example red blood cells, thereby producing anaemia; in cells derived from bone marrow, leading to leucopenia and thrombocytopenia; and in cells in the lining of the gastrointestinal tract. Taken together, the effects caused by the reduction in the DNA cycle result in an increased susceptibility to infection, a decrease in blood coagulation, and intestinal malabsorption. Folate deficiency will also decrease the flux through the methylation cycle but the DNA cycle may be the more sensitive. The most obvious expression of the decrease in the methylation cycle is an elevation in plasma homocysteine. This is due to a decreased availability of new methyl groups provided as 5-methyltetrahydrofolate, necessary for the remethylation of plasma homocysteine. Previously it was believed that a rise in plasma homocysteine was nothing more than a biochemical marker of possible folate deficiency. However, there is increasing evidence that elevations in plasma homocysteine are implicated in the etiology of cardiovascular disease (7). Moreover, this moderate elevation of plasma homocysteine occurs in subjects with a folate status previously considered adequate (8).

Interruption of the methylation cycle resulting from impaired folate status or decreased vitamin B_{12} or vitamin B_6 status may have serious long-term risks.

Such interruption, as seen in vitamin B_{12} deficiency (e.g. pernicious anaemia), causes a very characteristic demyelination and neuropathy known as subacute combined degeneration of the spinal cord and peripheral nerves. If untreated, this leads to ataxia, paralysis, and ultimately death (see also Chapter 14). Such neuropathy is not usually associated with folate deficiency but is seen if folate deficiency is very severe and prolonged (9). The explanation for this observation may lie in the well-established ability of nerve tissue to concentrate folate to a level of about five times that in the plasma. This may ensure that nerve tissue has an adequate level of folate when folate being provided to the rapidly dividing cells of the marrow has been severely compromised for a prolonged period. The resultant anaemia will thus inevitably present clinically earlier than the neuropathy.

15.2 Populations at risk for folate deficiency

Nutritional deficiency of folate is common in people consuming a limited diet (10). This can be exacerbated by malabsorption conditions, including coeliac disease and tropical sprue. Pregnant women are at risk for folate deficiency because pregnancy significantly increases the folate requirement, especially during periods of rapid fetal growth (i.e. in the second and third trimester) (6). During lactation, losses of folate in milk also increase the folate requirement.

During pregnancy, there is an increased risk of fetal neural tube defects (NTDs), with risk increasing 10-fold as folate status goes from adequate to poor (11). Between days 21 and 27 post-conception, the neural plate closes to form what will eventually be the spinal cord and cranium. Spina bifida, anencephaly, and other similar conditions are collectively called NTDs. They result from improper closure of the spinal cord and cranium, respectively, and are the most common congenital abnormalities associated with folate deficiency (12).

15.3 Dietary sources of folate

Although folate is found in a wide variety of foods, it is present in a relatively low density (10) except in liver. Diets that contain adequate amounts of fresh green vegetables (i.e. in excess of three servings per day) will be good folate sources. Folate losses during harvesting, storage, distribution, and cooking can be considerable. Similarly, folate derived from animal products is subject to loss during cooking. Some staples, such as white rice and unfortified corn, are low in folate (see Chapter 17).

In view of the increased requirement for folate during pregnancy and lactation and by select population groups, and in view of its low bioavailability, it may be necessary to consider fortification of foods or selected supplementation of diets of women of childbearing years.

15.4 Recommended nutrient intakes for folate

In 1988, a FAO/WHO Expert Consultation (*13*) defined three states of folate nutrition: folate adequacy, impending folate deficiency, and overt folate deficiency, and concluded that it would be appropriate to increase intake in those with impending folate deficiency, or more importantly in those with overt folate deficiency, but that nothing was to be gained by increasing the intake of those who already had an adequate status. In addition, it was suggested that adequate folate status is reflected in a red cell folate level of greater than 150 μg/l. Of less relevance was a liver folate level of greater than 7.5 μg/g, because such values only occur in rare circumstances. A normal *N*-formino-L-glutamate test was also cited as evidence of sufficiency, but this test has since been largely discredited and abandoned as not having any useful function (*10*). Red cell folate, however, continues to be used as an important index of folate status (*14*). Plasma folate is also used but is subject to greater fluctuation. Indicators of haematologic status such as raised mean corpuscular volume, hypersegmentation of neutrophils, and, eventually, the first stages of anaemia also remain important indicators of reduced folate status (*15*).

More recently, the biomarker plasma homocysteine has been identified as a very sensitive indicator of folate status and must be added to the list of possible indicators of folate adequacy (*16*). This applies not only to the deficient range of red blood cell folate but also to normal and even above-normal levels of red cell folate (*14*). There is also very strong evidence that plasma homocysteine is an independent risk factor for cardiovascular disease (*8, 17, 18*). Thus any elevation in plasma homocysteine, even at levels where overt folate deficiency is not an issue, may be undesirable because it is a risk factor for chronic disease. Formerly acceptable levels of red cell folate may moreover, be associated with an increased rise of cardiovascular disease and stroke (*18*). Thus, this new information requires the consideration of a folate intake that would reduce plasma homocysteine to a minimum level of less than 7.0 μmol/l. The possible benefit of lowering plasma homocysteine through increased folate intake can be proven only by an intervention trial with folic acid supplementation in large populations. Using plasma homocysteine as a biomarker for folate adequacy can only be done on an individual basis after the possibility of a genetic mutation or an inadequate supply of vitamin B_6 or vitamin B_{12} has been eliminated.

There is now conclusive evidence that most NTDs can be prevented by the ingestion of folic acid near the time of conception (*8, 12*). Levels of red cell folate previously considered to be in the adequate or normal range, are now associated with an increased risk of spina bifida and other NTDs (*19*). Red cell folate levels greater than 150 μg/l, which are completely adequate to prevent anaemia, are nevertheless associated with increased risk of NTDs (*11*).

In addition, low folate status has been associated with an increased risk of colorectal cancer (*20, 21*), even if such subjects were not folate deficient in the conventional clinical sense.

In 1998, the United States National Academy of Sciences (NAS) (*22*) exhaustively reviewed the evidence regarding folate intake, status, and health for all age groups, including pregnant and lactating women. On the basis of their review, the NAS calculated estimated average requirements (EARs) and recommended dietary allowances (RDAs), taken to be the EAR plus 2 standard deviations, for folate. The present Expert Consultation agreed that the values published by the NAS were the best available estimates of folate requirements based on the current literature, and thus adopted the RDAs of the NAS as the basis for their RNIs (Table 15.1). The definition of the NAS RDA accords with that of the RNI agreed by the present Consultation, that is to say the RNI is the daily intake which meets the nutrient requirements of almost all (97.5%) apparently healthy individuals in an age- and sex-specific population group (see Chapter 1).

TABLE 15.1
Estimated average requirements (EARs) and recommended nutrient intakes (RNIs) for folic acid expressed as dietary folate equivalents, by group

Group	EAR (μg/day)	RNI (μg/day)
Infants and children		
0–6 months[a]	65	80
7–12 months	65	80
1–3 years	120	150
4–6 years	160	200
7–9 years	250	300
Adolescents		
10–18 years	330	400
Adults		
19–65 years	320	400
65+ years	320	400
Pregnant women	520	600
Lactating women	450	500

[a] Based on a human milk intake of 0.75 l/day.
Source: adapted from reference (*22*).

15.5 Differences in bioavailability of folic acid and food folate: implications for the recommended intakes

The RNIs suggested for groups in Table 15.1 assume that food folate is the sole source of dietary folate because most societies in developing countries consume folate from naturally-occurring sources. As discussed in the introduction (section 15.1), natural folates are found in a conjugated form in food, which reduces their bioavailability by perhaps as much as 50% (4). In addition, natural folates are much less stable. If chemically pure folic acid (pteroylmonoglutamate) is used to provide part of the RNI, by way of fortification or supplementation, the total dietary folate, which contains conjugated forms (pteroylpolyglutamates), could be reduced by an appropriate amount.

The recommended daily intake of naturally-occurring mixed forms of folate in the diet for adults is 400 µg/day. If for example 100 µg is consumed as pure folic acid, on the basis of the assumption that, on average, the conjugated folate in natural foods is only half as available as synthetic folic acid this would be considered to be equivalent to 200 µg of dietary mixed folate. Hence, only an additional 200 µg of dietary folate would be needed to meet the adult RNI.

The Consultation agreed with the following findings of the Food and Nutrition Board of the United States NAS (22):

> Since folic acid taken with food is 85% bioavailable but food folate is only about 50% bioavailable, folic acid taken with food is 85/50 (i.e. 1.7) times more available. Thus, if a mixture of synthetic folic acid plus food folate has been fed, dietary folate equivalents (DFEs) are calculated as follows to determine the EAR:
>
> µg of DFE provided = [µg of food folate + (1.7 × µg of synthetic folic acid)].
>
> To be comparable to food folate, only half as much folic acid is needed if taken on an empty stomach, i.e. 1 µg of DFE = 1 µg of food folate = 0.5 µg of folic acid taken on an empty stomach = 0.6 µg of folic acid with meals.

The experts from the NAS went on to say that the required estimates for the dietary folate equivalents could be lowered if future research indicates that food folate is more than 50% bioavailable (22).

15.6 Considerations in viewing recommended intakes for folate

15.6.1 Neural tube defects

It is now agreed that a supplement of 400 µg of folic acid taken near the time of conception will prevent most NTDs (23, 24). The recommendation to prevent recurrence in women with a previous NTD birth remains 4.0 mg/day because of the high increase in risk in such cases and because that was the amount used in the most definitive trial (25). Because of the poorer bioavailability and stability of food folate, a diet based on food folate will not be optimum in the prevention of NTDs. One study determined that risk of NTD is 10-fold higher in people with poor folate status than in those with high normal folate status, as reflected by a red cell folate level greater than 400 µg/l (11). A further study suggests that an extra 200 µg/day or possibly 100 µg/day, if taken habitually in fortified food, would prevent most, if not all, folate-preventable NTDs (26). Ideally, an extra 400 µg/day should be provided because this is the amount used in various intervention trials (12) and that can be achieved by supplementation. This amount could not be introduced by way of fortification because exposure to high intakes of folic acid by people consuming a large intake of flour would run the risk of preventing the diagnosis of pernicious anaemia in the elderly. It is likely that depending on the staple chosen it would be possible to increase intake in most women by 100 µg/day without exposing other groups to an amount that might mask diseases such as pernicious anaemia. It is suggested that this amount, although not optimal, will prevent most NTDs.

15.6.2 Cardiovascular disease

Plasma homocysteine concentration, if only moderately elevated, is an independent risk factor for cardiovascular disease (7, 8, 17) and stroke (18). Increased risk has been associated with values higher than 11 µmol/l (8), which is well within what is generally considered to be the normal range (5–15 µmol/l) of plasma homocysteine levels (27). In addition, even in populations that are apparently normal and consuming diets adequate in folate, there is a range of elevation of plasma homocysteine (14) that could be lowered by an extra 100 or 200 µg/day of folic acid (8, 27). Large-scale intervention trials regarding the significance of interrelationships among folate levels, plasma homocysteine levels, and cardiovascular disease have not been completed and therefore it would be premature to introduce public health measures in this area.

15.6.3 Colorectal cancer

Evidence suggests a link between colorectal cancer and dietary folate intake and folate status (20, 21). One study reported that women who take multivitamin supplements containing folic acid for prolonged periods have a significantly reduced risk of colorectal cancer (28). Currently however, the scientific evidence is not sufficiently clear for recommending increased folate intake in populations at risk for colorectal cancer.

15.7 Upper limits

There is no evidence to suggest that it is possible to consume sufficient natural folate to pose a risk of toxicity (*22*). However, this clearly does not apply to folic acid given in supplements or fortified foods. The main concern with fortification of high levels of folic acid is the masking of the diagnosis of pernicious anaemia, because high levels of folic acid correct the anaemia, allowing the neuropathy to progress undiagnosed to a point where it may become irreversible, even upon treatment with vitamin B_{12} (*1, 29*). Consumption of large amounts of folic acid might also pose other less well-defined risks. Certainly, consumption of milligram amounts of folic acid would be undesirable except in cases of pregnant women with a history of children with NTD. Savage and Lindenbaum (*30*) suggest that even at levels of the RNI given here, there is a decreased opportunity to diagnose pernicious anaemia in subjects.

The United States NAS (*22*), after reviewing the literature, has suggested an upper level of 1000 µg. Thus, 400 µg/day of folic acid, in addition to dietary folate, would seem safe. There is probably no great risk of toxicity at a range of intakes between 400 and 1000 µg of folic acid per day, with the exception of some increased difficulty in diagnosing pernicious anaemia.

15.8 Recommendations for future research

There are many areas for future research, including:

* Folate status may be related to birth weight. Therefore, it is important to study the relationship between folate status and birth weight, especially in populations where low birth weight is prevalent.
* Folate status probably differs widely in different developing countries. Red cell folate levels are an excellent determinant of status. Such estimates in representative populations would determine whether some communities are at risk for folate deficiency.
* Some evidence indicates that elevated plasma homocysteine is a risk factor for cardiovascular disease and stroke. Elevated plasma homocysteine is largely related to poor folate status, with poor vitamin B_6 status, poor vitamin B_{12} status, or both, also contributing. Having a genetic polymor-

phism, namely the C → T 677 variant in the enzyme 5,10-methylenete-trahydrofolate reductase, is also known to significantly increase plasma homocysteine (*31*). The prevalence of elevated plasma homocysteine and its relationship to cardiovascular disease should be established in different developing countries.

- The relationship between folate deficiency and the incidence of NTDs in developing countries needs further investigation.

- More data should be generated on the bioavailability of natural folate from diets consumed in developing countries.

- Because the absorption of folate may be more efficient in humans with folate deficiency, folate absorption in these populations requires additional research.

- Quantification of the folate content of foods typically consumed in developing countries should be established for the different regions of the world.

References

1. Scott JM, Weir DG. Folate/vitamin B_{12} interrelationships. *Essays in Biochemistry*, 1994, 28:63–72.
2. Blakley R. *The biochemistry of folic acid and related pteridines*. Amsterdam, North Holland Publishing Company, 1969.
3. Kelly P et al. Unmetabolized folic acid in serum: acute studies in subjects consuming fortified food and supplements. *American Journal of Clinical Nutrition*, 1997. 69:1790–1795.
4. Gregory JF. Bioavailability of folate. *European Journal of Clinical Nutrition*, 1997, 51:554–559.
5. Cuskelly CJ, McNulty H, Scott JM. Effect of increasing dietary folate on red-cell folate : implications for prevention of neural tube defects. *Lancet*, 1996, 347:657–659.
6. McPartlin J et al. Accelerated folate breakdown in pregnancy. *Lancet*, 1993, 341:148–149.
7. Scott JM, Weir DG. Homocysteine and cardiovascular disease. *Quarterly Journal of Medicine*, 1996, 89:561–563.
8. Wald NJ et al. Homocysteine and ischaemic heart disease: results of a prospective study with implications on prevention. *Archives of Internal Medicine*, 1998, 158:862–867.
9. Manzoor M, Runcie J. Folate-responsive neuropathy: report of 10 cases. *British Medical Journal*, 1976, 1:1176–1178.
10. Chanarin I. *The megaloblastic anaemias*, 2nd ed. Oxford, Blackwell Scientific Publications, 1979.
11. Daly LE et al. Folate levels and neural tube defects. Implications for prevention. *Journal of the American Medical Association*, 1995, 274:1698–1702.
12. Scott JM et al. The role of folate in the prevention of neural tube defects. *Proceedings of the Nutrition Society*, 1994, 53:631–636.
13. *Requirements of vitamin A, iron, folate and vitamin B_{12}. Report of a*

Joint FAO/WHO Expert Consultation. Rome, Food and Agriculture Organization of the United Nations, 1988 (FAO Food and Nutrition Series, No. 23).

14. Sauberlich H. Folate status in the US population groups. In: Bailey LB, ed. *Folate in health and disease.* New York, NY, Marcel Dekker, 1995:171–194.

15. Lindenbaum J et al. Diagnosis of cobalamin deficiency. II. Relative sensitivities of serum cobalamin, methylmalonic acid, and total homocysteine concentrations. *American Journal of Hematology,* 1990, 34: 99–107.

16. Selhub J et al. Vitamin status and intake as primary determinants of homocysteinemia in an elderly population. *Journal of the American Medical Association,* 1993, 270:2693–2698.

17. Boushey CJ et al. A quantitative assessment of plasma homocysteine as a risk factor for vascular disease. *Journal of the American Medical Association,* 1995, 274:1049–1057.

18. Perry IJ et al. Prospective study of serum total homocysteine concentrations and risk of stroke in middle aged British men. *Lancet,* 1995, 346: 1395–1398.

19. Kirke PM et al. Maternal plasma folate and vitamin B12 are independent risk factors for neural tube defects. *Quarterly Journal of Medicine,* 1993, 86: 703–708.

20. Mason JB. Folate status: effect on carcinogenesis. In: Bailey LB, ed. *Folate in health and disease.* New York, NY, Marcel Dekker, 1995:361–378.

21. Kim YI et al. Colonic mucosal concentrations of folate correlate well with blood measurements of folate in persons with colorectal polyps. *American Journal of Clinical Nutrition,* 1998, 68:866–872.

22. Food and Nutrition Board. *Dietary reference intakes for thiamin, riboflavin, niacin, vitamin B₆, folate, vitamin B₁₂, pantothenic acid, biotin, and choline.* Washington, DC, National Academy Press, 1998.

23. Department of Health. *Folic acid and the prevention of neural tube defects. Report from an Expert Advisory Group.* London, Her Majesty's Stationery Office, 1992.

24. Centers for Disease Control and Prevention. Recommendations for the use of folic acid to reduce the number of cases of spina bifida and other neural tube defects. *Morbidity and Mortality Weekly Report,* 1992, 41:1–7.

25. MRC Vitamin Study Research Group. Prevention of neural tube defects: results of the Medical Research Council Vitamin Study. *Lancet,* 1991, 338:131–137.

26. Daly S et al. Minimum effective dose of folic acid for food fortification to prevent neural tube defects. *Lancet,* 1997, 350:1666–1669.

27. Refsum H et al. Homocysteine and cardiovascular disease. *Annual Review of Medicine,* 1998, 49:31–62.

28. Giovannucci E et al. Multivitamin use, folate and colorectal cancer in women in the Nurses' Health Study. *Annals of Internal Medicine,* 1998, 129:517–524.

29. Weir DG, Scott JM. Vitamin B12. In: Shils ME et al., eds. *Modern nutrition in health and disease.* Baltimore, MA, Williams & Wilkins, 1999:447–458.

30. Savage DG, Lindenbaum J. Neurological complications of acquired cobalamin deficiency: clinical aspects. In: Wickramasinghe SM, ed. *Bailliere's clinical*

haematology: megaloblastic anaemia. London, Bailliere Tindall, 1995, 8:657–678.

31. Whitehead AS et al. A genetic defect in 5,10-methylenetetrahydrofolate reductase in neural tube defects. *Quarterly Journal of Medicine*, 1995, 88:763–766.

16. Iodine

16.1 Role of iodine in human metabolic processes

At present, the only physiological role known for iodine in the human body is in the synthesis of thyroid hormones by the thyroid gland. Therefore, the dietary requirement of iodine is determined by normal thyroxine (T_4) production by the thyroid gland without stressing the thyroid iodide trapping mechanism or raising thyroid stimulating hormone (TSH) levels.

Iodine from the diet is absorbed throughout the gastrointestinal tract. Dietary iodine is converted into the iodide ion before it is absorbed. The iodide ion is 100% bioavailable and absorbed totally from food and water. This is, however, not true for iodine within thyroid hormones ingested for therapeutic purposes.

Iodine enters the circulation as plasma inorganic iodide, which is cleared from the circulation by the thyroid and kidney. The iodide is used by the thyroid gland for synthesis of thyroid hormones, and the kidney excretes excess iodine with urine. The excretion of iodine in the urine is a good measure of iodine intake. In a normal population with no evidence of clinical iodine deficiency either in the form of endemic goitre or endemic cretinism, urinary iodine excretion reflects the average daily iodine requirement. Therefore, for determining the iodine requirements and the iodine intake, the important indexes are serum T_4 and TSH levels (exploring thyroid status) and urinary iodine excretion (exploring iodine intake). A simplified diagram of the metabolic circuit of iodine is given in Figure 16.1.

All biological actions of iodide are attributed to the thyroid hormones. The major thyroid hormone secreted by the thyroid gland is T_4. T_4 in circulation is taken up by the cells and is de-iodinated by the enzyme 5'-monodeiodinase in the cytoplasm to convert it into triiodothyronine (T_3), the active form of thyroid hormone. T_3 traverses to the nucleus and binds to the nuclear receptor. All the biological actions of T_3 are mediated through the binding to the nuclear receptor, which controls the transcription of a particular gene to bring about the synthesis of a specific protein.

FIGURE 16.1
Summary of thyroid hormone production and regulation

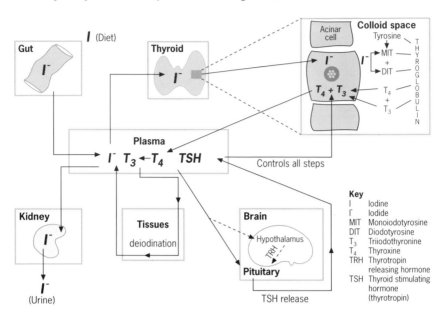

Source: reference (1).

The physiological actions of thyroid hormones can be categorized as 1) growth and development and 2) control of metabolic processes in the body. Thyroid hormones play a major role in the growth and development of the brain and central nervous system in humans from the 15th week of gestation to 3 years of age. If iodine deficiency exists during this period and results in thyroid hormone deficiency, the consequence is derangement in the development of the brain and central nervous system. These derangements are irreversible; the most serious form being that of cretinism. The effect of iodine deficiency at different stages of life is given in Table 16.1.

The other physiological role of thyroid hormones is to control several metabolic processes in the body. These include carbohydrate, fat, protein, vitamin, and mineral metabolism. For example, thyroid hormone increases energy production, increases lipolysis, and regulates neoglucogenesis, and glycolysis.

16.2 Populations at risk for iodine deficiency

Iodine deficiency affects all populations at all stages of life, from the intra-uterine stage to old age, as shown in Table 16.1. However, pregnant women, lactating women, women of reproductive age, and children younger than 3

TABLE 16.1
Effects of iodine deficiency, by life stage

Life stage	Effects
Fetus	Abortions Stillbirths Congenital anomalies Increased perinatal mortality Increased infant mortality Neurological cretinism: mental deficiency, deaf mutism, spastic diplegia, and squint Myxedematous cretinism: mental deficiency, hypothyroidism and dwarfism Psychomotor defects
Neonate	Neonatal goitre Neonatal hypothyroidism
Child and adolescent	Goitre Juvenile hypothyroidism Impaired mental function Retarded physical development
Adult	Goitre with its complications Hypothyroidism Impaired mental function Iodine-induced hyperthyroidism

Sources: adapted from references (2–4).

years of age are considered the most important groups in which to diagnose and treat iodine deficiency (2, 5), because iodine deficiency occurring during fetal and neonatal growth and development leads to irreversible damage of the brain and central nervous system and, consequently, to irreversible mental retardation.

16.3 Dietary sources of iodine

The iodine content of food depends on the iodine content of the soil in which it is grown. The iodine present in the upper crust of the earth is leached by glaciation and repeated flooding, and is carried to the sea. Seawater is, therefore, a rich source of iodine (6). The seaweed located near coral reefs has an inherent biological capacity to concentrate iodine from the sea. The reef fish which thrive on seaweed are also rich in iodine. Thus, a population consuming seaweed and reef fish will have a high intake of iodine, as is the case in Japan. Iodine intakes by the Japanese are typically in the range of 2–3 mg/day (6). In several areas of Africa, Asia, Latin America, and parts of Europe, iodine intake varies from 20 to 80 µg/day. In Canada and the United States and some parts of Europe, the intake is around 500 µg/day. The average iodine content

TABLE 16.2
Average iodine content of foods (μg/kg)

Food	Fresh basis		Dry basis	
	Mean	Range	Mean	Range
Fish (fresh water)	30	17–40	116	68–194
Fish (marine)	832	163–3180	3715	471–4591
Shellfish	798	308–1300	3866	1292–4987
Meat	50	27–97	—	—
Milk	47	35–56	—	—
Eggs	93	—	—	—
Cereal grains	47	22–72	65	34–92
Fruits	18	10–29	154	62–277
Legumes	30	23–36	234	223–245
Vegetables	29	12–201	385	204–1636

Source: reference (6).

TABLE 16.3
Iodine content of selected environmental media

Medium	Iodine content
Terrestrial air	1 μg/l
Marine air	100 μg/l
Terrestrial water	5 μg/l
Sea water	50 μg/l
Igneous rocks	500 μg/kg
Soils from igneous rocks	9000 μg/kg
Sedimentary rocks	1500 μg/kg
Soils from sedimentary rocks	4000 μg/kg
Metamorphic rocks	1600 μg/kg
Soils from metamorphic rocks	5000 μg/kg

Source: reference (6).

of foods (fresh and dry basis) as reported by Koutras et al. (6) is given in Table 16.2.

The iodine content of food varies with geographic location because there is a large variation in the iodine content of the various environmental media (Table 16.3) (6). Thus, the average iodine content of foods shown in Table 16.2 cannot be used universally for estimating iodine intake.

16.4 Recommended intakes for iodine

The daily intake of iodine recommended by the Food and Nutrition Board of the United States National Academy of Sciences in 1989 was 40 μg/day for young infants (0–6 months), 50 μg/day for older infants (7–12 months), 60–100 μg/day for children (1–10 years), and 150 μg/day for adolescents and adults (7). These values approximate to 7.5 µg/kg/day for infants aged 0–12 months, 5.4 µg/kg/day for children aged 1–10 years, and 2 µg/kg/day for adolescents and adults. These amounts are proposed to allow normal T$_4$ production without stressing the thyroid iodide trapping mechanism or raising TSH levels.

16.4.1 Infants

The recommendation of 40 µg/day for infants aged 0–6 months (or 8 µg/kg/day, 7 µg/100 kcal, or 50 µg/l milk) is probably based on the observation reported in the late 1960s that the iodine content of human milk was approximately 50 µg/l and the assumption that nutrition of the human-milk-fed infant growing at a satisfactory rate represents an adequate level of nutrient intake (8, 9). However, recent data indicate that the iodine content of human milk varies markedly as a function of the iodine intake of the population (10). For example, it ranges from 20 to 330 µg/l in Europe and from 30 to 490 µg/l in the United States (8, 10, 11). It is as low as 12 µg/l in populations experiencing severe iodine deficiency (8, 10). On this basis, an average human-milk intake of 750 ml/day would give an intake of iodine of about 60 µg/day in Europe and 120 µg/day in the United States. The upper United States value (490 µg/l) would provide 368 µg/day or 68 µg/kg/day for a 5-kg infant.

Positive iodine balance in the young infant, which is required for increasing the iodine stores of the thyroid, is achieved only when the iodine intake is at least 15 µg/kg/day in term infants and 30 µg/kg/day in pre-term infants (12). The iodine requirement of pre-term infants is twice that of term infants because of a much lower retention of iodine by pre-term infants (8, 12). Based on the assumption of an average body weight of 6 kg for a child of 6 months, 15 µg/kg/day corresponds approximately to an iodine intake and requirement of 90 µg/day. This value is twofold higher than the present United States recommendations.

On the basis of these considerations, The World Health Organization (WHO) in 2001 updated its 1996 recommendations (13) and proposed, together with the United Nations Children's Fund (UNICEF) and the International Council for Control of Iodine Deficiency Disorders (ICCIDD), an iodine intake of 90 µg/day from birth onwards (14). To reach this objective, and based on an intake of milk of about 150 ml/kg/day, it was further proposed that the iodine content of formula milk be increased from 50 µg/l, the former recommendation, to 100 µg/l for term infants and to 200 µg/l for pre-term infants.

For a urine volume of about 4–6 dl/day, the urinary concentration of iodine indicating iodine repletion should be in the range of 150–220 µg/l

(1.18–1.73 µmol/l) in infants aged 0–3 years. Such values have been observed in iodine-replete infants in Europe (*15*), Canada (*16*), and the United States (*16*). Under conditions of moderate iodine deficiency, as seen in Belgium for example, the average urinary iodine concentration is only 100 µg/l (0.80 µmol/l) in this age group. It reaches a stable normal value of about 200 µg/l (1.57 µmol/l) only from the 30th week of daily iodine supplementation with a physiological dose of 90 µg/day (*17, 18*) (Figure 16.2).

When the urinary iodine concentration in neonates and young infants is below a threshold of 50–60 µg/l (0.39–0.47 µmol/l), corresponding to an intake of 25–35 µg/day, there is a sudden increase in the prevalence of neonatal serum TSH values in excess of 50 mU/ml, indicating subclinical hypothyroidism, eventually complicated by transient neonatal hypothyroidism (*19*). When the urinary iodine concentration is in the range of 10–20 µg/l (0.08–0.16 µmol/l), as observed in populations with severe endemic goitre, up to 10% of the neonates have overt severe hypothyroidism, with serum TSH levels above 100 mU/ml and serum T_4 values below 30 µg/l (39 nmol/l) (*19*). Left untreated, these infants will develop myxedematous endemic cretinism (*20*).

FIGURE 16.2

Changes over time in the median urinary concentration of iodine in healthy Belgian infants aged 6–36 months and supplemented with iodine at 90 µg/kg/day for 44 weeks (each point represents 32–176 iodine determinations)

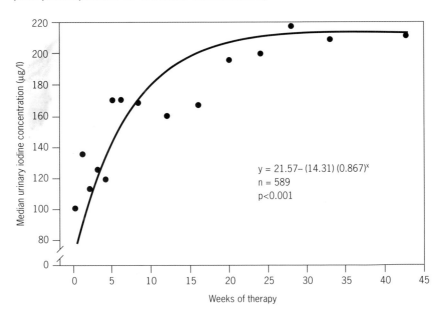

$$y = 21.57 - (14.31)(0.867)^x$$
$$n = 589$$
$$p < 0.001$$

Source: reference (*18*).

Overall, existing data point to an iodine requirement of the young infant of 15 µg/kg/day (30 µg/kg/day in pre-term infants). Hyperthyrotropinaemia (high levels of serum TSH), indicating subclinical hypothyroidism with the risk of brain damage, occurs when the iodine intake is about one third of this value, and dramatic neonatal hypothyroidism, resulting in endemic cretinism, occurs when the intake is about one tenth of this value.

16.4.2 Children

The daily iodine requirement on a body weight basis decreases progressively with age. A study by Tovar and colleagues (21) correlating 24-hour thyroid radioiodine uptake and urinary iodine excretion in 9–13-year-old school-children in rural Mexico suggested that an iodine intake in excess of 60 µg/day is associated with a 24-hour thyroidal radioiodine uptake below 30%. Lower excretion values are associated with higher uptake values. An iodine intake of 60 µg/day is equivalent to 3 µg/kg/day in an average size 10-year-old child (approximate body weight of 20 kg). An intake of 60–100 µg/day for a child of 1–10 years thus seems appropriate. These requirements are based on the body weight of Mexican children who participated in this study. The Food and Agriculture Organization of the United Nations calculates the average body weight of a 10-year-old child as being 25 kg. Using the higher average body weight, the iodine requirement for a 1–10-year-old child would be 90–120 µg/day.

16.4.3 Adults

A requirement for iodine of 150 µg/day for adolescents and adults is justified by the fact that it corresponds to the daily urinary excretion of iodine and to the iodine content of food in non-endemic areas (i.e. in areas where iodine intake is adequate) (22, 23). It also provides the iodine intake necessary to maintain the plasma iodide level above the critical limit of 0.10 µg/dl, which is the average level likely to be associated with the onset of goitre (24). More-over, this level of iodine intake is required to maintain the iodine stores of the thyroid above the critical threshold of 10 mg, below which an insufficient level of iodination of thyroglobulin leads to disorders in thyroid hormone synthesis (23).

Data reflecting either iodine balance or its effect on thyroid physiology can help to define optimal iodine intake. In adults and adolescents who consume adequate amounts of iodine, most dietary iodine eventually appears in the urine; thus, the urinary iodine concentration is a useful measure for assessing iodine intake (1, 23). For this, casual samples are sufficient if enough are col-lected and if they accurately represent a community (14, 25). A urinary iodine concentration of 100 μg/l corresponds to an intake of about 150 μg/day in the adult. Median urinary iodine concentrations below 100 μg/l in a population are associated with increases in median thyroid size and possibly in increases in serum TSH and thyroglobulin values. Correction of the iodine deficiency will bring all these measures back into the normal range. Recent data from the Thyro-Mobil project in Europe have confirmed these relationships by showing that the largest thyroid sizes are associated with the lowest urinary iodine concentrations (26). Once a median urinary iodine excretion of about 100 μg/l is reached, the ratio of thyroid size to body size remains fairly constant. Moulopoulos et al. (27) reported that a urinary iodine excretion between 151 and 200 μg/g creatinine (1.18–1.57 μmol/g creatinine), corresponding to a concentration of about 200 μg/l (1.57 μmol/l), correlated with the lowest values for serum TSH in a non-goitrous population. Similarly, recent data from Australia show that the lowest serum TSH and thyroglobulin values were associated with urine containing 200–300 μg iodine/g creatinine (1.57–2.36 μmol iodine/g creatinine) (28).

Other investigations followed serum TSH levels in adult subjects without thyroid glands who were given graded doses of T_4 and found that an average daily dose of 100 μg T_4 would require at least 65 μg of iodine to be used with maximal efficiency by the thyroid in order to establish euthyroidism. In practice, such maximal efficiency is never obtained and therefore considerably more iodine is necessary. Data from controlled observations associated a low urinary iodine concentration with a high goitre prevalence, high radioiodine uptake, and low thyroidal organic iodine content (12). Each of these measures reached a steady state once the urinary iodine excretion was 100 μg/l (0.78 μmol/l) or greater.

16.4.4 Pregnant women

The iodine requirement during pregnancy is increased to provide for the needs of the fetus and to compensate for the increased loss of iodine in the urine resulting from an increased renal clearance of iodine during pregnancy (29). Previously, requirements have been derived from studies of thyroid function during pregnancy and in the neonate under conditions of moderate iodine deficiency. For example, in Belgium, where the iodine intake is estimated to be 50–70 μg/day (30), thyroid function during pregnancy is characterized by a progressive decrease in the serum concentrations of free-thyroid hormones and an increase in serum TSH and thyroglobulin. Thyroid volume progressively increases and is above the upper limit of normal in 10% of the women by the end of pregnancy. Serum TSH and thyroglobulin are higher in the neonates than in the mothers (31). These abnormalities are prevented only

TABLE 16.4
Daily iodine intake recommendations by the World Health Organization, United Nations Children's Fund, and International Council for Control of Iodine Deficiency Disorders

	Iodine intake	
Group	(μg/day)	(μg/kg/day)
Infants and children, 0–59 months	90	6.0–30.0
Children, 6–12 years	120	4.0
Adolescents and adults, from 13 years of age through adulthood	150	2.0
Pregnant women	200	3.5
Lactating women	200	3.5

Source: reference (*14*).

when the mother receives a daily iodide supplementation of 161 μg/day during pregnancy (derived from 131 μg potassium iodide and 100 μg T$_4$ given daily) (*32*). T$_4$ was administered with iodine to the pregnant women to rapidly correct subclinical hypothyroidism, which would not have occurred if iodine had been administered alone. These data indicate that the iodine intake required to prevent the onset of subclinical hypothyroidism of mother and fetus during pregnancy, and thus to prevent the possible risk of brain damage of the fetus, is approximately 200 μg/day.

On the basis of the above considerations for the respective population groups, the Expert Consultation concluded that the WHO/UNICEF/ICCIDD recommendations for daily iodine intakes (*14*) were the best available and saw no grounds for altering them at the present time. The current intake recommendations for iodine are summarized in Table 16.4.

16.5 Upper limits

While a physiological amount of iodine is required for insuring a normal thyroid function, a large excess of iodine can be harmful to the thyroid by inhibiting the process of synthesis and release of thyroid hormones (Wolff-Chaikoff effect) (*33*). The threshold upper limit of iodine intake (the intake beyond which thyroid function is inhibited) is not easy to define because it is affected by the level of iodine intake before exposure to iodine excess. Indeed, long-standing moderate iodine deficiency is accompanied by an accelerated trapping of iodide and by a decrease in the iodine stores within the thyroid (*23*). Under these conditions, the critical ratio between iodide and total iodine within the thyroid, which is the starting point of the Wolff-Chaikoff effect, is more easily reached in conditions of insufficient dietary supply of iodine than under normal conditions. In addition, the neonatal thyroid is particularly sensitive to the Wolff-Chaikoff effect because the immature thyroid gland is unable to reduce the uptake of iodine from the plasma to compensate for increased iodine ingestion (34). Consequently, the upper limit of iodine intake will depend on both basal status of iodine intake and age.

16.5.1 Iodine intake in areas of moderate iodine deficiency

In a study in Belgium, iodine overload of mothers (caused by use of cutaneous povidone iodine for epidural anaesthesia or caesarean section) increased the milk iodine concentration of women and increased urinary iodine excretion in their term newborn infants (mean weight about 3 kg) (35). In the absence of iodine overload, the mean iodine content of breast milk was 9 µg/dl (0.63 µmol/l) and the urinary iodine of the infant at 5 days of life was 12 µg/dl (0.94 µmol/l). After the use of povidone iodine in the mother for epidural anaesthesia or for caesarean section, the mean milk iodine concentrations were 18 and 128 µg/dl, and were associated with average infant urinary iodine excretion levels of 280 and 1840 µg/l (2.20–14.48 µmol/l), respectively (35). Based on an intake of some 6.5 dl of breast milk per day, the estimated average iodine intakes in the babies of iodine overload mothers were 117 and 832 µg/day, or 39 and 277 µg/kg/day, respectively. The lower dose significantly increased the peak TSH response to exogenous thyroid-releasing hormone but did not increase the (secretory) area under the TSH response curve. The higher dose increased the peak response and secretory area as well as the baseline TSH concentration. Serum T_4 concentrations were not altered, however (35). Thus, these infants had a mild and transient, compensated hypothyroid state. More generally, the use of povidone iodine in mothers at the time of delivery increased neonatal TSH and the recall rate at the time of screening for congenital hypothyroidism (36). These data indicate that modest iodine overloading of term infants in the neonatal period in an area of relative dietary iodine deficiency (Belgium) can impair thyroid hormone formation.

Similarly, studies in France and Germany indicated that premature infants exposed to cutaneous povidone iodine or fluorescinated alcohol-iodine solutions, and excreting iodine in urine in excess of 100 µg/day, manifested decreased T_4 and increased TSH concentrations in serum (37, 38). The extent of these changes was more marked in premature infants with less than 34 weeks gestation than in those with 35–37 weeks gestation. The term infants were not affected.

These studies suggest that in Europe, the upper limit of iodine intake which predisposes to blockage of thyroid secretion in neonates and especially in premature infants (i.e. from about 120 µg/day, 40 µg/kg/day) is only 1.5 to 3 times higher than the average intake from normal human milk and roughly equivalent to the upper range of recommended intake.

16.5.2 Iodine intake in areas of iodine sufficiency

Similar studies have not been conducted in the United States, where transient hypothyroidism is eight times lower than in Europe because iodine intake is much higher in the United States (*39*). For example, urinary concentrations of 50 µg/dl and above in neonates, which can correspond to a Wolff-Chaikoff effect in Europe, are frequently seen in healthy neonates in North America (*15, 16*).

The average iodine intake of infants in the United States in 1978, including infants fed whole cow milk, was estimated by the market-basket approach (*40*) to be 576 µg/day (standard deviation [SD], 196); that of toddlers, 728 µg/day (SD, 315) and that of adults, 952 µg/day (SD, 589). The upper range for infants (968 µg/day) would provide a daily intake of 138 µg/kg for a 7-kg infant, and the upper range for toddlers (1358 µg/day) would provide a daily intake of 90 µg/kg for a 15-kg toddler.

Table 16.5 summarizes the recommended upper limits of dietary intake of iodine by group, which did not appear to impair thyroid function in the group of Delange infants in European studies; in adults in loading studies in the United States; or during ingestion of the highest estimates of dietary intake in the United States (*40*). Except for the value for premature infants who appear hypersensitive to iodine excess, the probable safe upper limits listed in Table 16.5 are 15–20 times higher than the recommended intakes. These data

TABLE 16.5
Recommended dietary intakes of iodine and upper limits, by group

Group	Recommended intake (µg/kg/day)	Upper limit[a] (µg/kg/day)
Infants and children		
Premature	30	100
0–6 months	15	150
7–12 months	15	140
1–6 years	6	50
7–12 years	4	50
Adolescents and adults (13+ years)	2	30
Pregnant women	3.5	40
Lactating women	3.5	40

[a] Probably safe.
Source: adapted from reference (*18*).

refer to all sources of iodine intake. The average iodine content of infant formulas is approximately 5 µg/dl. The upper limit probably should be one that
provides a daily iodine intake of no more than 100 µg/kg. For this limit — with
the assumption that the total intake is from infant formula — and with a daily
milk intake of 150 ml/kg (100 kcal/kg), the upper limit of the iodine content
of infant formula would be about 65 µg/dl. The current suggested upper limit
of iodine in infant formula of 75 µg/100 kcal (89 µg/500 kJ or 50 µg/dl), therefore, seems reasonable.

16.5.3 Excess iodine intake

Excess iodine intake in healthy adults in iodine-replete areas is difficult to
define. Many people are regularly exposed to huge amounts of iodine — in the
range 10–200 mg/day — without apparent adverse effects. Common sources
are medicines (e.g. amiodarone contains 75 mg iodine per 200-mg capsule),
foods (particularly dairy products), kelp (eaten in large amounts in Japan),
and iodine-containing dyes (for radiologic procedures). Occasionally, each of
these may have significant thyroid effects, but generally, they are tolerated
without difficulty. Braverman et al. (41) showed that people without evidence
of underlying thyroid disease almost always remain euthyroid in the face
of large amounts of excess iodine and escape the acute inhibitory effects of
excess intrathyroidal iodide on the organification (i.e. attachment of
oxidized iodine species to tyrosil residues in the thyroid gland for the synthesis of thyroid hormones) of iodide and on subsequent hormone synthesis
(escape from, or adaptation to, the acute Wolff-Chaikoff effect). This adaptation most likely involves a decrease in thyroid iodide trapping, perhaps corresponding to a decrease in the thyroid sodium-iodide transporter recently
cloned (42).

This tolerance to huge doses of iodine in healthy iodine-replete adults is
the reason why WHO stated in 1994 that, "Daily iodine intakes of up to
1 mg, i.e. 1000 µg, appear to be entirely safe" (43). This statement, of course,
does not include neonates and young infants (due to factors previously discussed). In addition, it has to be considered that iodine excess can induce
hypothyroidism in patients affected by thyroiditis (44) and can induce hyperthyroidism in cases of a sudden and excessive increment of iodine supply in
patients with autonomous thyroid nodules (3, 4, 45). Finally, iodine excess
can trigger thyroid autoimmunity in genetically susceptible animals and individuals and may modify the pattern of thyroid cancer by increasing the ratio
of papillary–follicular thyroid cancers (46).

In conclusion, it clearly appears that the benefits of correcting iodine deficiency far outweigh the risks of iodine supplementation (46, 47).

References

1. Stanbury JB. Physiology of endemic goitre. In: *Endemic goitre*. Geneva, World Health Organization, 1960:261–262.
2. Hetzel BS. Iodine deficiency disorders (IDD) and their eradication. *Lancet*, 1983, 2:1126–1129.
3. Stanbury JB et al. Iodine-induced hyperthyroidism: occurrence and epidemiology. *Thyroid*, 1998, 8:83–100.
4. Delange F et al. Risks of iodine-induced hyperthyroidism following correction of iodine deficiency by iodized salt. *Thyroid*, 1999, 9:545–556.
5. Dunn JT. The use of iodized oil and other alternatives for the elimination of iodine deficiency disorders. In: Hetzel BS, Pandav CS, eds. *SOS for a billion. The conquest of iodine deficiency disorders*. New Delhi, Oxford University Press, 1996:119–128.
6. Koutras DA, Matovinovic J, Vought R. The ecology of iodine. In: Stanbury JB, Hetzel BS, eds. *Endemic goitre and endemic cretinism. Iodine nutrition in health and disease*. New Delhi, Wiley Eastern Limited, 1985:185–195.
7. Subcommittee on the Tenth Edition of the Recommended Dietary Allowances, Food and Nutrition Board. *Recommended dietary allowances*, 10th ed. Washington, DC, National Academy Press, 1989.
8. Delange F et al. Physiopathology of iodine nutrition during pregnancy, lactation and early postnatal life. In: Berger H, ed. *Vitamins and minerals in pregnancy and lactation*. New York, NY, Raven Press, 1988:205–214 (Nestlé Nutrition Workshop Series, No. 16).
9. Gushurst CA et al. Breast milk iodide: reassessment in the 1980s. *Pediatrics*, 1984, 73:354–357.
10. Semba RD, Delange F. Iodine in human milk: perspectives for human health. *Nutrition Reviews*, 2001, 59:269–278.
11. Bruhn JA, Franke AA. Iodine in human milk. *Journal of Dairy Sciences*, 1983, 66:1396–1398.
12. Delange F. Requirements of iodine in humans. In: Delange F, Dunn JT, Glinoer D, eds. *Iodine deficiency in Europe. A continuing concern*. New York, NY, Plenum Press, 1993:5–16.
13. *Trace elements in human nutrition and health*. Geneva, World Health Organization, 1996.
14. *Assessment of the iodine deficiency disorders and monitoring their elimination*. Geneva, World Health Organization, 2001 (WHO/NHD/01.1).
15. Delange F et al. Regional variations of iodine nutrition and thyroid function during the neonatal period in Europe. *Biology of the Neonate*, 1986, 49:322–330.
16. Delange F et al. Increased risk of primary hypothyroidism in preterm infants. *Journal of Pediatrics*, 1984, 105:462–469.
17. Delange F et al. Iodine deficiency during infancy and early childhood in Belgium: does it pose a risk to brain development? *European Journal of Pediatrics*, 2001, 160:251–254.
18. Fisher DA, Delange F. Thyroid hormone and iodine requirements in man during brain development. In: Stanbury JB et al., eds. *Iodine in pregnancy*. New Delhi, Oxford University Press, 1998:1–33.
19. Delange F. Iodine nutrition and congenital hypothyroidism. In: Delange F, Fisher DA, Glinoer D, eds. *Research in congenital hypothyroidism*. New York, NY, Plenum Press, 1989:173–185.
20. Delange F. Endemic cretinism. In: Braverman LE, Utiger RD, eds. *The

thyroid. A fundamental and clinical text, 8th ed. Philadelphia, PA, Lippincott, 2000:743–754.

21. Tovar E, Maisterrena JA, Chavez A. Iodine nutrition levels of school children in rural Mexico. In: Stanbury JB, ed. *Endemic goitre*. Washington, DC, Pan American Health Organization, 1969:411–415 (PAHO Scientific Publication, No. 193).

22. Bottazzo GF et al. Thyroid growth-blocking antibodies in autoimmune (AI) atrophic thyroiditis. *Annales d'Endocrinologie* (Paris), 1981, 42:13A.

23. Delange F. The disorders induced by iodine deficiency. *Thyroid*, 1994, 4:107–128.

24. Wayne EJ, Koutras DA, Alexander WD. *Clinical aspects of iodine metabolism*. Oxford, Blackwell, 1964:1–303.

25. Bourdoux P et al. A new look at old concepts in laboratory evaluation of endemic goitre. In: Dunn JT et al., eds. *Towards the eradication of endemic goitre, cretinism, and iodine deficiency*. Washington, DC, Pan American Health Organization, 1986:115–129 (PAHO Scientific Publication, No. 502).

26. Delange F et al. Thyroid volume and urinary iodine in European school-children. Standardization of values for assessment of iodine deficiency. *European Journal of Endocrinology*, 1997, 136:180–187.

27. Moulopoulos DS et al. The relation of serum T_4 and TSH with the urinary iodine excretion. *Journal of Endocrinological Investigation*, 1988, 11:437–439.

28. Buchinger W et al. Thyrotropin and thyroglobulin as an index of the optimal iodine intake: correlation with iodine excretion of 39913 euthyroid patients. *Thyroid*, 1997, 7:593–597.

29. Aboul-Khair SA et al. The physiological changes in thyroid function during pregnancy. *Clinical Sciences*, 1964, 27:195–207.

30. Glinoer D et al. Regulation of maternal thyroid during pregnancy. *Journal of Clinical Endocrinology and Metabolism*, 1990, 71:276–287.

31. Glinoer D et al. Maternal and neonatal thyroid function at birth in an area of marginally low iodine intake. *Journal of Clinical Endocrinology and Metabolism*, 1992, 75:800–805.

32. Glinoer D et al. A randomized trial for the treatment of excessive thyroidal stimulation in pregnancy: maternal and neonatal effects. *Journal of Clinical Endocrinology and Metabolism*, 1995, 80:258–269.

33. Roti E, Vagenakis G. Effect of excess iodide: clinical aspects. In: Braverman LE, Utiger RD, eds. *The thyroid. A fundamental and clinical text*, 8th ed. Philadelphia, PA, Lippincott, 2000:316–329.

34. Sherwin J. Development of the regulatory mechanisms in the thyroid: failure of iodide to suppress iodide transport activity. *Proceedings of the Society for Experimental Biology and Medicine*, 1982, 169:458–462.

35. Chanoine JP et al. Increased recall rate at screening for congenital hypothyroidism in breast fed infants born to iodine overloaded mothers. *Archives of Diseases in Childhood*, 1988, 63:1207–1210.

36. Chanoine JP et al. Iodinated skin disinfectants in mothers at delivery and impairment of thyroid function in their breast-fed infants. In: Medeiros-Neto GA, Gaitan E, eds. *Frontier of thyroidology*. New York, NY, Plenum Press, 1986:1055–1060.

37. Castaing H et al. Thyroïde du nouveau-né et surcharge en iode après la naissance. [The thyroid gland of the newborn infant and postnatal iodine overload]. *Archives Francaises de Pédiatrie*, 1979, 36:356–368.

38. Gruters A et al. Incidence of iodine contamination in neonatal transient hyper-thyrotropinemia. *European Journal of Pediatrics*, 1983, 140:299–300.
39. Burrow GN, Dussault JH. *Neonatal thyroid screening.* New York, NY, Raven Press, 1980.
40. Park YK et al. Estimation of dietary iodine intake of Americans in recent years. *Journal of the American Dietetic Association*, 1981, 79:17–24.
41. Braverman LE. Iodine and the thyroid—33 years of study. *Thyroid*, 1994, 4:351–356.
42. Dai G, Levy O, Carraco N. Cloning and characterisation of the thyroid iodide transporter. *Nature*, 1996, 379:458–460.
43. *Iodine and health. Eliminating iodine deficiency disorders safely through salt iodization.* Geneva, World Health Organization, 1994.
44. Paris J et al. The effect of iodide on Hashimoto's thyroiditis. *Journal of Clinical Endocrinology*, 1961, 21:1037–1043.
45. Todd CH et al. Increase in thyrotoxicosis associated with iodine supplements in Zimbabwe. *Lancet*, 1995, 346:1563–1564.
46. Delange F, Lecomte P. Iodine supplementation: benefits outweigh risks. *Drug Safety*, 2000, 22:89–95.
47. Braverman LE. Adequate iodine intake—the good far outweighs the bad. *European Journal of Endocrinology*, 1998, 139:14–15.

17. Food as a source of nutrients

17.1 Importance of defining food-based recommendations

Dietary patterns have varied over time. Changes in these patterns are dependent on such things as agricultural practices and climatic, ecologic, cultural, and socioeconomic factors, which in turn, determine which foods are available. At present, virtually all dietary patterns show that the nutritional needs of population groups are adequately satisfied or even exceeded. This is true except where socioeconomic conditions limit the capacity to produce and purchase food or aberrant cultural practices restrict the choice of foods. It is thought that if people have access to a sufficient quantity and variety of foods, they will meet, in large part, their nutritional needs. However, for certain groups of people because of economic restrictions, levels of certain micronutrients may not be met from food alone. Thus, micronutrient adequacy must be included in evaluating the nutritive value of diets alongside energy and protein adequacy.

A healthful diet can be attained through the intake of multiple combinations of a variety of foods. Given this, it is difficult to define the ranges of intake for a specific food, which should be included in a given combination with other foods to comply with nutritional adequacy. In practice, the set of food combinations which provide nutritional adequacy are limited by the level of food production sustainable in a given ecological setting. In addition, there are economic constraints that limit food supply at the household level. The development of food-based dietary guidelines (FBDGs) (1) recognizes this and focuses on how a combination of foods can meet nutrient requirements rather than on how each specific nutrient is provided in adequate amounts.

The first step in the process of setting dietary guidelines is defining the significant diet-related public health problems in a community. Once these are defined, the adequacy of the diet is evaluated by comparing the information available on dietary intake with the established recommended nutrient intakes (RNIs). Nutrient intake goals are specific for a given setting, and their purpose is to promote overall health, control specific nutritional diseases (whether they are induced by an excess or deficiency of nutrient intake), and reduce the risk of diet-related multifactorial diseases. Dietary guidelines represent the practical way to reach the nutritional goals for a given population. They take into account customary dietary patterns and indicate what aspects of each should be modified. They consider the ecological setting in which the population lives, as well as the socioeconomic and cultural factors that affect nutritional adequacy.

The alternative approach to defining nutritional adequacy of diets relies on the biochemical and physiological basis of human nutritional requirements in health and disease. The quantitative definition of nutrient needs and its expression as RNIs have been important instruments of food and nutrition policy in many countries and have focused the attention of international bodies on this critical issue. This nutrient-based approach has served many purposes but has not always fostered the establishment of nutritional and dietary priorities consistent with the broad public health priorities at the national and international levels. It has permitted a more precise definition of requirements for essential nutrients but unfortunately has often been too narrowly focused, concentrating on the precise nutrient requirement amount, and not on solving the nutritional problems of the world.

In contrast to RNIs, FBDGs are based on the fact that people eat food, not nutrients. Defining nutrient intakes alone is only part of the task of dealing with nutritional adequacy. As will be illustrated in this chapter, the notion of nutrient density is helpful for defining FBDGs and evaluating the adequacy of diets. However, unlike RNIs, FBDGs can be used to educate the public through the mass media and provide a practical guide to selecting foods by defining dietary adequacy (1).

Advice for a healthful diet should provide both a quantitative and qualitative description of the diet for it to be understood by individuals, who should be given information on both size and number of servings per day. The quantitative aspects include the estimation of the amount of nutrients in foods and their bioavailability in the form they are actually consumed. Unfortunately, available food composition data for most foods currently consumed in the world are incomplete, outdated, or insufficient for evaluating true bioavailability. The qualitative aspects relate to the biological utilization of nutrients in the food as consumed by humans and explore the potential for interaction among nutrients. Such an interaction may enhance or inhibit the bioavailability of a nutrient from a given food source.

The inclusion of foods in the diet which have high micronutrient density— such as pulses or legumes, vegetables (including green leafy vegetables), and fruits—is the preferred way of ensuring optimal nutrition, including micronutrient adequacy, for most population groups. Most population groups who are deficient in micronutrients subsist largely on refined cereal grain- or tuber-based diets, which provide energy and protein (with an improper amino acid balance) but insufficient levels of critical micronutrients. There is a need for a broadening of the food base and a diversification of diets. Figures 17.1–17.4 illustrate how addition of a variety of foods to four basic diets (i.e. a white rice-based diet; a corn-tortilla-based diet; a refined couscous-based diet; and a potato-based diet) can increase the nutrient density of a cereal- or tuber-based diet. Adding reasonable amounts of these foods will add micronutrient density to the staple diet and in doing so could reduce the prevalence of diseases resulting from a micronutrient deficiency across populations groups.

The recent interest in the role of phytochemicals and antioxidants on health, and their presence in plant foods, lends further support to the recommendation for increasing the consumption of vegetables and fruit in the diet. The need for dietary diversification is supported by the knowledge of the interrelationships of food components, which may enhance the nutritional value of foods and prevent undesirable imbalances which may limit the utilization of some nutrients. For example, fruits rich in ascorbic acid will enhance the absorption of non-haem iron.

If energy intake is low (< 8.368 MJ/day), for example, in the case of young children, sedentary women, or the elderly, the diet may not provide sufficient amounts of vitamins and minerals to meet RNIs. This situation may be of special relevance to the elderly, who are inactive, have decreased lean body mass, and typically decrease their energy intake. Young children, pregnant women, and lactating women who have greater micronutrient needs relative to their energy needs will also require an increased micronutrient density.

The household is the basic unit in which food is consumed in most settings. If there is sufficient food, individual members of the household can consume a diet with the recommended nutrient densities (RNDs) and meet their specific RNIs. However, appropriate food distribution within the family must be considered to ensure that children and women receive adequate food with high micronutrient density. Household food distribution must be considered when establishing general dietary guidelines and addressing the needs of vulnerable groups in the community. In addition, education detailing the appropriate storage and processing of foods to reduce micronutrient losses at the household level is important.

FIGURE 17.1

Impact of the addition of selected micronutrient-rich foods to a white rice-based diet on the recommended nutrient density (RND) of vitamin A, vitamin C, folate, iron (Fe) and zinc (Zn)

a. White rice-based diet

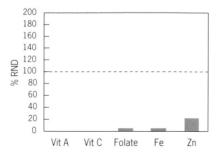

b. White rice + carrots

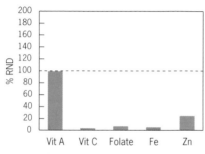

c. White rice + carrots and an orange

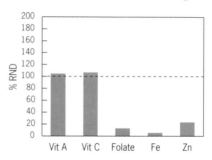

d. White rice + carrots, an orange and lentils

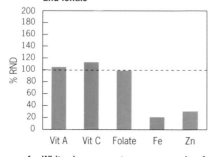

e. White rice + carrots, an orange and beef

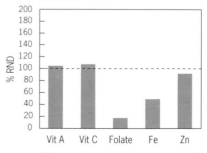

f. White rice + carrots, an orange, beef and spinach

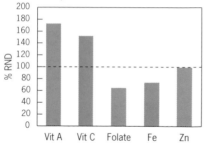

g. White rice + carrots, an orange, beef, spinach and lentils

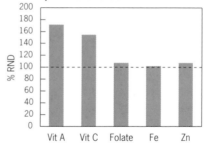

Source: adapted from reference (2).

FIGURE 17.2

Impact of the addition of selected micronutrient-rich foods to a corn-tortilla-based diet on the recommended nutrient density (RND) of vitamin A, vitamin C, folate, iron (Fe) and zinc (Zn)

a. **Corn-tortilla-based diet**

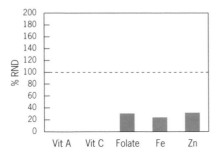

b. **Corn-tortilla + carrots**

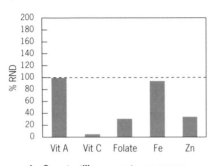

c. **Corn-tortilla + carrots and an orange**

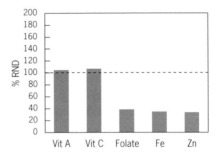

d. **Corn-tortilla + carrots, an orange and lentils**

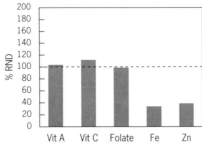

e. **Corn-tortilla + carrots, an orange and beef**

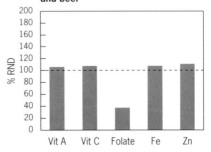

f. **Corn-tortilla + carrots, an orange, beef and spinach**

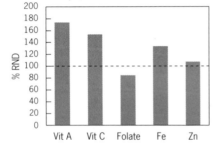

g. **Corn-tortilla + carrots, an orange, beef, spinach and black beans**

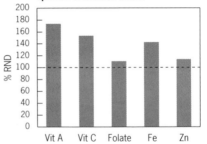

Source: adapted from reference (2).

FIGURE 17.3

Impact of the addition of selected micronutrient-rich foods to a refined couscous-based diet on the recommended nutrient density (RND) of vitamin A, vitamin C, folate, iron (Fe) and zinc (Zn)

a. Refined couscous-based diet

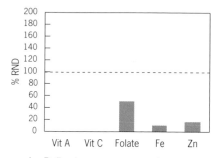

b. Refined couscous + carrots

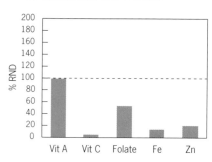

c. Refined couscous + carrots and an orange

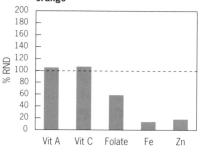

d. Refined couscous + carrots, an orange and lentils

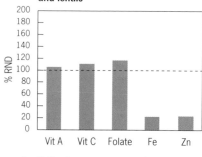

e. Refined couscous + carrots, an orange and beef

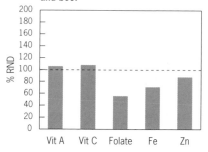

f. Refined couscous + carrots, an orange, beef and spinach

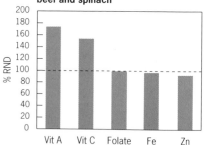

g. Refined couscous + carrots, an orange, beef, spinach and black beans

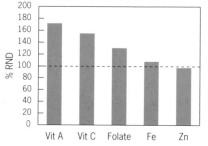

Source: adapted from reference (2).

FIGURE 17.4

Impact of the addition of selected micronutrient-rich foods to a potato-based diet on the recommended nutrient density (RND) of vitamin A, vitamin C, folate, iron (Fe) and zinc (Zn)

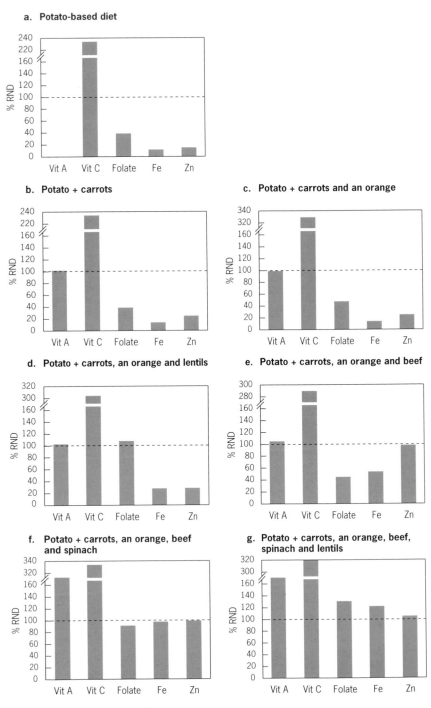

a. Potato-based diet

b. Potato + carrots

c. Potato + carrots and an orange

d. Potato + carrots, an orange and lentils

e. Potato + carrots, an orange and beef

f. Potato + carrots, an orange, beef and spinach

g. Potato + carrots, an orange, beef, spinach and lentils

Source: adapted from reference (2).

17.2 Dietary diversification when consuming cereal- and tuber-based diets

Dietary diversification is important to improve the intake of critical nutrients. How this can be achieved is illustrated below with reference to five micronutrients, which are considered to be of public health relevance or serve as markers for overall micronutrient intake. The nutrients selected for discussion include those that are among the most difficult to obtain in cereal- and tuber-based diets (i.e. diets based on rice, corn, wheat, potato or cassava). Moreover, nutrient deficiencies of vitamin A, iron, and zinc are widespread.

17.2.1 Vitamin A

The vitamin A content of most staple diets can be significantly improved with the addition of a relatively small portion of plant foods rich in carotenoids, the precursors of vitamin A. For example, a typical portion of cooked carrots (50 g) added to a daily diet, or 21 g of carrots per 4.184 MJ, provides 500 μg retinol equivalents, which is the recommended nutrient density for this vitamin. The biological activity of provitamin A varies among different plant sources; fruits and vegetables such as carrots, mango, papaya, and melon contain large amounts of nutritionally active carotenoids (3, 4). Green leafy vegetables such as ivy gourd have been successfully used in Thailand as a source of vitamin A, and carotenoid-rich red palm oil serves as an easily available and excellent source of vitamin A in other countries. Consequently, a regular portion of these foods included in an individual's diet may provide 100% or more of the daily requirement for retinol equivalents (Figures 17.1–17.4b). Vitamin A is also present in animal food sources in a highly bioavailable form. Therefore, it is important to consider the possibility of meeting vitamin A needs by including animal foods in the diet. For example, providing minor amounts of fish or chicken liver (20–25 g) in the diet provides more than the recommended vitamin A nutrient density for virtually all population groups.

17.2.2 Vitamin C

An increased vitamin C intake can be achieved by including citrus fruit or other foods rich in ascorbic acid in the diet. For example, an orange or a small amount of other vitamin C-rich fruit (60 g of edible portion) provides the recommended ascorbic acid density (Figures 17.1–17.3c). Adding an orange per day to a potato-based diet increases the level of vitamin C threefold (Figure 17.4c). Other good vitamin C food sources are guava, amla, kiwi, cranberries, strawberries, papaya, mango, melon, cantaloupe, spinach, Swiss chard, tomato, asparagus, and Brussels sprouts. All these foods, when added to a diet or meal in regular portion sizes, will significantly improve the vitamin C density. Because ascorbic acid is heat labile, minimal cooking (steaming or stir-frying) is recommended to maximize the bioavailable nutrient. The significance of consuming vitamin C with meals is discussed relative to iron absorption below (see also Chapter 13).

17.2.3 Folate

Folate is now considered significant not only for the prevention of macrocytic anaemia, but also for normal fetal development. Recently, this vitamin was implicated in the maintenance of cardiovascular health and cognitive function in the elderly. Staple diets consisting largely of cereal grains and tubers are very low in folate but can be improved by the addition of legumes or green leafy vegetables. For example, a regular portion of cooked lentils (95 g) added to a rice-based diet can provide an amount of folate sufficient to meet the desirable nutrient density for this vitamin (Figure 17.1d). Other legumes such as beans and peas are also good sources of this vitamin, but larger portions are needed for folate sufficiency (100 g beans and 170 g peas). Cluster bean and colacasia leaves are excellent folate sources used in the Indian diet. Another good source of folate is chicken liver; only one portion (20–25 g) is sufficient to meet the desirable nutrient density for folate and vitamin A simultaneously. The best sources of folate are organ meats, green leafy vegetables, and Brussels sprouts. However, 50% or more of food folate is destroyed during cooking. Prolonged heating in large volumes of water should be avoided, and it is advisable to consume the water used in the cooking of vegetables.

17.2.4 Iron and zinc

Minerals such as iron and zinc are found in low amounts in cereal- and tuber-based diets. The addition of legumes slightly improves the iron content of such diets. However, the bioavailability of this non-haem iron source is low. Therefore, it is not possible to meet the recommended levels of iron in the staple-based diets through a food-based approach unless some meat or fish is included. For example, adding a small portion (50 g) of flesh food will increase the total iron content of the diet as well as the amount of bioavailable iron. For zinc, the presence of a small portion (50 g) of flesh food will secure dietary sufficiency of most staple diets (Figures 17.1–17.4e).

The consumption of ascorbic acid along with food rich in iron will enhance iron's absorption. There is a critical balance between enhancers and inhibitors of iron absorption. Nutritional status can be improved significantly by educating households about food preparation practices that minimize the consumption of inhibitors of iron absorption; for example, the fermentation of phytate-containing grains before the baking of breads to enhance iron absorption.

17.3 How to accomplish dietary diversity in practice

It is essential to create strategies which promote and facilitate dietary diversification in order to achieve complementarity of cereal- or tuber-based diets with foods rich in micronutrients in populations with limited financial resources or access to food. A recent FAO/International Life Sciences Institute publication (5) proposed strategies to promote dietary diversification as part of food-based approaches to preventing micronutrient malnutrition. These strategies, which are listed below, have been further adapted or modified by the present Expert Consultation:

- *Community or home vegetable and fruit gardens.* Support for small-scale vegetable and fruit growing should lead to increased production and consumption of micronutrient-rich foods (e.g. legumes, green leafy vegetables, and fruits) at the household level. The success of such projects depends on a good knowledge and understanding of local conditions as well as the involvement of women and the community in general. These are key elements for supporting, achieving, and sustaining beneficial nutritional change at the household level. Land availability and water supply are often constraints, and may require local government support before they are overcome. The educational effort should be directed towards securing appropriate within-family distribution, which considers the needs of the most vulnerable members of the family, especially infants and young children.
- *Raising of fish, poultry, and small animals (rabbits, goats, and guinea pigs).* Flesh foods are excellent sources of highly bioavailable essential micronutrients such as vitamin A, iron, and zinc. Raising animals at the local level may permit communities to access foods which otherwise would not be available because of their high costs. These types of projects also need some support from local governments or nongovernmental organizations to overcome cost constraints of programme implementation, including education and training on how to raise animals.
- *Implementation of large-scale commercial vegetable and fruit production.* The objective of such initiatives is to provide micronutrient-rich foods at

reasonable prices through effective and competitive markets which lower consumer prices without reducing producer prices. This will serve predominantly the urban and non-food-producing rural areas.

- *Reduction of post-harvest losses of the nutritional value of micronutrient-rich foods, such as fruits and vegetables.* Improvement of storage and food-preservation facilities significantly reduces post-harvest losses. At the household level, the promotion of effective cooking methods and practical ways of preserving foods (e.g. solar drying of seasonal micronutrient-rich foods such as papaya, grapes, mangoes, peaches, tomatoes, and apricots) may preserve significant amounts of micronutrients in foods, which in turn will lead to an increase of these nutrients in the diet. At the commercial level, appropriate grading, packing, transport, and marketing practices can reduce losses, stimulate economic growth, and optimize income generation.
- *Improvement of micronutrient levels in soils and plants, which will improve the composition of plant foods and enhance yields.* Current agricultural practices can improve the micronutrient content of foods by correcting soil quality and pH and by increasing soil mineral content where it has been depleted by erosion and poor soil conservation practices. Long-term food-based solutions to micronutrient deficiencies will require improvement of agricultural practices, seed quality, and plant breeding (by means of a classical selection process or genetic modification).

The green revolution made important contributions to cereal supplies, and it is time to address the need for improvements in the production of legumes, vegetables, fruits, and other micronutrient-rich foods. FBDGs can serve to re-emphasize the need for these crops.

It is well recognized that the proposed strategies for promoting dietary diversity need a strong community-level commitment. For example, the increase in the price of legumes associated with decreased production and lower demand needs to be corrected. The support of local authorities and government may facilitate the implementation of such projects because these actions require economic resources, which are sometimes beyond the reach of those most in need of dietary diversity.

17.4 Practices which will enhance the success of food-based approaches

To achieve dietary adequacy of vitamin A, vitamin C, folate, iron, and zinc by using food-based approaches, food preparation and dietary practices must be considered. For example, it is important to recommend that vegetables rich in vitamin C, folate, and other water-soluble or heat-labile vitamins are minimally cooked in small amounts of water. In the case of iron, it is essential to reduce the intake of inhibitors of iron absorption and to increase the intake of enhancers of absorption in a given meal. Following this strategy, it is recommended to increase the intake of germinated seeds; fermented cereals; heat-processed cereals; meats; and fruits and vegetables rich in vitamin C. In addition, the consumption of tea, coffee, chocolate, or herbal infusions should be encouraged at times other than with meals (see Chapter 13). Consumption of flesh foods improves zinc absorption whereas it is inhibited by consumption of diets high in phytate, such as diets based on unrefined cereals. Zinc availability can be estimated according to the phytate–zinc molar ratio of the meal (6) (see Chapter 12).

This advice is particularly important for people who consume cereal-based and tuber-based diets. These foods constitute the main staples for most populations of the world, populations which are also most at risk for micronutrient deficiencies. Other alternatives—fortification and supplementation—have been proposed as stopgap measures when food-based approaches are not feasible or are still under development. There is a definite role for fortification in meeting iron, folate, iodine, and zinc needs. Fortification and supplementation should be seen as complementary to food-based strategies and not as a replacement. Combined implementation of these strategies can lead to substantial improvements in normalizing the micronutrient status of populations at risk. Food-based approaches usually take longer to implement than supplementation programmes, but once established they are truly sustainable.

17.5 Delineating the role of supplementation and food fortification for micronutrients which cannot be supplied by food

Under ideal conditions of food access and availability, food diversity should satisfy micronutrient and energy needs of the general population. Unfortunately, for many people in the world, the access to a variety of micronutrient-rich foods is not possible. As demonstrated in the analysis of cereal- and tuber-based diets (see Figures 17.1–17.4), micronutrient-rich foods, including small amounts of flesh foods and a variety of plant foods (vegetables and fruits), are needed daily. This may not be realistic at present for many communities living under conditions of poverty. Food fortification and food supplementation are important alternatives which complement food-based approaches to satisfy the nutritional needs of people in developing and developed countries.

17.5.1 Fortification

Fortification refers to the addition of nutrients to a commonly eaten food (the vehicle). It is possible for a single nutrient or group of micronutrients (the fortificant) to be added to the vehicle, which has been identified through a process in which all stakeholders have participated. This approach is accepted as sustainable under most conditions and is often cost effective on a large scale when successfully implemented. Both iron fortification of wheat flour and iodine fortification of salt are examples of fortification strategies that have produced excellent results (7).

There are at least three essential conditions which must be met in any fortification programme (7, 8): the fortificant should be effective, bioavailable, acceptable, and affordable; the selected food vehicle should be easily accessible and a specified amount of it should be regularly consumed in the local diet; and detailed production instructions and monitoring procedures should be in place and enforced by law.

Iron fortification

Food fortification with iron is recommended when dietary iron is insufficient or the dietary iron is of poor bioavailability, which is the reality for most people in the developing world and for vulnerable population groups in the developed world. Moreover, the prevalence of iron deficiency and anaemia in vegetarians and in populations of the developing world which rely on cereal or tuber foods is significantly higher than in omnivorous populations.

Iron is present in foods in two forms, as haem iron, which is derived from flesh foods (meats and fish), and as non-haem iron, which is the inorganic form present in plant foods such as legumes, grains, nuts, and vegetables (9, 10). Haem iron is the more readily absorbed (20–30%) and its bioavailability is relatively unaffected by dietary factors. Non-haem iron has a lower rate of absorption (2–10%), depending on the balance between iron absorption inhibitors (e.g. phytates, polyphenols, calcium, and phosphate) and iron absorption enhancers (e.g. ascorbic and citric acids, cysteine-containing peptides, ethanol, and fermentation products) present in the diet (9, 10). Because staple foods around the world provide predominantly non-haem iron sources of low bioavailability, the traditionally eaten staple foods represent an excellent vehicle for iron fortification. Examples of foods that have been fortified are wheat flour, corn (maize) flour, rice, salt, sugar, cookies, curry powder, fish sauce, and soy sauce (9). Nevertheless, the beneficial effects of consumption of iron absorption enhancers have been extensively proven and should always be promoted (i.e. consumption of a vitamin C-rich food together with the non-haem iron source).

Iodine fortification

Iodine is sparsely distributed in the Earth's surface and foods grown in soils with little or no iodine lack an adequate amount of this micronutrient. This situation had made iodine deficiency disorders exceedingly common in most of the world and highly prevalent in many countries before the introduction of salt iodination (*11*). Only foods of marine origin are naturally rich sources of iodine. Salt is a common food used by most people worldwide, and the establishment of a well-implemented permanent salt-iodination programme has been proven to eradicate iodine deficiency disorders. Universal salt iodination is the best way to virtually eliminate iodine deficiency disorders (*5*).

However, salt iodination is not simply a matter of legislating the mandatory iodination of salt. It is important to determine the best fortification technique, coordinate the implementation at all salt production sites, establish effective monitoring and quality control programmes, and measure the iodine fortification level periodically. The difficulties in implementing salt iodination programmes arise primarily when the salt industry is widely dispersed among many small producers. The level of iodine fortification usually lies between 25 and 50 mg/kg salt. The actual amount should be specified according to the level of salt intake and the magnitude of the deficit at the country level, because iodine must be added within safe and effective ranges. Thus, it is very important to implement a monitoring plan to control the amount of iodine in the salt at the consumer's table (*11*, *12*). Additionally, United Nations agencies responsible for assisting governments in establishing iodination programmes should provide technical support for programme implementation, monitoring, and evaluation to ensure sustainability.

Zinc fortification

The body depends on a regular zinc supply provided by the daily diet because stores are quite limited. Food diversity analysis demonstrates that it is virtually impossible to achieve zinc adequacy in the absence of a flesh food source (see Figures 17.1–17.4). Among flesh foods, beef is the best source of zinc, followed by poultry and then fish. Zinc fortification programmes are being studied, especially for populations that consume predominately plant foods. Fortification of cereal staple foods is a potentially attractive intervention which could benefit the whole population as well as target the vulnerable population groups, namely children and pregnant women. Such addition of zinc

331

to the diet would decrease the prevalence of stunting in many developing countries with low-zinc diets, because linear growth is affected by zinc supply in the body.

Folic acid fortification

The recommended nutrient density for folic acid is 200 μg/4.184 MJ (1). Although this value is higher than other standards of reference, the increase in folic acid consumption by women of childbearing age is very important: it may improve birth weight and reduce the prevalence of neural tube defects (see Chapter 15). Elevated plasma homocysteine levels are considered to be an independent risk factor for heart disease; a higher intake of folic acid may also benefit the rest of the population because it may lower homocysteine levels in adults (see Chapter 15). In addition, folate may improve the mental condition of the elderly population (13, 14).

Although the desirable folic acid density may be achieved through dietary diversity, it requires the daily presence of organ meats, green leafy vegetables, pulses, legumes, or nuts in the diet (15). Most population groups may not easily reach the appropriate level of folic acid consumption; therefore, folic acid fortification has been recommended. The United States initiated mandatory folic acid fortification of cereal-grain products in January 1998. The fortification level approved in the United States is 140 μg/100 g of product, which will increase the average woman's intake by 100 μg/day. This amount is considered safe (a dose that will not mask pernicious anaemia, which results from vitamin B_{12} deficiency) and though not optimal in most settings, should contribute to the prevention of neural tube defects (16).

17.5.2 Supplementation

Supplementation refers to periodic administration of pharmacologic preparations of nutrients as capsules or tablets, or by injection when substantial or immediate benefits are necessary for the group at risk. As established at the International Conference on Nutrition (17), nutritional supplementation should be restricted to vulnerable groups which cannot meet their nutrient needs through food (e.g. women of childbearing age, infants and young children, elderly people, low socioeconomic groups, displaced people, refugees, and populations experiencing other emergency situations). For example, iron supplementation is recognized as the only effective option to control or prevent iron deficiency anaemia in pregnant women. Supplementation with folic acid must be considered for women of childbearing age who have had a child with a neural tube defect to prevent recurrence.

17.6 Food-based dietary guidelines

FBDGs are an instrument and an expression of food and nutrition policy and should be based directly on diet and disease relationships of particular relevance to an individual country and/or group, such as pregnant and lactating women, children, and the elderly. Their primary purpose is to educate health-care professionals and consumers about health promotion and disease prevention. In this way, priorities in establishing dietary guidelines can address the relevant public health concerns whether they are related to dietary insufficiency or excess. In this context, meeting the nutritional needs of populations takes its place as one of the components of food and nutrition policy goals along with the priorities included in the FBDGs for improved health and nutrition for a given population.

The world nutrition and health situation demonstrates that the major causes of death and disability have been traditionally related to malnutrition in developing countries and to the imbalance between energy intake and expenditure (which lead to obesity and other chronic diseases—diabetes, cardiovascular disease, hypertension, and stroke) in industrialized countries. The tragedy is that many suffer from too little food while others have diseases resulting from too much food; both, however, would benefit from a more balanced distribution of food and other resources. Although the nature of the health and nutrition problems in these two contrasting groups is very different, the dietary guidelines required to improve both situations are not. Most countries presently have the combined burden of malnutrition from deficit and increasing prevalence of obesity and other chronic diseases from over-consumption. The approaches to address the problems, however, should be country and population specific.

Although two thirds of the world's population depends on cereal-based or tuber-based diets, the other one third consumes significant amounts of animal food products. The latter group places an undue demand on land, water, and other resources required for intensive food production, which makes the typical Western diet not only undesirable from the standpoint of health but also environmentally unsustainable. If energy intake is balanced with the expenditure required for basal metabolism, physical activity, growth, and cellular repair, the dietary quality required for health is essentially the same across population groups.

Efforts in nutrition education and health promotion should include a strong encouragement for active lifestyles. Improving energy balance for rural populations in developing countries may mean increasing energy intake to normalize low body mass index (BMI, weight/height^2, calculated as kg/m^2), ensuring adequate energy stores for daily living. In sedentary urban populations, improving energy balance will mean increasing physical activity to decrease energy stores (body fat mass) and thus normalize BMI. Thus, the apparent conflicting goals—eradicating malnutrition while preventing overnutrition—are resolved by promoting an appropriate energy balance, which will lead to a normal BMI. Moreover, given that FBDGs should be ecologically sustainable, the types and amounts of foods included in a balanced diet are not very different for promoting adequate nutrition in the impoverished and preventing overnutrition in the affluent.

This is well exemplified by the similarities in the FBDGs across countries, whether represented by pyramids, rainbows, dishes or pots. It is obvious that consumption of excess energy will induce an increase in energy stores, which may lead to obesity and related health complications. Populations should consume nutritionally adequate and varied diets, based primarily on foods of plant origin with small amounts of added flesh foods. Households across all regions should select predominantly plant-based diets rich in a variety of vegetables and fruits, pulses or legumes, and minimally processed starchy staple foods. The evidence that such diets will prevent or delay a significant proportion of noncommunicable chronic diseases is consistent. A predominantly plant-based diet has a low energy density, which may protect against obesity. This should not exclude small amounts of animal foods, which make an important nutritional contribution to plant-food-based diets, as illustrated in the examples presented earlier (Figures 17.1–17.4). Inadequate diets occur when food is scarce or when food traditions change rapidly, as is seen in societies undergoing demographic transitions or rapid urbanization. Traditional diets, when adequate and varied, are likely to be generally healthful and more protective against chronic noncommunicable diseases than the typical Western diet, consumed predominantly in industrialized societies (18).

Reorienting food production, agricultural research, and commercialization policies needs to take into consideration FBDGs, which increase the demand for a variety of micronutrient-rich foods and thus stimulate production to meet consumption needs. Prevailing agricultural policies encourage research on production and importation of foods, which do not necessarily meet the requirements of FBDG implementation. For example, great emphasis is placed on cereals, horticultural crops for export, legumes for export, non-food cash crops, and large livestock. Necessary policy reorientation is required to ensure increased availability of micronutrient-rich foods within the local food system. Norway has successfully implemented agricultural and food production policies based on a national nutrition plan of action, providing economic incentives for the producer and consumer in support of healthful diets. The results speak for themselves, as Norway has experienced a sustained improvement in life expectancy and a reduction in deaths from cardiovascular disease and other chronic noncommunicable conditions.

17.7 Recommendations for the future

The Consultation acknowledged the limitations in its knowledge of the important factors which affect nutrient utilization, and recommended that the International Food Data System (INFoods) effort, led by FAO and the United Nations University (UNU), be strengthened. Special emphasis should be placed on the micronutrient composition of local diets as affected by the ecological setting by including an analysis of food components (nutrients or bioactive components), which may affect the bioavailability and utilization of critical micronutrients, and an analysis of cooked foods and typical food combinations as actually consumed by population groups. In addition, the development of FBDGs at the country level should be supported by United Nations agencies.

17.8 Future research needs

To facilitate the implementation of a food-based approach in the prevention of micronutrient deficiencies the following research needs were identified:

- food data system development, which includes development of a methodology for micronutrient composition of foods, organizing data retrieval, and reporting and dissemination through electronic means; this effort should include phytochemicals, antioxidants, and other components which may affect health and nutrition, with special emphasis on local foods which may be important for given cultures;
- identification and evaluation of optimal methods for cooking foods to preserve the nutrient value and enhance the bioavailability of micronutrients;
- development of better methods to preserve foods, especially micronutrient-rich foods, at the household and community levels;
- identification and propagation of agricultural methods which will enhance the yield, content, and biological value of micronutrient-rich foods;
- identification of optimal food combinations and serving size which will be most effective in preventing micronutrient deficits and methods of promotion for these food combinations at the community level;
- development of agricultural research to support the implementation of FBDGs;

- evaluation of the nutritional impact and cost–benefit of food-based approaches in combating micronutrient deficiencies.

References

1. *Preparation and use of food-based dietary guidelines. Report of a Joint FAO/WHO Consultation.* Geneva, World Health Organization, 1996 (WHO Technical Report Series, No. 880).
2. Oyarzun MT, Uauy R, Olivares S. Food-based approaches to improve vitamin and mineral nutrition adequacy. *Archivos Latinoamericanos de Nutricion* (Guatemala), 2001, 51:7–18.
3. *Requirements of vitamin A, iron, folate and vitamin B$_{12}$. Report of a Joint FAO/WHO Expert Consultation.* Rome, Food and Agriculture Organization of the United Nations, 1988 (FAO Food and Nutrition Series, No. 23).
4. Olson JA. Needs and sources of carotenoids and vitamin A. *Nutrition Reviews*, 1994, 52(Suppl. 2):S67–S73.
5. *Preventing micronutrient malnutrition: a guide to food-based approaches.* Washington, DC, International Life Sciences Institute Press, 1997.
6. *Trace elements in human nutrition.* Geneva, World Health Organization, 1996.
7. Lotfi M et al. *Micronutrient fortification of foods. Current practices, research, and opportunities.* Ottawa, The Micronutrient Initiative, and Wageningen, International Development Research Center/International Agricultural Center, 1996.
8. Viteri FE. Prevention of iron deficiency. In: Howson CP, Kennedy ET, Horwitz A, eds. *Prevention of micronutrient deficiencies. Tools for policy-makers and public health workers.* Washington, DC, National Academy Press, 1998, 3:45–102.
9. Hallberg L, Hulthén L, Gramatkovski E. Iron absorption from the whole diet in men: how effective is the regulation of iron absorption? *American Journal of Clinical Nutrition*, 1997, 66:347–356.
10. Allen LH, Ahluwalia N. *Improving iron status through diet. The application of knowledge concerning dietary iron bioavailability in human populations.* Arlington, VA, John Snow, and Opportunities for Micronutrient Interventions Project, 1997.
11. Stanbury JB. Prevention of iodine deficiency. In: Howson CP, Kennedy ET, Horwitz A, eds. *Prevention of micronutrient deficiencies. Tools for policy-makers and public health workers.* Washington, DC, National Academy Press, 1998, 5:167–201.
12. Sullivan KM et al., eds. *Monitoring universal salt iodization programs.* Ottawa, The Micronutrient Initiative, 1995.
13. Tucker KL et al. Folic acid fortification of the food supply. Potential benefits and risk for the elderly population. *Journal of the American Medical Association*, 1996, 2776:1879–1885.
14. Oakley GP, Adams MJ, Dickinson CM. More folic acid for everyone, now. *Journal of Nutrition*, 1996, 126(Suppl.):S751–S755.
15. Bower C. Folate and neural tube defects. *Nutrition Reviews*, 1995, 53(Suppl. 2):S33–S38.
16. Daly S et al. Minimum effective dose of folic acid for food fortification to prevent neural-tube defects. *Lancet*, 1997, 350:1666–1669.

17. *International Conference on Nutrition. World Declaration and Plan of Action for Nutrition, 1992.* Rome, Food and Agriculture Organization of the United Nations, 1992.
18. *Diet, nutrition, and the prevention of chronic diseases. Report of a WHO Study Group.* Geneva, World Health Organization, 1990 (WHO Technical Report Series, No. 797).

Annex 1
Recommended nutrient intakes[a] — minerals

Group	Calcium[b] (mg/day)	Selenium (µg/day)	Magnesium (mg/day)	Zinc[c] (mg/day) High bioavailability	Moderate bioavailability	Low bioavailability
Infants						
0–6 months	300[d] 400[g]	6	26[d] 36[h]	1.1[d]	2.8	6.6
7–12 months	400	10	54	0.8[d] 2.5[j]	4.1	8.4
Children						
1–3 years	500	17	60	2.4	4.1	8.3
4–6 years	600	22	76	2.9	4.8	9.6
7–9 years	700	21	100	3.3	5.6	11.2
Adolescents						
Females						
10–18 years	1300[k]	26	220	4.3	7.2	14.4
Males						
10–18 years	1300[k]	32	230	5.1	8.6	17.1
Adults						
Females						
19–50 years (premenopausal)	1000	26	220	3.0	4.9	9.8
51–65 years (menopausal)	1300	26	220	3.0	4.9	9.8
Males						
19–65 years	1000	34	260	4.2	7.0	14.0
Elderly						
Females						
65+ years	1300	25	190	3.0	4.9	9.8
Males						
65+ years	1300	33	224	4.2	7.0	14.0
Pregnant women						
First trimester	m	m	220	3.4	5.5	11.0
Second trimester	m	28	220	4.2	7.0	14.0
Third trimester	1200	30	220	6.0	10.0	20.0
Lactating women						
0–3 months	1000	35	270	5.8	9.5	19.0
3–6 months	1000	35	270	5.3	8.8	17.5
7–12 months	1000	42	270	4.3	7.2	14.4

[a] Recommended nutrient intake (RNI) is the daily intake which meets the nutrient requirements of almost all (97.5%) apparently healthy individuals in an age- and sex-specific population.
[b] See Chapter 4 for details.
[c] See Chapter 12 for details.
[d] Breastfed.
[e] Neonatal iron stores are sufficient to meet the iron requirement for the first 6 months in full-term infants. Premature infants and low birth weight infants require additional iron.
[f] Recommendation for the age group 0–4.9 years.
[g] Cow milk-fed.
[h] Formula-fed.

Iron (mg/day)				Iodine
15% Bioavailability	12% Bioavailability	10% Bioavailability	5% Bioavailability	(μg/day)
e	e	e	e	90[f]
6.2[i]	7.7[i]	9.3[i]	18.6[i]	90[f]
3.9	4.8	5.8	11.6	90[f]
4.2	5.3	6.3	12.6	90[f]
5.9	7.4	8.9	17.8	120 (6–12 yrs)
9.3 (11–14 yrs)[l]	11.7 (11–14 yrs)[l]	14.0 (11–14 yrs)[l]	28.0 (11–14 yrs)[l]	150 (13–18 yrs)
21.8 (11–14 yrs)	27.7 (11–14 yrs)	32.7 (11–14 yrs)	65.4 (11–14 yrs)	
20.7 (15–17 yrs)	25.8 (15–17 yrs)	31.0 (15–17 yrs)	62.0 (15–17 yrs)	
9.7 (11–14 yrs)	12.2 (11–14 yrs)	14.6 (11–14 yrs)	29.2 (11–14 yrs)	150 (13–18 yrs)
12.5 (15–17 yrs)	15.7 (15–17 yrs)	18.8 (15–17 yrs)	37.6 (15–17 yrs)	
19.6	24.5	29.4	58.8	150
7.5	9.4	11.3	22.6	150
9.1	11.4	13.7	27.4	150
7.5	9.4	11.3	22.6	150
9.1	11.4	13.7	27.4	150
n	n	n	n	200
n	n	n	n	200
n	n	n	n	200
10.0	12.5	15.0	30.0	200
10.0	12.5	15.0	30.0	200
10.0	12.5	15.0	30.0	200

[i] Bioavailability of dietary iron during this period varies greatly.
[j] Not applicable to infants exclusively breastfed.
[k] Particularly during the growth spurt.
[l] Pre-menarche.
[m] Not specified.
[n] It is recommended that iron supplements in tablet form be given to all pregnant women because of the difficulties in correctly assessing iron status in pregnancy. In non-anaemic pregnant women, daily supplements of 100 mg of iron (e.g. as ferrous sulphate) given during the second half of pregnancy are adequate. In anaemic women higher doses are usually required.

Annex 2
Recommended nutrient intakes[a] — water- and fat-soluble vitamins

Group	Water-soluble vitamins					
	Vitamin C[b] (mg/day)	Thiamine (mg/day)	Riboflavin (mg/day)	Niacin[c] (mg NE/day)	Vitamin B$_6$ (mg/day)	Pantothenate (mg/day)
Infants						
0–6 months	25	0.2	0.3	2[i]	0.1	1.7
7–12 months	30	0.3	0.4	4	0.3	1.8
Children						
1–3 years	30	0.5	0.5	6	0.5	2.0
4–6 years	30	0.6	0.6	8	0.6	3.0
7–9 years	35	0.9	0.9	12	1.0	4.0
Adolescents						
Females						
10–18 years	40	1.1	1.0	16	1.2	5.0
Males						
10–18 years	40	1.2	1.3	16	1.3	5.0
Adults						
Females						
19–50 years (premenopausal)	45	1.1	1.1	14	1.3	5.0
51–65 years (menopausal)	45	1.1	1.1	14	1.5	5.0
Males						
19–65 years	45	1.2	1.3	16	1.3 (19–50 yrs) 1.7 (50+ yrs)	5.0
Elderly						
Females						
65+ years	45	1.1	1.1	14	1.5	5.0
Males						
65+ years	45	1.2	1.3	16	1.7	5.0
Pregnant women	55	1.4	1.4	18	1.9	6.0
Lactating women	70	1.5	1.6	17	2.0	7.0

[a] Recommended nutrient intake (RNI) is the daily intake which meets the nutrient requirements of almost all (97.5%) apparently healthy individuals in an age- and sex-specific population.
[b] See Chapter 7 for details.
[c] NE = Niacin equivalents.
[d] DFE = Dietary folate equivalents; μg of DFE provided = [μg of food folate + (1.7 × μg of synthetic folic acid)].
[e] Vitamin A values are "recommended safe intakes" instead of RNIs. See Chapter 2 for further details.
[f] Recommended safe intakes as μg retinol equivalent (RE)/day; conversion factors are as follows:
    1 μg retinol = 1 RE
    1 μg β-carotene = 0.167 μg RE
    1 μg other provitamin A carotenoids = 0.084 μg RE.

Water-soluble vitamins			Fat-soluble vitamins			
Biotin (µg/day)	Vitamin B_{12} (µg/day)	Folate[d] (µg DFE/day)	Vitamin A[e,f] (µg RE/day)	Vitamin D (µg/day)	Vitamin E[g] (mg α-TE/day)	Vitamin K[h] (µg/day)
5	0.4	80	375	5	2.7[j]	5[k]
6	0.7	80	400	5	2.7[j]	10
8	0.9	150	400	5	5.0[j]	15
12	1.2	200	450	5	5.0[j]	20
20	1.8	300	500	5	7.0[j]	25
25	2.4	400	600	5	7.5	35–55
25	2.4	400	600	5	10.0	35–55
30	2.4	400	500	5	7.5	55
30	2.4	400	500	10	7.5	55
30	2.4	400	600	5 (19–50 yrs) 10 (51–65 yrs)	10.0	65
	2.4	400	600	15	7.5	55
[l]	2.4	400	600	15	10.0	65
30	2.6	600	800	5	[j]	55
35	2.8	500	850	5	[j]	55

[g] Data were not strong enough to formulate recommendations. The figures in the table therefore represent the best estimate of requirements.
[h] See Chapter 6 for details.
[i] Preformed niacin.
[j] See Chapter 5 for details.
[k] This intake cannot be met by infants who are exclusively breastfed. To prevent bleeding due to vitamin K deficiency, all breast-fed infants should receive vitamin K supplementation at birth according to nationally approved guidelines.
[l] Not specified.

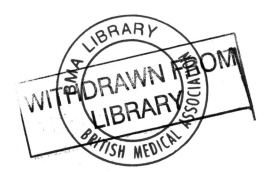